临床解剖学实物图谱丛书
Serial Objective Atlas of Clinical Anatomy

头颈部临床解剖实物图谱（第2版）

Objective Atlas of Clinical Anatomy of the Head and Neck (2nd Edition)

总 主 编 纪荣明　杨向群

主　　编 李玉泉　王玉海

副 主 编 刘　镇　李　强　章建全　李军辉　周义德

编　　者（按姓氏笔画为序）

于　永　解放军火箭军总医院神经外科
王玉海　江苏省无锡市解放军第一零一医院神经外科
生　晶　第二军医大学长海医院影像科
刘　镇　第二军医大学人体解剖学教研室
纪荣明　第二军医大学人体解剖学教研室
李　骁　第二军医大学长海医院影像科
李　强　第二军医大学长海医院神经外科
李玉泉　第二军医大学人体解剖学教研室
李军辉　第二军医大学长海医院整形外科
杨向群　第二军医大学人体解剖学教研室
杨理坤　江苏省无锡市解放军第一零一医院神经外科
张煜辉　第二军医大学长海医院神经外科
陈　磊　江苏省无锡市解放军第一零一医院神经外科
周义德　第二军医大学长海医院耳鼻咽喉科
章建全　第二军医大学长征医院超声科
彭　旭　北京回龙观医院临床心理科

秘　书（兼） 蔺海燕　第二军医大学人体解剖学教研室

人民卫生出版社

图书在版编目（CIP）数据

头颈部临床解剖实物图谱/李玉泉,王玉海主编. —2 版.
—北京:人民卫生出版社,2017
　ISBN 978-7-117-24795-5

Ⅰ.①头…　Ⅱ.①李…②王…　Ⅲ.①头部-人体解剖-
图谱②颈-人体解剖-图谱　Ⅳ.①R323.1-64

中国版本图书馆 CIP 数据核字(2017)第 163669 号

人卫智网　www.ipmph.com　医学教育、学术、考试、健康,
　　　　　　　　　　　　　　购书智慧智能综合服务平台
人卫官网　www.pmph.com　人卫官方资讯发布平台

头颈部临床解剖实物图谱
第 2 版

总　主　编:纪荣明　杨向群
主　　　编:李玉泉　王玉海
出版发行:人民卫生出版社(中继线 010-59780011)
地　　　址:北京市朝阳区潘家园南里 19 号
邮　　　编:100021
E - mail:pmph @ pmph.com
购书热线:010-59787592　010-59787584　010-65264830
印　　　刷:北京画中画印刷有限公司
经　　　销:新华书店
开　　　本:889×1194　1/16　印张:24
字　　　数:743 千字
版　　　次:2010 年 5 月第 1 版　　2017 年 10 月第 2 版
　　　　　　2017 年 10 月第 2 版第 1 次印刷(总第 2 次印刷)
标准书号:ISBN 978-7-117-24795-5/R · 24796
定　　　价:179.00 元

总主编简介

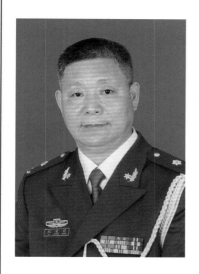

纪荣明,第二军医大学人体解剖学教研室副教授,曾任《中国临床解剖学杂志》编委,中国解剖学会临床解剖学专业委员会委员、护理临床专业委员会委员、大体解剖学专业委员会委员。享受国务院政府特殊津贴。

从事人体解剖学教学42年,临床应用解剖学研究36年,为临床实践的发展提供了大量应用解剖学资料。"臂丛神经损伤诊断与治疗的新方法"获国家发明四等奖;"心脏二尖瓣装置的应用基础研究""严重手外伤修复重建的实验与应用研究"等6个项目获军队科技进步二等奖,"415例原发性三叉神经痛手术治疗的经验"等2个项目获军队医疗成果二等奖。此外,获上海市医疗成果一等奖1项、三等奖2项。

发表科研论文130余篇,其中第一作者52篇。系《临床解剖学实物图谱丛书》第一版主编,此外还主编了《颅底外科临床应用解剖图谱》《常用皮瓣、肌瓣、骨瓣和神经瓣解剖学图谱》《心脏临床应用解剖学图谱》《麻醉解剖学实物图谱》《人体解剖学标本彩色图谱》《口腔种植应用解剖实物图谱》《人体解剖学与组织胚胎学》及《护理临床解剖学》等专著和教材。副主编《心胸外科临床应用解剖学图谱》《口腔种植手术学图解》《人体系统解剖学》等专著和教材。

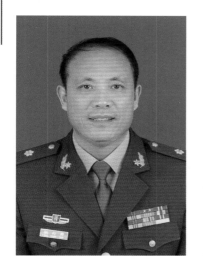

杨向群,医学博士、教授、博士生导师,现任第二军医大学人体解剖学教研室主任。中国解剖学会人体解剖和数字解剖学分会、科技开发与咨询工作委员会、体质调查工作委员会委员,中国力学会/中国生物医学工程学会生物力学专业委员会委员,中国生物医学工程学会组织工程和再生医学专业委员会委员,中华医学会工程学分会干细胞工程学组委员,国家医师资格考试临床类别试题开发专家委员会委员,军队医学科学技术委员会解剖组织胚胎专业委员会副主任委员,上海市力学会生物力学专业委员会委员,上海市解剖学会理事,《解剖学杂志》等3部杂志编委。

从事解剖学教学和科研工作30年,获军队院校育才银奖、上海市育才奖、第二军医大学特级优秀教员、"最受学员喜爱的老师"等荣誉。主要科研方向为心血管再生医学和临床解剖学,曾主持多项国家和上海市自然科学基金面上项目,获军队科技进步二等奖、三等奖、美国生理学会职业机会奖。发表教学和科研论文100余篇,主编《人体系统解剖学》《导学式教学-人体局部解剖学》《人体系统解剖学实物图谱》,副主编《人体局部解剖学》《模块法教学-人体系统解剖学》和《人体局部解剖学实物图谱》等,参编教材和专著20余部。

主编简介

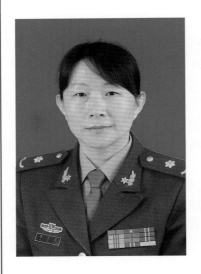

李玉泉,医学博士,第二军医大学人体解剖学教研室副教授,硕士生导师。从事人体解剖学教学 20 年,从事临床应用解剖学研究 16 年。发表教学论文近 20 篇,副主编《人体系统解剖学》《导学式教学-人体局部解剖学》教材 2 部,参编《外科及断层影像应用解剖学(第 2 版)》《模块法教学-人体系统解剖学》等教材 10 余部。获第二军医大学教学成果二等奖 1 项。主要科研方向是心血管再生医学,主持国家自然科学基金项目 2 项,参研国家自然科学基金重点项目 1 项,面上项目 6 项;参研上海市自然科学基金重点项目 1 项,《军队十一五规划》项目 1 项。发表科研论文 40 余篇,其中临床解剖相关研究论文 10 余篇;获得国家发明专利授权 2 项,国家实用新型专利授权 1 项。副主编《麻醉解剖学实物图谱》《人体解剖学标本彩色图谱》专著 2 部,参编《胸心外科临床应用解剖学图谱》等专著 6 部。

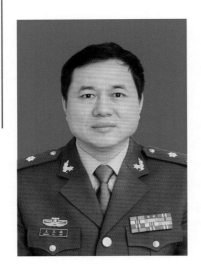

王玉海,主任医师,教授,医学博士,博士生导师。解放军第 101 医院副院长、脑科医院院长、神经外科主任。任中华创伤学会神经创伤专业委员会常委,中国神经外科重症管理协作组委员,江苏省神经外科专业委员会常委,江苏省神经外科重症学组组长,全军神经外科专业委员会委员,南京军区科学技术委员会委员,南京军区神经外科专业委员会副主任委员,《中华神经外科杂志》审稿专家。曾赴比利时安特卫普大学进修。长期从事颅底肿瘤及脑动脉瘤的临床及解剖研究,尤其擅长岩斜区及颈静脉孔区肿瘤的显微手术。先后获得军队医疗成果二等 6 项,承担各类课题 9 项,其中全军课题 2 项,军区重点课题 6 项,累计科研经费 200 余万元。发表论文 50 余篇,被 SCI 收录 20 篇,参编专著 4 部。培养硕士生 12 名、博士生 4 名。现为南京军区科技拔尖人才,南京军区科技英才,享受军队优秀专业技术人才津贴。多次被评为优秀党员和优秀党支部书记,荣立三等功 1 次。

第一版　序

"书如其人，人如其书"，见到这套宏浩的书稿，让我联系起纪荣明教授其人。他是一位从基层起步，一步一个脚印走过来的学者，是既动手实践，又动脑思考的专家。"应知学问难，在乎点滴勤"，这里选用的1300余幅实物标本照片，是经历了"铁杵磨成针"的艰辛历程，是作者集教学、科研和临床应用为一体的心血结晶。

"操千曲而后晓声，观千剑而后识器"，这批数量巨大的实物标本照片，集腋成裘，来之不易。经作者匠心编排，以局部为序，参照手术入路，由浅入深，逐层揭示人体的奥秘，阐明位置、毗邻、血供和神经支配等有关问题。针对临床上的要点和难点（如海绵窦、颅底、翼腭窝、纵隔、甲状腺和直肠会阴等区），采用了在体、离体等不同处理的手段和多方位、不同剖面显示的方法。部分重要器官，还配备了组织学切片（光镜、电镜）和影像学图片（CT、MRI）；宏观与微观相结合，实视与透视相对照，相得益彰。专著作者，经过实践和思考，努力阐明复杂结构，分析其客观规律。有如"庖丁解牛"，目无全牛、游刃有余，能帮助手术医师，得心应手，运用自如，迎刃而解。

书中许多科研资料，是作者的获奖成果（包括国家发明奖、军队科技进步奖、军队医疗成果奖和上海市医疗成果奖多项）。这些成果已应用于临床，为伤病患者带来过福音。作为临床解剖学园地里的老园丁，我十分珍视园地里的新品奇葩，望其苗壮成长，通过著书立说，将能扩大效应的覆盖面，是为之序。

中国工程院资深院士、南方医科大学教授

钟世镇

2009 年秋于广州

丛书 前言

　　"临床解剖学实物图谱丛书"第一版自 2010 年由人民卫生出版社出版以来,不仅为临床医生和解剖同行及医学生认识人体形态结构提供了新视角,也为临床开展新手术提供了很好的解剖学参考,受到了广大医生和解剖同行的认可和好评。

　　此次,应人民卫生出版社之邀,对"临床解剖学实物图谱丛书"进行修订再版,目的在于使解剖学内容与临床应用结合更加紧密,更好地为临床服务。因此,在广泛听取和吸收临床医生的意见和建议之上,我们对本丛书各分册从内容到编排上都作了较大的调整,并邀请各相关临床学科经验丰富的专家与解剖学老师担任共同主编和副主编,以便更好地把握本丛书的临床应用内容。

　　为了突出本书的临床应用特色,第二版新增加图片 278 幅。我们增加了外科常用手术切口的部位和手术入路层次,以便更好地为基层医院医生、年轻医生提供更加实用的解剖学知识。我们还增加了一些高难度手术区域的解剖结构图,例如在头颈部增加了"蝶鞍区""海绵窦区""颈静脉孔区",以及颈内动脉、椎动脉在颅底的正常行程和毗邻等解剖内容,以期临床医生对这些区域的解剖有更深入的了解,并在此基础上敢于突破手术禁区,开展新的手术。此外,第二版还增加了介入治疗相关的解剖结构,以及部分内镜手术图、MRI 图等,为临床医生提供更多的参考资料。

　　临床手术各种各样,但同一部位的手术涉及的解剖结构往往大同小异。因此,这一版我们未能按手术入路编排相关的解剖结构,依旧按照人体局部、区域或器官来进行编排,但在图片的排列顺序上力求做到符合临床应用的实际,读者可以根据手术部位查找相应的解剖结构。

　　为了规范解剖学名词,本书采用了"全国科学技术名词审定委员会"公布的《人体解剖学名词》(第二版)中规定的名词,但我们深知临床医生们喜欢的名词往往与解剖学名词有一定的差异,望读者们能自行克服这种"不适应"感。

　　虽然此次再版是在前一版的基础上进行的,但部分第一版编者由于种种原因未能参加再版工作,在此我们对他们以前的工作表示深深的谢意。此次再版,还得到了第二军医大学基础部领导的大力支持,对此我们表示由衷的感谢!尽管我们一直尽力将自己的所知奉献给广大的临床医生和解剖界同行,但由于水平有限,错误和不当之处恳请大家不吝赐教,以便在以后的再版中改正。

纪荣明　杨向群

2017.3

本册 前言

　　头部、颈部是人体重要器官较为集中的部位，且诸器官间排列紧密、毗邻关系十分复杂，血管和神经纵横交错。某一器官的微小损伤，都会给人体带来严重的功能障碍，因而有一些部位的疾病（如颅底）曾被视为手术禁区。随着临床诊疗技术的飞速发展，如 CT 和 MRI 的广泛应用，使以前诊断不明确的疾病现在不仅可以明确诊断并且能显示出病变（如肿瘤）的具体部位和形态，给手术治疗提供了有价值的参考。

　　头颈外科医生在设计手术入路和实施手术时都希望能有一本正常人体实物图谱作参考。一本结构清晰、毗邻关系明确、立体感强的临床应用解剖学图谱，再结合临床的图像诊断（CT、MRI）资料，将会对诊断及随后的手术治疗有很大帮助。

　　目前已有不少正常人体实物标本图谱出版，但结合头颈外科临床应用的解剖实物图谱极少。我们在第一版的基础上，根据头颈外科发展的需要并结合本单位在头颈外科临床应用解剖研究方面的最新成果，对原书进行了再版。此次再版作者对本书的章节编排进行了大幅度调整，全书分为头部和颈部两章，其中头部分为 9 节，颈部分为 8 节。特别是，此次再版新增了大量实物及相关影像学图片，图片数量由原来的 400 幅左右增加至近 500 幅。对一些重要的、难点局部的结构尽量按照手术入路层次的方式进行呈现，这些改变将更有利于临床医生和解剖学工作者参考。

　　该书在标本制作、图像处理等工作进行时，得到第二军医大学解剖学教研室的领导和许多老师的指导和帮助，在此一并表示感谢。

　　限于作者的水平和条件，在本书的编排、内容的取舍特别是临床应用要点的撰写方面仍有很大的局限性，诚恳希望各位读者，特别是头颈外科医生和解剖学同行们指出该书的问题、不足或错误，以便我们今后进一步完善，在此深表谢意。

李玉泉　　王玉海

2017 年 3 月于上海

目　录

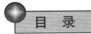

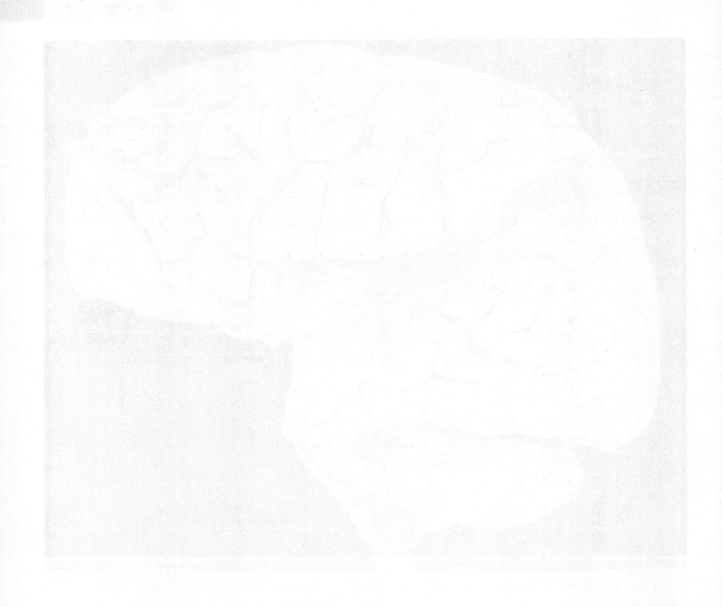

第一章 头 部

第一节 概 述

头部通常可分为颅部、面部等区域。颅部可分为颅盖部、颅底部和颅腔内容物等。颅顶部包括顶部的软组织、颅盖骨。颅腔内容物主要有脑膜、脑血管、脑组织和脑神经。颅底承托颅内容物,凹凸不平,自前向后可分为颅前、中、后窝。

一、颅部常用的骨性标志及临床应用要点

1. 眉弓 位于眶上缘上方约1.5cm处的隆嵴,其深面为额窦。
2. 枕外隆凸 位于枕鳞中央的骨性隆起,项韧带的附着处,隆凸的内面为窦汇所在之处。
3. 颧弓 位于眶下缘与枕外隆凸之间的水平连线上,是腮腺及腮腺导管、面神经等在面部的定位标志。
4. 乳突 位于耳垂的后下方,其深面的后半部为乙状窦沟。乳突根部前缘有茎乳孔,为面神经的出颅点。
5. 道上三角 位于外耳道口后上方的一个小凹陷,其上界为乳突上嵴,前界为外耳道后上缘,后界为通外耳道口所作的垂直线。此三角构成鼓窦的外侧壁。
6. 翼点 为蝶骨大翼、顶骨、额骨及颞骨鳞部相接处,其中心位于颧弓中点上方4cm及额骨颧突后方3cm处,该处骨质较薄,其深面有脑膜中动脉额支通过。

二、颅顶区的软组织层次

1. 额、顶、枕区 由浅至深为皮肤→浅筋膜→颅顶肌和帽状腱膜→腱膜下疏松结缔组织→颅骨外膜。
2. 颞区 颞区的上界为颞线,下界为颧弓上缘,前界为颧骨额突和额骨颧突,后界为乳突基部和外耳门。该区由浅至深分为六层:分别为皮肤→浅筋膜→耳外肌和帽状腱膜的延续部→颞筋膜→颞肌→颅骨外膜。
3. 颅顶部的神经 由前向后分别有:①滑车上神经;②眶上神经;③面神经;④耳颞神经;⑤耳大神经;⑥枕小神经;⑦枕大神经。上述神经均行于皮下组织内,彼此间相吻合,使相邻的神经分布区域有重叠。因此,手术时在一处施行单纯局部麻醉很难获得满意的效果。
4. 颅顶部的动脉 在耳的前方有滑车上动脉、眶上动脉和颞浅动脉;在耳的后方有耳后动脉和枕动脉。上述动脉直接来自于颈外动脉或间接地发自颈内动脉,它们均从下方走向颅顶,相互吻合成网。故头皮创伤出血较多,而结扎1支或一侧的动脉很难彻底止血。

三、颅底结构

(一) 颅前窝

位于眼眶和鼻腔的上方,构成两者的顶,其前方与额窦仅以一骨板相隔,其下方与筛窦相邻,颅前窝的骨板极薄,是颅底骨折的好发部位,骨折后可出现向鼻腔和眼眶流血及脑脊液鼻漏等。大脑的额叶、嗅神经、嗅球和嗅束均位于颅前窝。视交叉、垂体及大脑颞叶前端与颅前窝相邻。这些结构的手术有时须经颅前窝方可到达。

(二) 颅中窝

颅中窝位于颅底中部,覆盖有硬脑膜的颅中窝平均长度为123mm,从前岩床襞至颅外侧壁的横径左侧

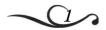

为51mm,右侧为53mm。

1. 眶上裂 上界为蝶骨小翼的下面,下界为蝶骨大翼,内侧界为蝶骨体的一部分,全长约20.8mm,内有眼神经、动眼神经、滑车神经、展神经和眼动脉通过。

2. 圆孔 直径为3.1mm,外侧缘与下颌关节结节处颧弓上缘的距离为44mm,内有上颌神经通过。

3. 卵圆孔 与圆孔相距约12mm,卵圆孔外侧缘与关节结节附近颧弓上缘之间的距离为35mm,内有下颌神经通过。

4. 棘孔 棘孔前缘与卵圆孔相距2.6mm,内有脑膜中动脉通过。

5. 破裂孔 构成颈动脉管内口的外侧界。

6. 三叉神经压迹 位于颞骨岩尖部。

7. 脑膜中动脉沟。

8. 行经颅中窝的神经

（1）动眼神经、滑车神经和展神经,它们行经海绵窦,经眶上裂入眶。

（2）三叉神经。

9. 颅中窝的血管

（1）大脑中动脉,长15mm,外径3.0mm。

（2）大脑后动脉。

（3）大脑深静脉。

10. 海绵窦 海绵窦位于蝶鞍两旁,呈前后狭长的不规则形,前方达眶上裂的内侧部,后方至颞骨岩尖部、上内侧抵中床突与后床突的连线,下外侧距圆孔与卵圆孔内缘连线3～4mm。海绵窦长20mm,宽约10mm,窦腔内有颈内动脉和展神经,外侧壁有动眼神经、滑车神经、眼神经和上颌神经通过。

（三）颅后窝

颅后窝是颅腔的一个特殊重要的部分:第一,它是颅腔内被硬脑膜分隔出来的另一个腔,窝底由蝶骨、颞骨和枕骨构成,窝顶为小脑幕;第二,颅后窝向下经枕骨大孔与椎管相通,向上经小脑幕切迹与颅腔的其他部分相通,这些交通之口均是危险点。因为颅后窝内的占位性病变可使其内容物推压向下经枕骨大孔,或推向上经小脑幕切迹形成脑疝;相反幕上间隙的病灶可使幕上内容物经小脑幕切迹疝入颅后窝;第三,颅后窝内容纳小脑、脑干、后6对脑神经的全部行程和动眼神经、滑车神经的部分行程,因此颅后窝疾病可产生脑干受累的症状,或导致第3～12对脑神经中任何一对脑神经的功能障碍。

颅后窝的境界:颅后窝的前界为鞍背,其外上端为呈结节状的后床突。前外侧界为颞骨岩部上缘。后外侧界为横窦沟。

颅后窝各壁及其主要结构:

1. 前壁 为斜坡。斜坡由上向下由鞍背、蝶骨体背面和枕骨基底部构成,斜坡全长约34mm,中部宽为28mm。斜坡上部(鞍背)与大脑脚的基底部、脚间窝相邻,中部与脑桥、下部与延髓腹侧相邻。斜坡前方邻垂体窝和蝶窦,故垂体瘤可侵蚀鞍背而累及颅后窝。蝶窦的肿瘤和感染也可累及颅后窝内的脑桥和中脑的连接部。

2. 外侧壁 由颞骨岩部后面构成,其后方与小脑中脚及小脑半球相邻。外侧壁上有内耳门,内有面神经和前庭蜗神经通过。内耳道下后方有颈静脉孔,孔的颅外端为颈内静脉的起端,孔的前内侧部有舌咽神经、副神经和迷走神经通过。枕骨大孔前外侧缘有舌下神经管,内有舌下神经通过。

颅后窝内脑神经的行程和毗邻:

颅后窝内占位性病变,如肿瘤、脓肿和动脉瘤等可压迫脑神经产生相应的临床症状。因此脑神经的局部位置、行程和毗邻有着重要的临床应用意义。

1. 舌下神经 起自延髓腹侧面的橄榄前沟,约12～15条根丝。出脑区上端距桥延沟约4.0mm,长度约13mm,绕橄榄前沟向前外侧走行,通常在蛛网膜下腔内合成两束,分别穿过蛛网膜及硬脑膜,在舌下神经管外或内合成一干。

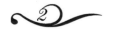

2. 舌咽、迷走和副神经 这3对脑神经从下向上以一系列根丝附着于延髓的橄榄后沟,向外侧走行,至颈静脉孔处形成独立的脑神经。颈静脉孔区骨折、肿瘤、炎症等病变均可引起上述神经的损伤而产生相应的症状,即颈静脉孔区综合征,患者同时出现患侧软腭、咽喉肌、胸锁乳突肌和斜方肌瘫痪,当病变侵及颈内动脉周围的交感神经丛时,还可并发 Horner 综合征。

3. 面神经和前庭蜗神经 面神经出脑处距正中矢状面12mm,最大直径为1.8mm,其中枢段长约2mm,为易损伤段,从脑干至内耳门的长度为15.5mm。中间神经较细小,紧贴前庭蜗神经。前庭神经和蜗神经在连脑处紧密相贴,形成一单干,入脑处距正中平面为15mm,前庭蜗神经中枢端长8~12mm,由脑干至内耳门的长度为14mm。由于前庭蜗神经位于面神经的外侧和稍下方,故小脑手术入路时,面神经被遮挡而难以看到。

4. 前庭蜗神经与面神经及小脑的位置关系密切 在脑桥小脑角处,前庭蜗神经瘤及蛛网膜炎症时,首先可产生前庭神经受损症状,如耳鸣、耳聋、眩晕和眼球震颤,当病变累及小脑时,可产生小脑共济失调。面神经也常受累及,出现同侧面瘫,同侧舌前2/3味觉丧失,泪液和唾液分泌减少等症状。

5. 展神经 展神经在脑桥下缘锥体外侧距前正中裂6mm处出脑。展神经由起点至进入眼眶的长度为59mm。

面部位于脑颅部的前下方,上为眶上缘和颧弓上缘,下为下颌骨下缘,两侧为下颌角至乳突的连线。面部血管丰富,神经分布较密集,腔隙繁多,结构复杂。根据其解剖学特点与临床应用的需要,可将面部分为鼻区、眶区、眶下区、颞区、唇区、颏区、颊区、腮腺咬肌区、耳区和面侧深区等。

面部的皮肤具有不同走行的皮纹,它是由真皮内的胶原纤维按抵抗该皮肤区所受最大张力的方向平行排列而成,故称张力线。

面部浅筋膜由疏松结缔组织构成,与皮肤间有皮下支持带及肌束相连。浅筋膜内有表情肌、血管、神经及淋巴管,脂肪组织较少。

表情肌为皮肌,肌薄,肌纤维细,位于浅筋膜内,一般起自骨或筋膜,止于皮肤,收缩时牵动皮肤,可使面部呈现各种表情,并参与咀嚼、语言运动。表情肌按所在部位分为口、鼻、眶、耳与颅顶肌五组。

面部的动脉极为丰富,除眼内眦部、鼻背及颧部由颈内动脉分支供应外,面部的其他部分均直接或间接由颈外动脉分支供应,其中面浅部主要由面动脉供应,面深部由上颌动脉供应。

面部的静脉按所在的位置分浅、深两组,它们分别与同名动脉伴行,收集面浅、深部的静脉血,浅、深两组静脉可借交通支相互交通,也可借交通支与颅内静脉交通。

面部的淋巴管、淋巴结较为丰富,主要的淋巴结有:腮腺淋巴结、面淋巴结、下颌下淋巴结、颏下淋巴结。

腮腺呈一尖向内侧、底向外侧的不规则锥体形,位于外耳道的前下方,其尖向内侧称下颌后突或咽突,此突在咬肌后部浅面与胸锁乳突肌前缘及乳突间,经下颌后窝突向内侧,达咽旁间隙。腮腺的底朝向外侧,借腮腺鞘与浅面的浅筋膜和皮肤相隔。腮腺实质内有面神经、颈外动脉、面后静脉等重要血管、神经穿过。

第二节 颅 骨

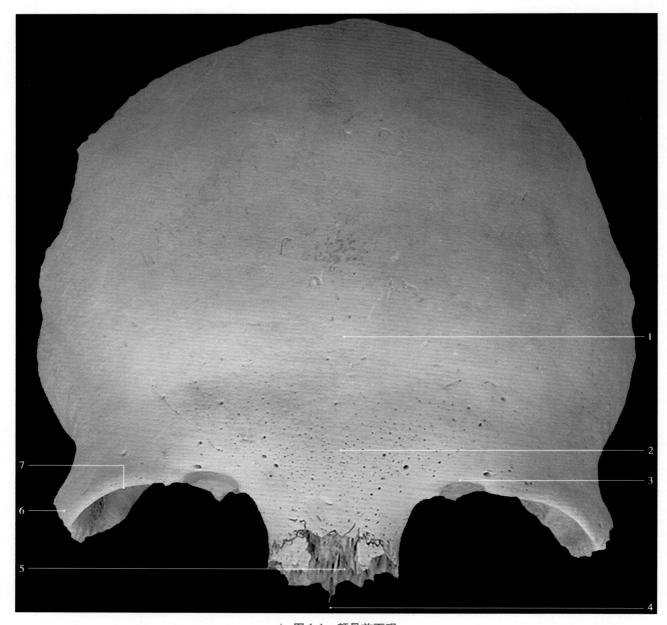

▲ 图 1-1　额骨前面观
Fig. 1-1　Anterior aspect of the frontal bone

1. 额结节 frontal tuber
2. 眉间 glabella
3. 眶上切迹 supraorbital notch
4. 鼻棘 nasal spine
5. 鼻缘 nasal margin
6. 颧突 zygomatic process
7. 眶缘 orbital margin

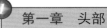

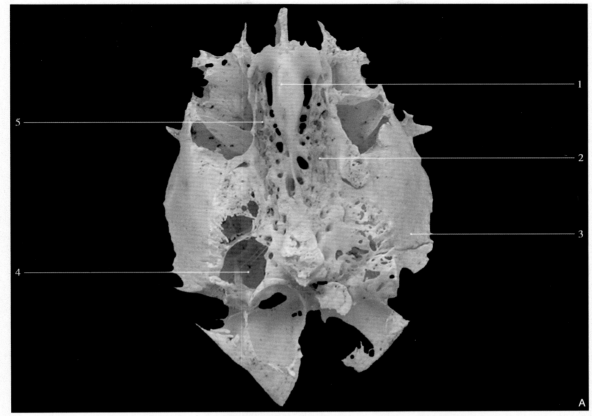

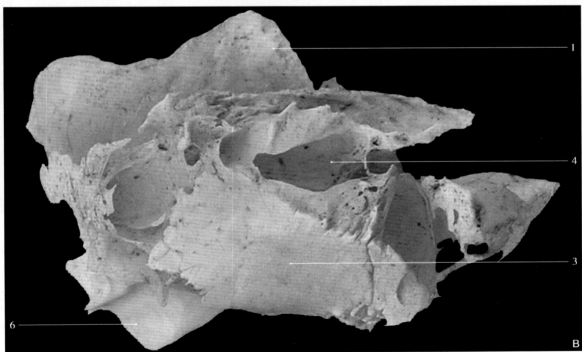

▲ 图1-2　筛骨

Fig. 1-2　Ethmoid bone

A：上面观　B：侧面观

1. 鸡冠 crista galli　　　　　3. 眶板 orbital plate　　　　　5. 筛板 cribriform plate

2. 筛孔 cribriform foramina　　4. 筛窦 ethmoidal sinus　　　6. 垂直板 perpendicular plate

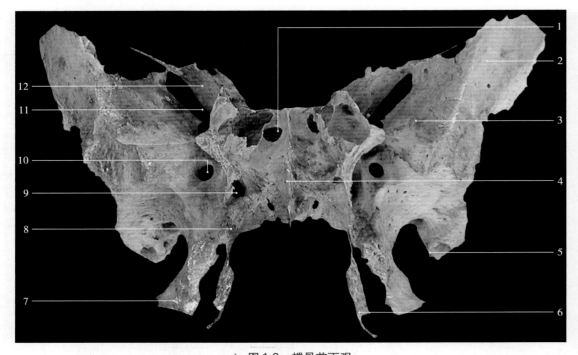

▲ 图1-3　蝶骨前面观

Fig. 1-3　Anterior aspect of the sphenoid bone

1. 蝶窦口 aperture of sphenoidal sinus
2. 颞面 temporal surface
3. 大翼 greater wing
4. 蝶骨体 body of sphenoid bone
5. 颞下嵴 infratemporal crest
6. 翼突内侧板 medial pterygoid plate
7. 翼突外侧板 lateral pterygoid plate
8. 翼突 pterygoid process
9. 翼管 pterygoid canal
10. 圆孔 foramen rotundum
11. 眶上裂 superior orbital fissure
12. 小翼 lesser wing

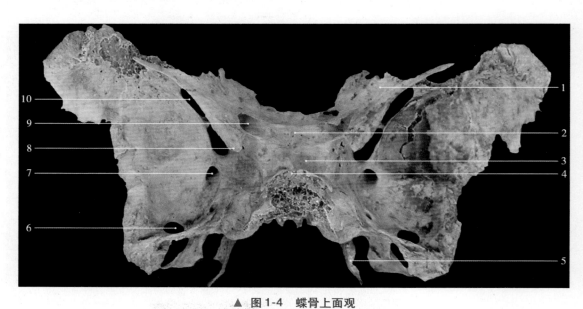

▲ 图1-4　蝶骨上面观

Fig. 1-4　Superior aspect of the sphenoid bone

1. 小翼 lesser wing
2. 交叉前沟 sulcus prechiasmaticus
3. 垂体窝 hypophysial fossa
4. 后床突 posterior clinoid process
5. 翼突内侧板 medial pterygoid plate
6. 卵圆孔 foramen ovale
7. 圆孔 foramen rotundum
8. 前床突 anterior clinoid process
9. 视神经孔 optic foramen
10. 眶上裂 superior orbital fissure

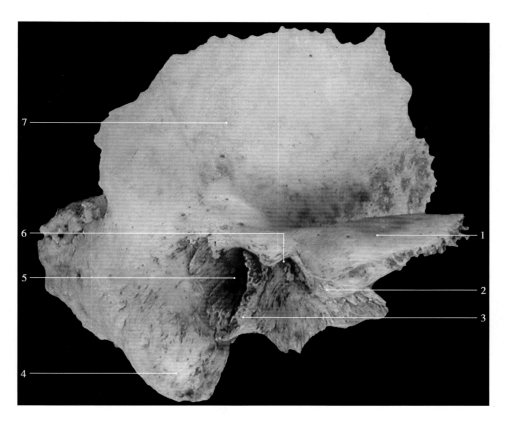

◀ 图1-5 颞骨外面观
Fig. 1-5 External aspect
of the temporal bone

1. 颧突 zygomatic process
2. 关节结节 articular tubercle
3. 鼓部 tympanic part
4. 乳突 mastoid process
5. 外耳门 external acoustic pore
6. 下颌窝 mandibular fossa
7. 鳞部 squamous part

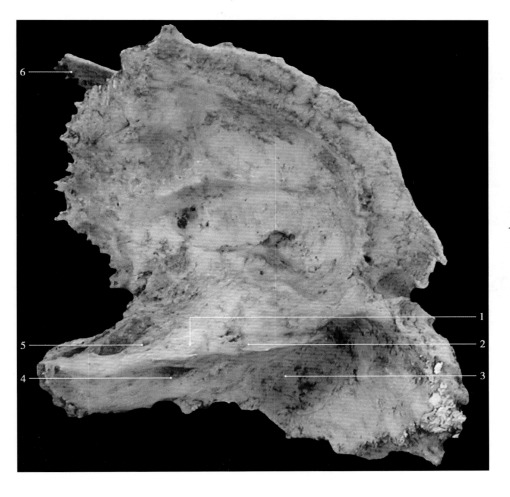

◀ 图1-6 颞骨内面观
Fig. 1-6 Internal aspect
of the temporal bone

1. 鼓室盖 tegmen tympani
2. 岩下窦沟 sulcus for inferior petrosal sinus
3. 乙状窦沟 sigmoid sulcus
4. 内耳门 internal acoustic pore
5. 三叉神经压迹 trigeminal impression
6. 颧突 zygomatic process

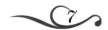

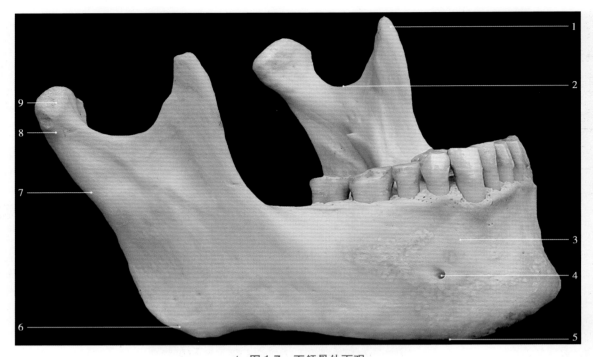

▲ 图 1-7 下颌骨外面观

Fig. 1-7 External aspect of the mandible

1. 冠突 coronoid process
2. 下颌切迹 mandibular notch
3. 下颌体 body of mandible
4. 颏孔 mental foramen
5. 下颌底 base of mandible
6. 下颌角 angle of mandible
7. 下颌支 ramus of mandible
8. 下颌颈 neck of mandible
9. 下颌头 head of mandible

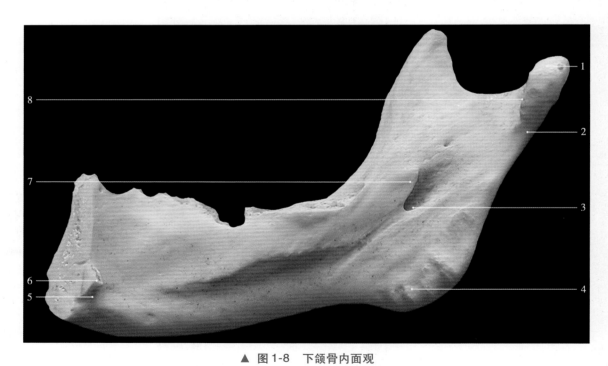

▲ 图 1-8 下颌骨内面观

Fig. 1-8 Internal aspect of the mandible

1. 下颌头 head of mandible
2. 下颌颈 neck of mandible
3. 下颌孔 mandibular foramen
4. 翼肌粗隆 pterygoid tuberosity
5. 二腹肌窝 digastric fossa
6. 颏棘 mental spine
7. 下颌小舌 mandibular lingula
8. 翼肌凹 pterygoid fovea

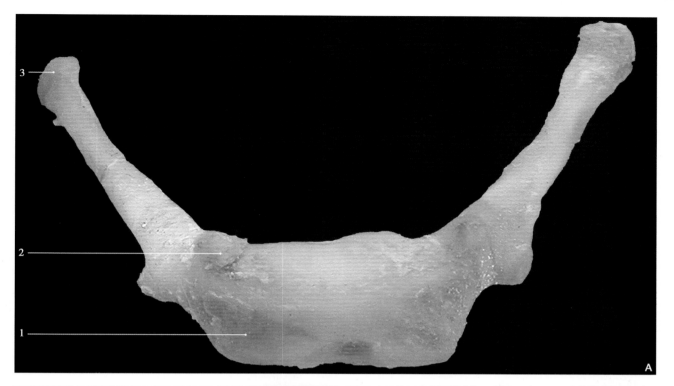

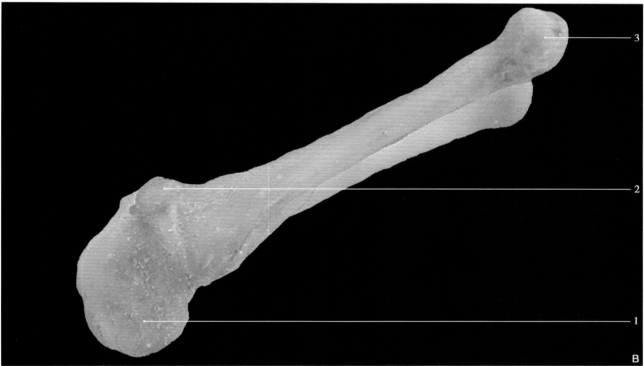

▲ 图 1-9　舌骨
Fig. 1-9　Hyoid bone

A：上面观　B：侧面观
1. 舌骨体 body of hyoid bone　　3. 大角 great cornu
2. 小角 lesser cornu

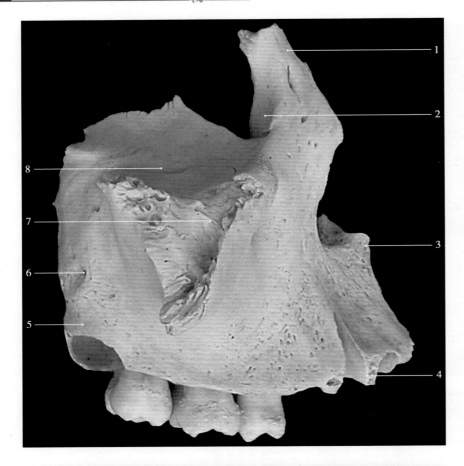

◀ 图 1-10　上颌骨外面观
Fig. 1-10　External aspect of the maxilla

1. 额突 frontal process
2. 泪沟 lacrimal sulcus
3. 鼻棘 nasal spine
4. 牙槽突 alveolar process
5. 上颌结节 maxillary tuberosity
6. 牙槽孔 alveolar foramina
7. 颧突 zygomatic process
8. 眶下沟 infraorbital groove

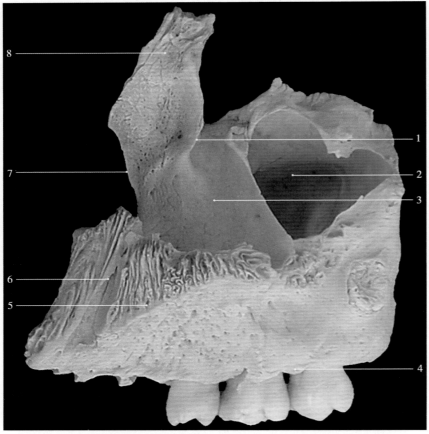

◀ 图 1-11　上颌骨内面观
Fig. 1-11　Internal aspect of the maxilla

1. 泪沟 lacrimal sulcus
2. 上颌窦 maxillary sinus
3. 上颌体 body of maxilla
4. 牙槽突 alveolar process
5. 腭突 palatine process
6. 切牙管 incisive canal
7. 鼻切迹 nasal notch
8. 额突 frontal process

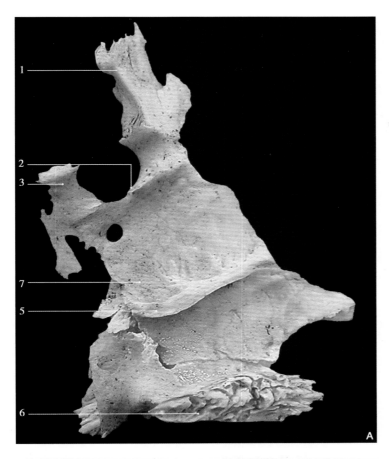

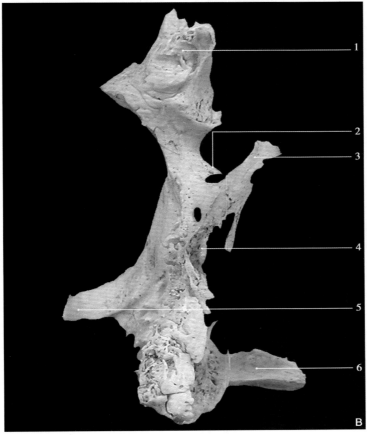

◀ 图 1-12　腭骨
Fig. 1-12　Palatine bone

A：内侧面观　B：后面观
1. 眶突 orbital process
2. 蝶腭切迹 sphenopalatine notch
3. 蝶突 sphenoidal process
4. 垂直板 perpendicular plate
5. 鼻甲嵴 conchal crest
6. 水平板 horizontal plate
7. 鼻面 nasal surface

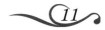

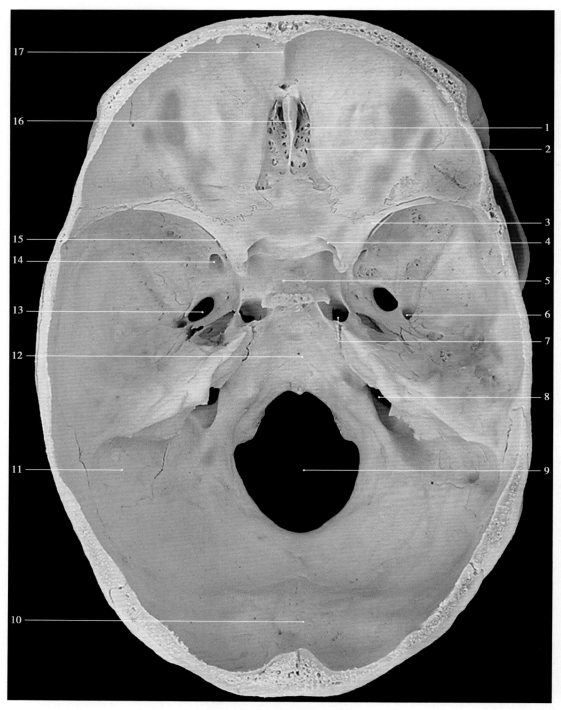

▲ 图 1-13 颅底内面观
Fig. 1-13 Internal aspect of the skull base

1. 筛板 cribriform plate
2. 筛孔 cribriform foramina
3. 蝶骨小翼 lesser wing of sphenoid bone
4. 视神经孔 optic foramen
5. 垂体窝 hypophysial fossa
6. 棘孔 foramen spinosum
7. 破裂孔 foramen lacerum
8. 颈静脉孔 jugular foramen
9. 枕骨大孔 foramen magnum of occipital bone

10. 枕内隆起 internal occipital protuberance
11. 乙状窦沟 sigmoid sulcus
12. 斜坡 clivus
13. 卵圆孔 foramen ovale
14. 圆孔 foramen rotundum
15. 眶上裂 superior orbital fissure
16. 鸡冠 crista galli
17. 额嵴 frontal crest

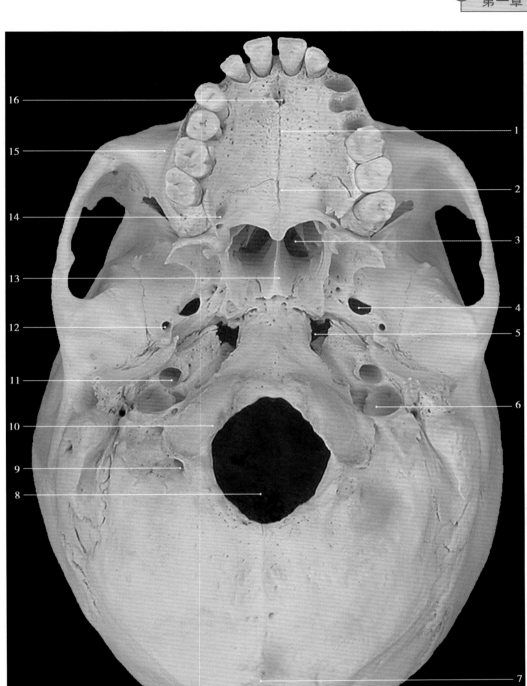

▲ 图 1-14　颅底外面观
Fig. 1-14　External aspect of the skull base

1. 腭正中缝 median palatine suture
2. 腭骨 palatine bone
3. 鼻后孔 posterior nare
4. 卵圆孔 foramen ovale
5. 破裂孔 foramen lacerum
6. 颈静脉孔 jugular foramen
7. 枕外隆凸 external occipital protuberance
8. 枕骨大孔 foramen magnum of occipital bone
9. 髁管 condylar canal
10. 枕髁 occipital condyle
11. 颈动脉管外口 external aperture of carotid canal
12. 棘孔 foramen spinosum
13. 犁骨 vomer
14. 腭大孔 greater palatine foramen
15. 上颌骨 maxilla
16. 切牙孔 incisive foramina

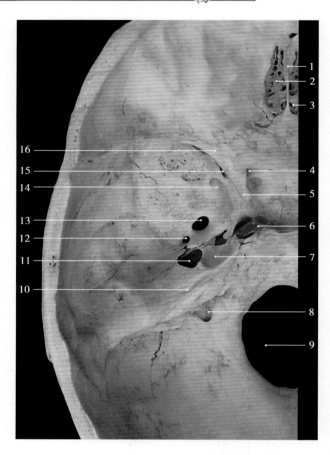

◀ 图 1-15　颈动脉管（上壁后段打开）
Fig. 1-15　Carotid canal（the posterior part of the superior wall was opened）

1. 鸡冠 crista galli
2. 筛板 cribriform plate
3. 筛孔 cribriform foramina
4. 视神经管 optic canal
5. 前床突 anterior clinoid process
6. 模拟颈内动脉 simulated internal carotid artery
7. 三叉神经压迹 trigeminal impression
8. 颈静脉孔 jugular foramen
9. 枕骨大孔 foramen magnum of occipital bone
10. 颞骨岩部 petrous part of temporal bone
11. 颈动脉管（上壁打开）carotid canal（the superior wall was opened）
12. 棘孔 foramen spinosum
13. 卵圆孔 foramen ovale
14. 圆孔 foramen rotundum
15. 眶上裂 superior orbital fissure
16. 蝶骨小翼 lesser wing of sphenoid bone

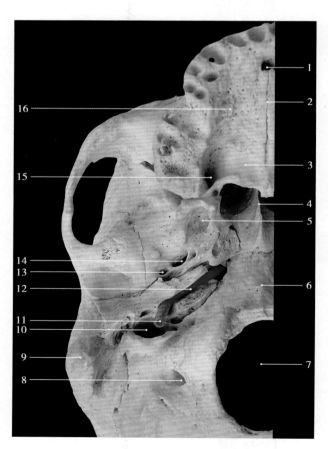

◀ 图 1-16　颈动脉管（下壁打开）
Fig. 1-16　Carotid canal（the inferior wall was opened）

1. 切牙孔 incisive foramina
2. 腭中缝 midline palatine suture
3. 腭骨水平板 horizontal plate of palatine bone
4. 犁骨 vomer
5. 蝶骨舟状窝 scaphoid fossa of sphenoid bone
6. 咽结节 pharyngeal tuberecle
7. 枕骨大孔 foramen magnum of occipital bone
8. 髁管 condylar canal
9. 乳突点 mastoideale
10. 颈静脉窝 jugular fossa
11. 模拟颈内动脉 simulated internal carotid artery
12. 颈动脉管（下壁打开）carotid canal（the inferior wall was opened）
13. 棘孔 foramen spinosum
14. 卵圆孔 foramen ovale
15. 腭大孔 greater palatine foramen
16. 硬腭 hard palate

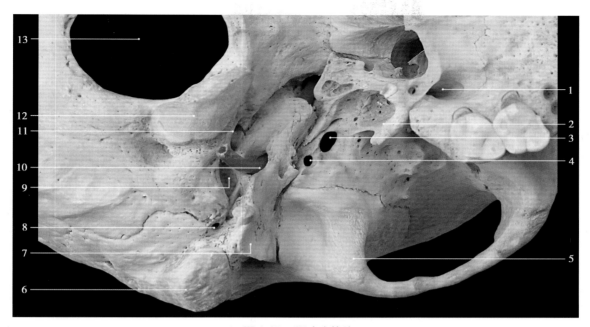

▲ 图 1-17　颈动脉管外口
Fig. 1-17　External aperture of the carotid canal

1. 腭大孔 greater palatine foramen
2. 翼突外侧板 lateral pterygoid plate
3. 卵圆孔 foramen ovale
4. 棘孔 foramen spinosum
5. 关节结节 articular tubercle
6. 乳突点 mastoideale

7. 颞骨鼓部 tympanic part of temporal bone
8. 茎乳孔 stylomastoid foramen
9. 颈静脉窝 jugular fossa
10. 颈动脉管外口 external aperture of carotid canal

11. 舌下神经管外口 external aperture of hypoglossal canal
12. 枕骨髁 occipital condyle
13. 枕骨大孔 foramen magnum of occipital bone

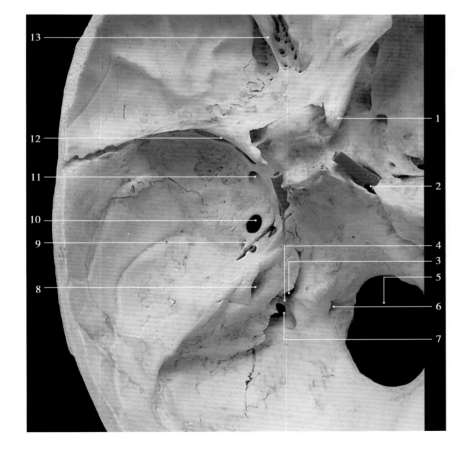

◀ 图 1-18　颈静脉孔骨间桥
Fig. 1-18　Bony bridge of the jugular foramen

1. 前床突 anterior clinoid process
2. 破裂孔 foramen lacerum
3. 颈静脉孔前部 anterior part of jugular foramen
4. 颈静脉孔骨间桥 bony bridge of jugular foramen
5. 枕骨大孔 foramen magnum of occipital bone
6. 舌下神经管内口 internal aperture of hypoglossal canal
7. 颈静脉孔后部 posterior part of jugular foramen
8. 内耳门 internal acoustic pore
9. 棘孔 foramen spinosum
10. 卵圆孔 foramen ovale
11. 圆孔 foramen rotundum
12. 眶上裂 superior orbital fissure
13. 鸡冠 crista galli

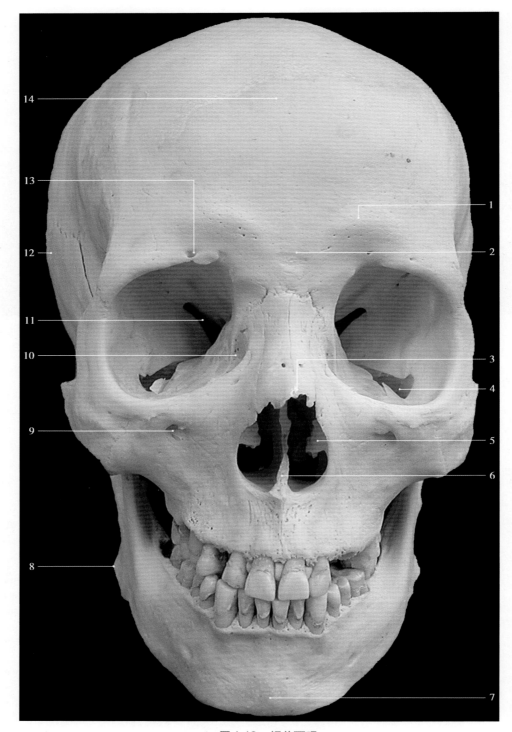

▲ 图 1-19　颅前面观
Fig. 1-19　Anterior aspect of the skull

1. 眉弓 superciliary arch
2. 眉间 glabella
3. 鼻骨 nasal bone
4. 眶下裂 inferior orbital fissure
5. 下鼻甲 inferior nasal concha
6. 骨鼻中隔 bony septum of nose
7. 颏隆凸 mental protuberance
8. 下颌角 angle of mandible
9. 眶下孔 infraorbital foramen
10. 泪囊窝 fossa for lacrimal sac
11. 眶上裂 superior orbital fissure
12. 颞骨 temporal bone
13. 眶上孔 supraorbital foramen
14. 额骨 frontal bone

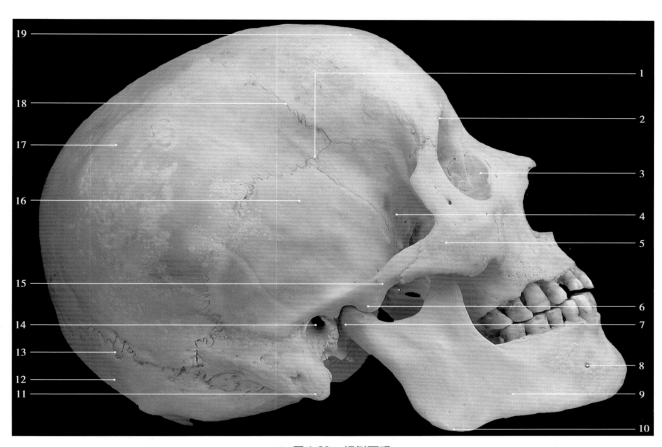

▲ 图 1-20　颅侧面观

Fig. 1-20　Lateral aspect of the skull

1. 翼点 pterion
2. 眶缘 orbital margin
3. 泪骨 lacrimal bone
4. 蝶骨大翼 greater wing of sphenoid bone
5. 颧骨 zygomatic bone
6. 关节结节 articular tubercle
7. 下颌头 head of mandible
8. 颏孔 mental foramen
9. 下颌骨 mandible
10. 下颌角 angle of mandible
11. 乳突 mastoid process
12. 枕骨 occipital bone
13. 人字缝 lambdoid suture
14. 外耳门 external acoustic pore
15. 颧弓 zygomatic arch
16. 颞骨 temporal bone
17. 顶骨 parietal bone
18. 冠状缝 coronal suture
19. 额骨 frontal bone

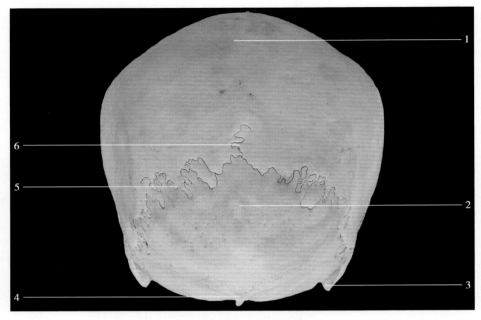

▲ 图 1-21　颅后面观

Fig. 1-21　Posterior aspect of the skull

1. 顶骨 parietal bone
4. 枕外隆凸 external occipital protuberance
2. 枕骨 occipital bone
5. 人字缝 lambdoid suture
3. 乳突 mastoid process
6. 矢状缝 sagittal suture

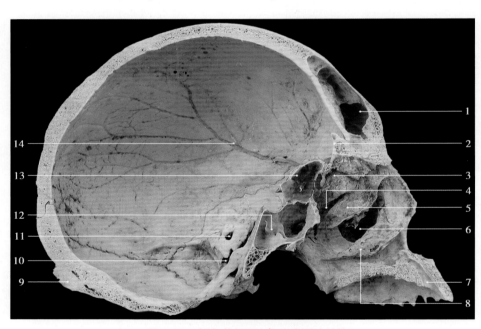

▲ 图 1-22　颅矢状切面（鼻腔外侧壁结构）

Fig. 1-22　Sagittal section of the skull（lateral wall of bony nasal cavity）

1. 额窦 frontal sinus
8. 下鼻甲 inferior nasal concha
2. 鸡冠 crista galli
9. 枕外隆凸 external occipital protuberance
3. 上鼻甲 superior nasal concha
10. 颈静脉孔 jugular foramen
4. 上鼻道 superior nasal meatus
11. 内耳门 internal acoustic pore
5. 中鼻甲 middle nasal concha
12. 蝶窦 sphenoidal sinus
6. 中鼻道 middle nasal meatus
13. 筛窦 ethmoidal sinus
7. 切牙管 incisive canal
14. 脑膜中动脉沟 sulcus for middle meningeal artery

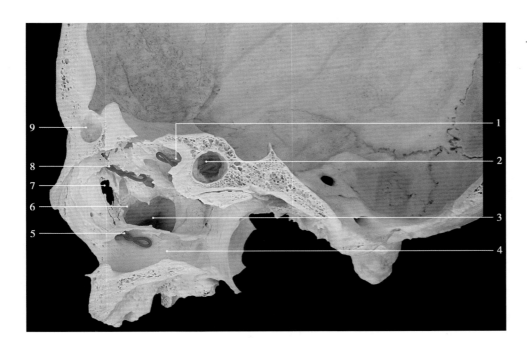

◀ 图 1-23 鼻旁窦及开口
Fig. 1-23 Paranasal sinuses and their debouch

1. 蝶窦口 aperture of sphenoidal sinus
2. 蝶窦 sphenoidal sinus
3. 上颌窦 maxillary sinus
4. 下鼻道 inferior nasal meatus
5. 鼻泪管口 orifice of nasolacrimal duct
6. 中鼻道 middle nasal meatus
7. 额窦开口 debouch of frontal sinus
8. 筛窦前组开口 aperture of anterior ethmoidal sinus
9. 额窦 frontal sinus

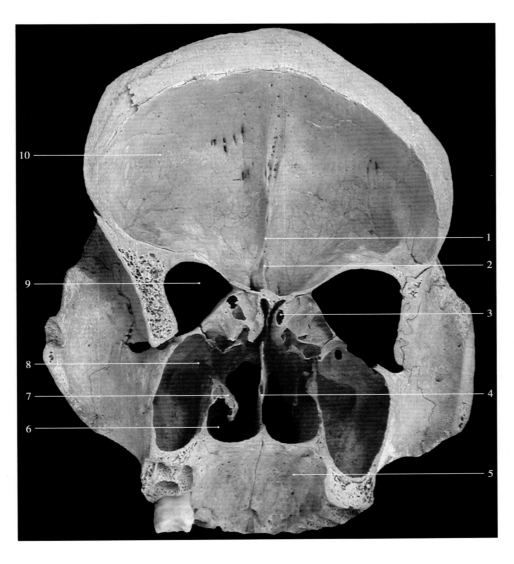

◀ 图 1-24 颅冠状切面
Fig. 1-24 Coronary section of the skull

1. 额嵴 frontal crest
2. 鸡冠 crista galli
3. 筛窦 ethmoidal sinus
4. 鼻中隔 nasal septum
5. 骨腭 bony palate
6. 下鼻道 inferior nasal meatus
7. 下鼻甲 inferior nasal concha
8. 上颌窦 maxilliary sinus
9. 眶 orbit
10. 额骨 frontal bone

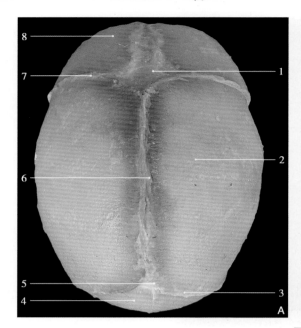
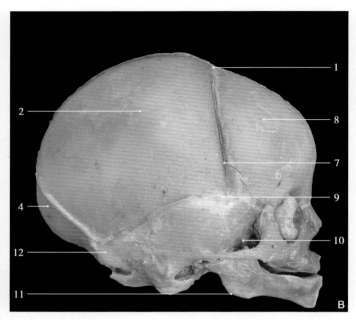

▲ 图 1-25　新生儿颅

Fig. 1-25　Skull of the newborn

A：上面观　B：侧面观

1. 前囟 anterior fontanelle
2. 顶骨 parietal bone
3. 人字缝 lambdoid suture
4. 枕骨 occipital bone
5. 后囟 posterior fontanelle
6. 矢状缝 sagittal suture

7. 冠状缝 coronal suture
8. 额骨 frontal bone
9. 蝶囟 sphenoidal fontanelle
10. 蝶骨 sphenoid bone
11. 下颌角 angle of mandible
12. 后外侧囟 posterolateral fontanelle

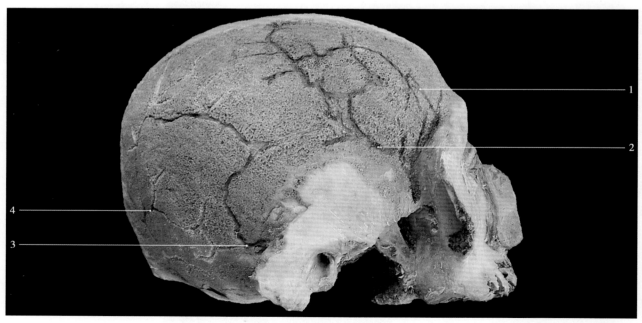

▲ 图 1-26　板障静脉

Fig. 1-26　Diploic vein

1. 额板障静脉 frontal diploic vein
2. 颞前板障静脉 anterior temporal diploic vein
3. 颞后板障静脉 posterior temporal diploic vein
4. 枕板障静脉 occipital diploic vein

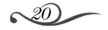

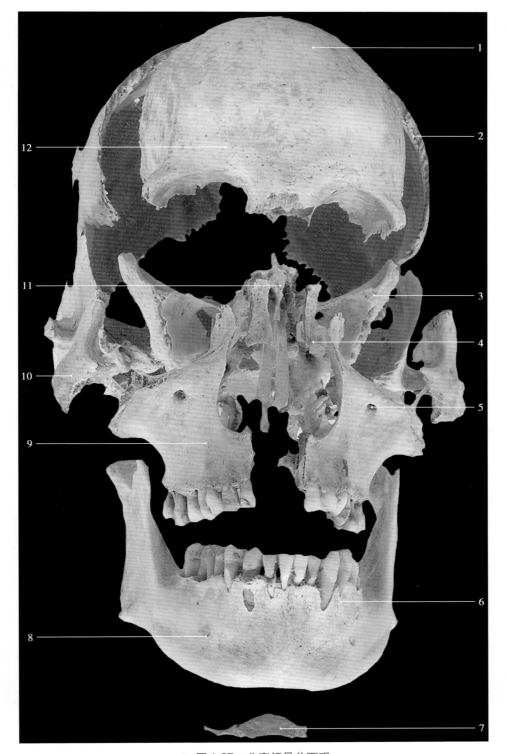

▲ 图 1-27　分离颅骨前面观
Fig. 1-27　Anterior aspect of the separated skull

1. 额骨 frontal bone
2. 顶骨 parietal bone
3. 蝶骨 sphenoid bone
4. 鼻骨 nasal bone
5. 眶下孔 infraorbital foramen
6. 下颌骨 mandible
7. 舌骨 hyoid bone
8. 颏孔 mental foramen
9. 上颌骨 maxilla
10. 颧骨 zygomatic bone
11. 筛骨 ethmoid bone
12. 眉弓 superciliary arch

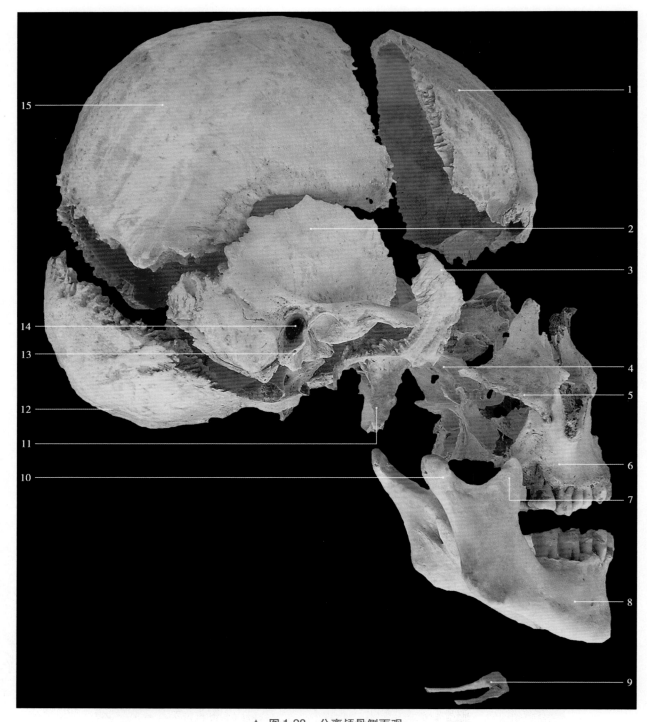

▲ 图 1-28　分离颅骨侧面观
Fig. 1-28　Lateral aspect of the separated skull

1. 额骨 frontal bone
2. 颞骨 temporal bone
3. 蝶骨大翼 great wing of sphenoid bone
4. 犁骨 vomer bone
5. 颧骨 zygomatic bone
6. 上颌骨 maxilla
7. 冠突 coronoid process
8. 下颌骨 mandible

9. 舌骨 hyoid bone
10. 髁突 condylar process
11. 蝶骨翼突 pterygoid process of sphenoid bone
12. 枕骨 occipital bone
13. 鼓部 tympanic part
14. 外耳门 external acoustic pore
15. 顶骨 parietal bone

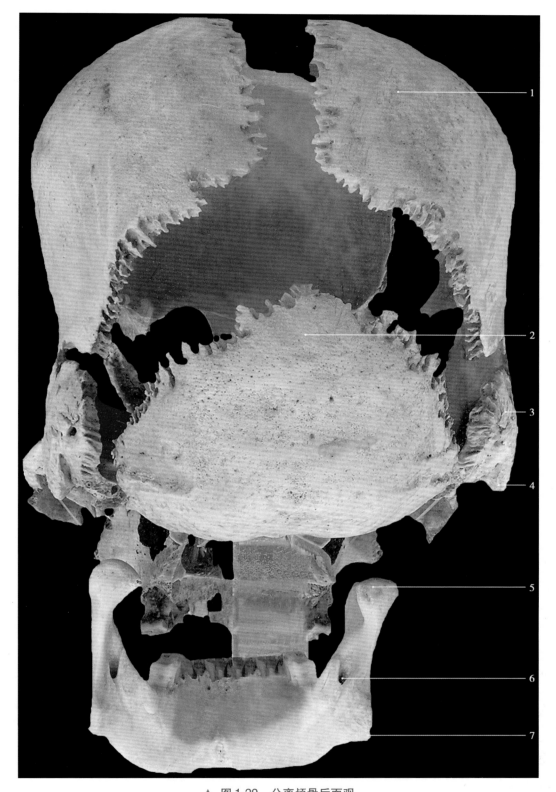

▲ 图 1-29　分离颅骨后面观
Fig. 1-29　Posterior aspect of the separated skull

1. 顶骨 parietal bone　　　5. 髁突 condylar process
2. 枕骨 occipital bone　　　6. 下颌孔 mandibular foramen
3. 颞骨 temporal bone　　　7. 下颌角 angle of mandible
4. 乳突 mastoid process

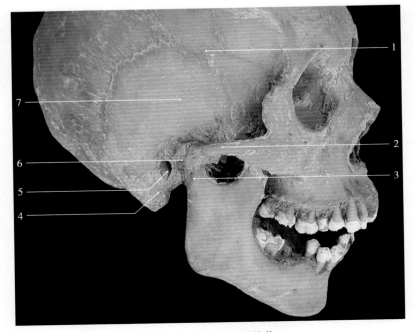

▲ 图1-30　颞下颌关节

Fig. 1-30　Temporomandibular joint

1. 翼点 pterion
2. 颧弓 zygomatic arch
3. 下颌颈 neck of mandible
4. 乳突 mastoid process
5. 外耳门 external acoustic pore
6. 关节囊 articular capsule
7. 颞骨 temporal bone

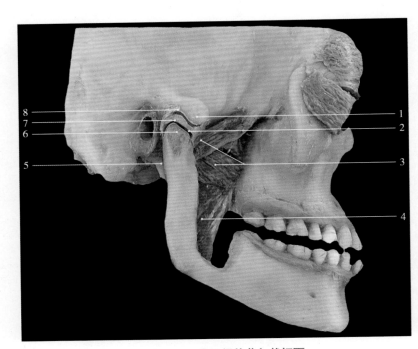

▲ 图1-31　颞下颌关节矢状切面

Fig. 1-31　Sagittal section through the temporomandibular joint

1. 关节结节 articular tubercle
2. 关节腔 articular cavity
3. 翼外肌 lateral pterygoid
4. 翼内肌 medial pterygoid
5. 茎突 styloid process
6. 下颌头 head of mandible
7. 关节盘 articular disc
8. 下颌窝 mandibular fossa

第三节 头面部的浅层结构

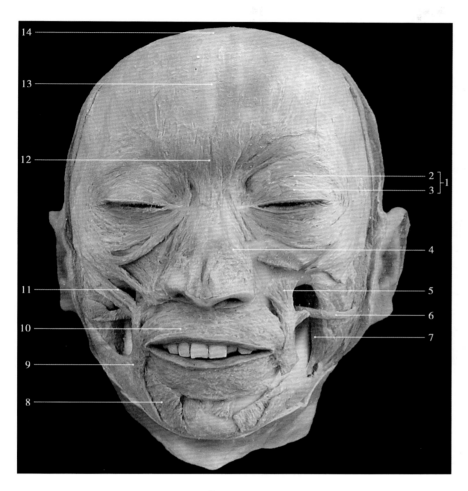

◄ 图 1-32 面肌前面观
Fig. 1-32 Anterior aspect of the facial muscle

1. 眼轮匝肌 orbicularis oculi
2. 眶部 orbital part
3. 睑部 palpebral part
4. 鼻肌 nasalis
5. 提上唇肌 levator labii superioris
6. 腮腺管 parotid duct
7. 咬肌 masseter
8. 降下唇肌 depressor labii inferioris
9. 降口角肌 depressor anguli oris
10. 口轮匝肌 orbicularis oris
11. 颧肌 zygomaticus
12. 皱眉肌 corrugator supercilii
13. 枕额肌额腹 frontal belly of occipitofrontalis
14. 帽状腱膜 epicranial aponeurosis

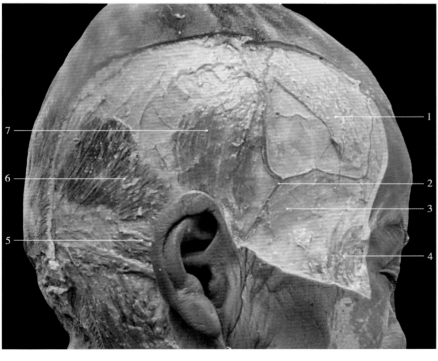

◄ 图 1-33 耳肌侧面观
Fig. 1-33 Lateral aspect of the auricular muscle

1. 颅顶肌额腹 frontal belly of epicranius
2. 颞浅动脉 superficial temporal artery
3. 耳前肌 auricularis anterior
4. 眼轮匝肌 orbicularis oculi
5. 耳后肌 auricularis posterior
6. 颅顶肌枕腹 occipital belly of epicranius
7. 耳上肌 auricularis superior

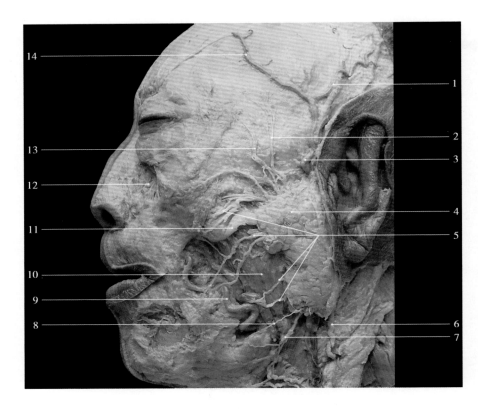

◀ 图 1-34　面部浅层结构左侧面观
Fig. 1-34　Left aspect of the superficial structures of the face

1. 颞浅动脉顶支 parietal branch of superficial temporal artery
2. 面神经颞支 temporal branch of facial nerve
3. 颞浅动脉 superficial temporal artery
4. 腮腺 parotid gland
5. 面神经颊支 buccal branch of facial nerve
6. 耳大神经 great auricular nerve
7. 面神经颈支 cervical branch of facial nerve
8. 面神经下颌缘支 marginal mandibular branch of facial nerve
9. 面动脉 facial artery
10. 咬肌 masseter
11. 腮腺管 parotid duct
12. 眶下神经 infraorbital nerve
13. 面神经颧支 zygomatic branch of facial nerve
14. 颞浅动脉额支 frontal branch of superficial temporal artery

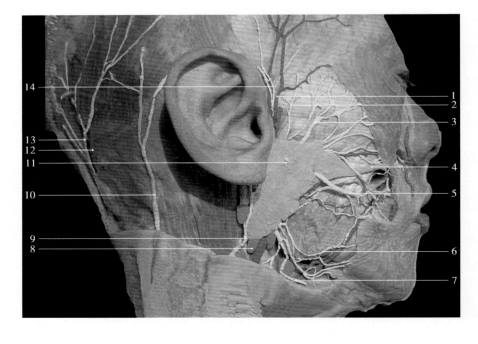

◀ 图 1-35　面部浅层结构右侧面观
Fig. 1-35　Right aspect of the superficial structures of the face

1. 颞浅动脉 superficial temporal artery
2. 面神经颞支 temporal branches of facial nerve
3. 面神经颧支 zygomatic branches of facial nerve
4. 腮腺管 parotid duct
5. 面神经颊支 buccal branches of facial nerve
6. 面神经下颌缘支 marginal mandibular branch
7. 面神经颈支 cervical branch of facial nerve
8. 腮腺淋巴结 parotid lymph node
9. 耳大神经 great auricular nerve
10. 枕小神经 lesser occipital nerve
11. 腮腺 parotid gland
12. 枕动脉 occipital artery
13. 枕大神经 greater occipital nerve
14. 耳颞神经 auriculotemporal nerve

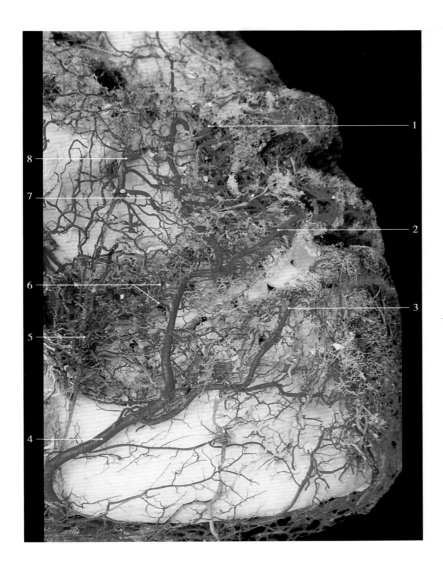

◀ 图 1-36 面部皮肤血管铸型
Fig. 1-36 Vascular cast of the facial skin

1. 鼻翼动脉 nasal alar artery
2. 上唇动脉 superior labial artery
3. 下唇动脉 inferior labial artery
4. 面动脉 facial artery
5. 面静脉 facial vein
6. 面颊皮动脉 cutaneous artery of cheek
7. 面横动脉 transverse facial artery
8. 眶下动脉 infraorbital artery

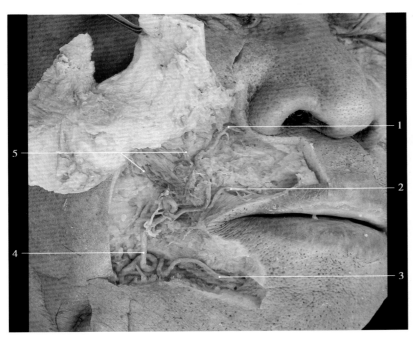

◀ 图 1-37 面颊部穿支皮瓣
Fig. 1-37 Perforator flap of the cheek

1. 鼻翼动脉 nasal alar artery
2. 上唇动脉 superior labial artery
3. 下唇动脉 inferior labial artery
4. 面动脉 facial artery
5. 面颊皮动脉 cutaneous artery of cheek

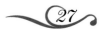

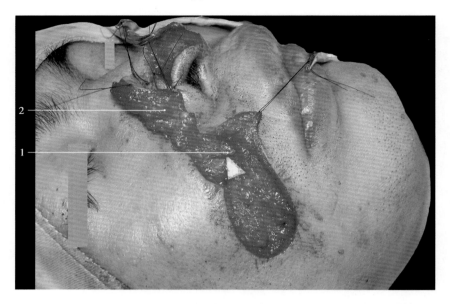

◀ 图 1-38　面颊部转移皮瓣
Fig. 1-38　Transfer flap in the cheek

1. 面颊皮动脉 cutaneous artery of cheek
2. 面颊部转移皮瓣 transfer flap in cheek

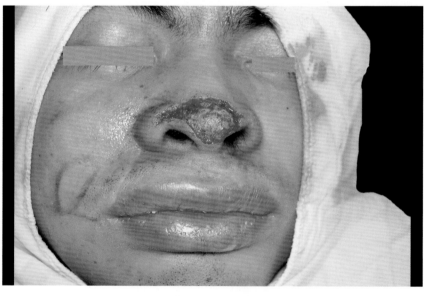

◀ 图 1-39　面颊部皮瓣受区
Fig. 1-39　Recipient site of the skin flap in the cheek

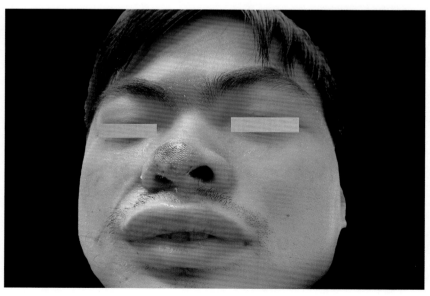

◀ 图 1-40　面颊部皮瓣的临床应用（术后）
Fig. 1-40　Clinical application of the skin flap in the cheek（after operation）

带血管蒂面颊部皮瓣移位修复鼻尖部缺损的应用解剖学要点

以内眦动脉为蒂的颊部轴型皮瓣逆行修复鼻尖部缺损,供区(面颊部)可Ⅰ期愈合。切口隐藏于鼻唇沟内而不显,供区及修复的鼻尖外形良好,是修复鼻尖部缺损的良好供区(图1-36~图1-40)。

应用解剖要点:

面动脉发出上唇动脉后,由其后壁向上发出1支至颊部的皮动脉,出现率为86.7%,皮支起始处外径为0.98mm,可游离的长度为15.0mm。皮支起点处的投影位于横线(为两侧口角的连线的延长线)上方者为76%,与横线的垂直距离为6.5mm。皮支起点处的体表投影点均位于垂线(为眶上孔和颏孔间的连线)外侧,与垂线的水平距离为26.4mm。

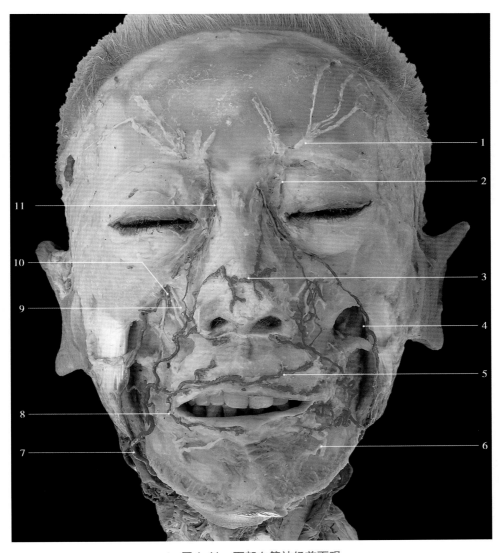

▲ 图1-41 面部血管神经前面观

Fig. 1-41 Anterior aspect of the facial vessels and nerves

1. 眶上神经 supraorbital nerve
2. 眶上动脉 supraorbital artery
3. 鼻翼动脉 nasal alar artery
4. 面静脉 facial vein
5. 上唇动脉 superior labial artery
6. 颏神经 mental nerve
7. 面动脉 facial artery
8. 下唇动脉 inferior labial artery
9. 眶下神经 infraorbital nerve
10. 眶下动脉 infraorbital artery
11. 内眦静脉 angular vein

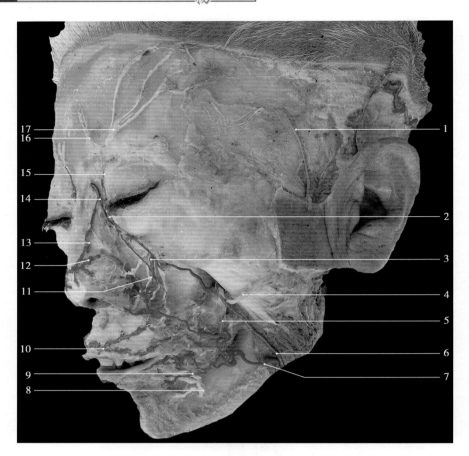

◀ 图 1-42   面部血管神经左侧面观

Fig. 1-42   Left aspect of the facial vessels and nerves

1. 颞浅动脉 superficial temporal artery
2. 内眦动脉 angular artery
3. 眶下动脉 infraorbital artery
4. 腮腺管 parotid duct
5. 颊肌 buccinator
6. 面静脉 facial vein
7. 面动脉 facial artery
8. 颏神经 mental nerve
9. 下唇动脉 inferior labial artery
10. 上唇动脉 superior labial artery
11. 眶下神经 infraorbital nerve
12. 鼻翼动脉 nasal alar artery
13. 鼻背动脉 dorsal nasal artery
14. 内眦静脉 angular vein
15. 眶上动脉 supraorbital artery
16. 滑车上神经 supratrochlear nerve
17. 眶上神经 supraorbital nerve

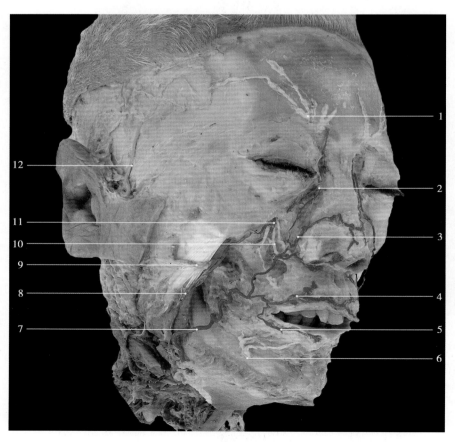

◀ 图 1-43   面部血管神经右侧面观

Fig. 1-43   Right aspect of the facial vessels and nerves

1. 眶上动脉 supraorbital artery
2. 内眦动脉 angular artery
3. 鼻翼动脉 nasal alar artery
4. 上唇动脉 superior labial artery
5. 下唇动脉 inferior labial artery
6. 颏神经 mental nerve
7. 面动脉 facial artery
8. 面静脉 facial vein
9. 腮腺管 parotid duct
10. 眶下神经 infraorbital nerve
11. 眶下动脉 infraorbital artery
12. 颞浅动脉 superficial temporal artery

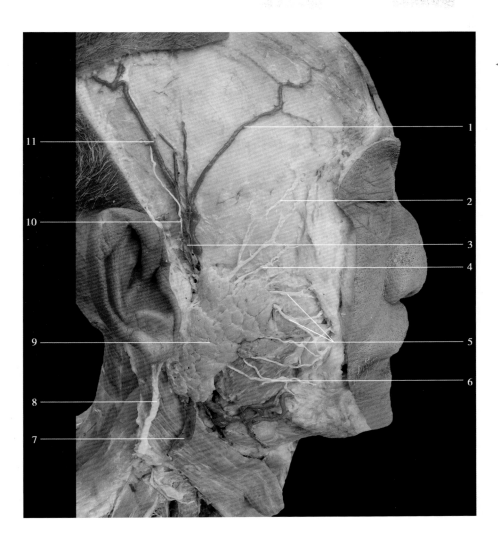

 图 1-44 腮腺的形态、毗邻
Fig. 1-44 Morphology and adjacent structures of the parotid gland

1. 颞浅动脉额支 frontal branch of superficial temporal artery
2. 面神经颞支 temporal branch of facial nerve
3. 颞浅静脉 superficial temporal vein
4. 面神经颧支 zygomatic branch of facial nerve
5. 面神经颊支 buccal branch of facial nerve
6. 面神经下颌缘支 marginal mandibular branch of facial nerve
7. 颈外静脉 external jugular vein
8. 耳大神经 great auricular nerve
9. 腮腺 parotid gland
10. 耳颞神经 auriculotemporal nerve
11. 颞浅动脉顶支 parietal branch of superficial temporal artery

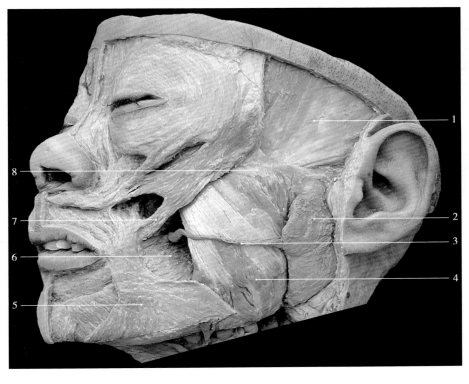

图 1-45 腮腺与腮腺管
Fig. 1-45 Parotid gland and parotid duct

1. 颞肌 temporalis
2. 腮腺 parotid gland
3. 腮腺管 parotid duct
4. 咬肌 masseter
5. 降口角肌 depressor anguli oris
6. 颊肌 buccinator
7. 颧大肌 zygomaticus major
8. 颧弓 zygomatic arch

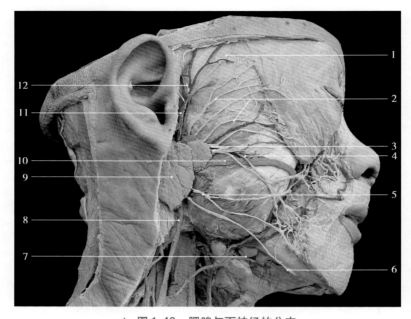

▲ 图 1-46 腮腺与面神经的分支
Fig. 1-46 Parotid gland and branches of the facial nerve

1. 颞支 frontal branch
2. 颧支 zygomatic branch
3. 颊支 buccal branch
4. 面横动脉 transverse facial artery
5. 下颌缘支 marginal mandibular branch
6. 颈支 cervical branch

7. 下颌下淋巴结 submandibular lymph node
8. 下颌后静脉 retromandibular vein
9. 腮腺 parotid gland
10. 腮腺管 parotid duct
11. 颞浅静脉 superficial temporal vein
12. 耳颞神经 auriculotemporal nerve

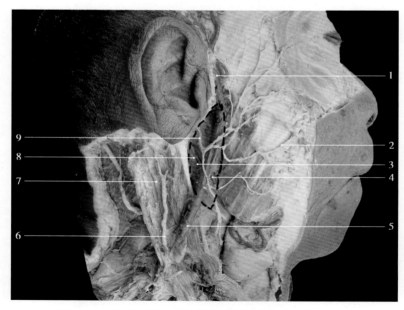

▲ 图 1-47 腮腺床浅层结构
Fig. 1-47 Superficial structures of the parotid bed

1. 颞浅静脉 superficial temporal vein
2. 面神经颊支 buccal branch of facial nerve
3. 腮腺床 parotid bed
4. 枕动脉 occipital artery
5. 颈外静脉 external jugular vein

6. 耳大神经 great auricular nerve
7. 胸锁乳突肌 sternocleidomastoid
8. 二腹肌后腹 posterior belly of digastric
9. 面神经 facial nerve

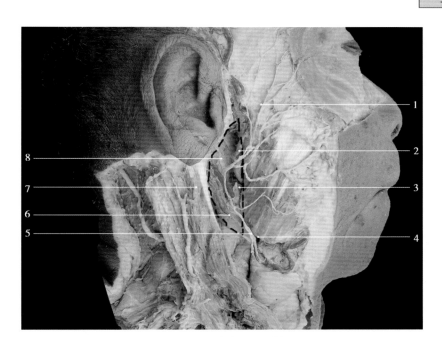

▲ 图 1-48 腮腺床深层结构（一）
Fig. 1-48 Deep structures of the parotid bed（1）

1. 面神经颧支 zygomatic branch of facial nerve
2. 颞浅动脉 superficial temporal artery
3. 腮腺床 parotid bed
4. 下颌角 angle of mandible
5. 面神经颈支 cervical branch of facial nerve
6. 二腹肌后腹 posterior belly of digastric
7. 胸锁乳突肌 sternocleidomastoid
8. 面神经 facial nerve

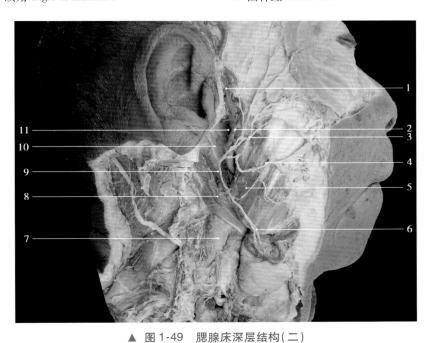

▲ 图 1-49 腮腺床深层结构（二）
Fig. 1-49 Deep structures of the parotid bed（2）

1. 颞浅静脉 superficial temporal vein
2. 颞浅动脉 superficial temporal artery
3. 面神经颧支 zygomatic branch of facial nerve
4. 面神经颊支 buccal branch of facial nerve
5. 咬肌 masseter
6. 面神经下颌缘支 marginal mandibular branch of facial nerve
7. 颈内静脉 internal jugular vein
8. 二腹肌后腹 posterior belly of digastric
9. 枕动脉 occipital artery
10. 面神经 facial nerve
11. 腮腺床 parotid bed

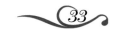

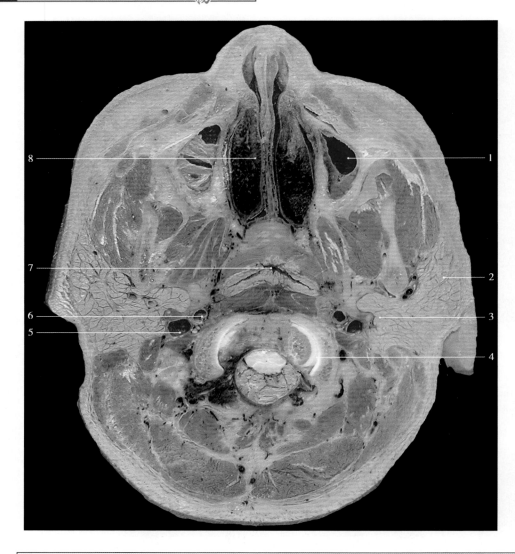

◄ 图 1-50 腮腺横切面
Fig. 1-50 Transverse section of the parotid gland

1. 上颌窦 maxillary sinus
2. 腮腺浅部 superficial part of parotid gland
3. 腮腺深部 deep part of parotid gland
4. 寰枕关节 atlantooccipital joint
5. 颈内静脉 internal jugular vein
6. 颈内动脉 internal carotid artery
7. 咽腔 pharyngeal cavity
8. 下鼻甲 inferior nasal concha

面神经阻滞术的应用解剖学要点

面神经在延髓脑桥沟外侧连于脑干,位于前庭蜗神经的前内侧,向前外侧经内耳门入内耳道,经内耳道底上方的面神经区进入颞骨岩部的面神经管内;在管内先向前外行至膝神经节处后转向后外,转折处称面神经膝,继而沿鼓室内侧壁上缘向后行,至乳突窦口处面神经转向下,经鼓室后壁下降从茎乳孔出颅,出茎乳孔后面神经向前进入腮腺,构成腮腺丛。至腮腺前缘自上而下分为颞支、颧支、颊支、下颌缘支和颈支,分布于面部表情肌和颈阔肌(图 1-47 ~ 图 1-49)。

应用解剖要点:

面神经阻滞术的进针点选在:

1. 颧弓根与下颌小头交界处(即颞下颌关节前缘)。

2. 外耳道正下方,乳突尖前 1 ~ 2cm 处至茎乳孔。

颞下颌关节前缘的阻滞术以阻滞面神经的颞支和颧支为主。穿刺针经过的结构为:皮肤→浅筋膜→深筋膜→颞支和颧支。

乳突尖前方 1 ~ 2cm 处的阻滞术是阻滞面神经主干。穿刺层次为:皮肤→浅筋膜→深筋膜→颈阔肌→腮腺→面神经。

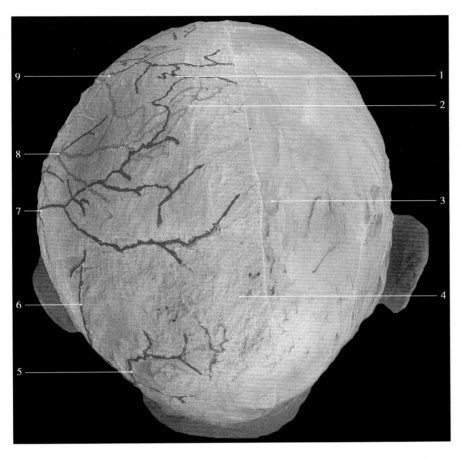

◀ 图 1-51 头皮血管上面观
Fig. 1-51 Superior aspect of the vessel of the scalp

1. 头皮动脉吻合支 anastomotic branch of scalp artery
2. 头皮静脉吻合支 anastomotic branch of scalp vein
3. 腱膜下组织 subaponeurotic tissue
4. 帽状腱膜 epicranial aponeurosis
5. 枕动脉 occipital artery
6. 耳后动脉 posterior auricular artery
7. 颞浅动脉 superficial temporal artery
8. 颞浅静脉 superficial temporal vein
9. 眶上动脉 supraorbital artery

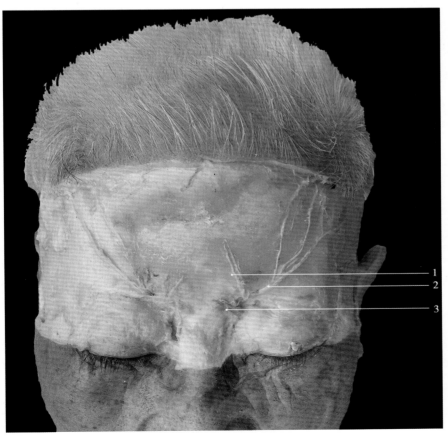

◀ 图 1-52 头皮血管神经前面观
Fig. 1-52 Anterior aspect of the vessel and nerve of the scalp

1. 滑车上神经 supratrochlear nerve
2. 眶上神经 supraorbital nerve
3. 滑车上动脉 supratrochlear artery

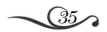

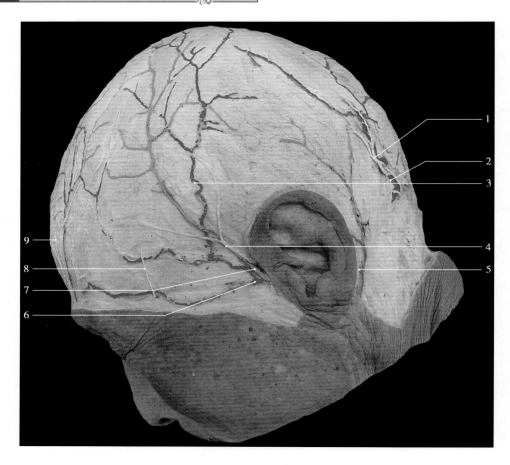

◀ 图 1-53　头皮血管神经左侧面观

Fig. 1-53　Left aspect of the vessel and nerve of the scalp

1. 枕大神经 greater occipital nerve
2. 枕动脉 occipital artery
3. 颞浅动脉顶支 parietal branch of superficial temporal arery
4. 耳颞神经 auriculotemporal nerve
5. 耳后静脉 posterior auricular vein
6. 颞浅动脉 superficial temporal artery
7. 颞浅静脉 superficial temporal vein
8. 面神经颞支 temporal branch of facial nerve
9. 眶上神经 supraorbital nerve

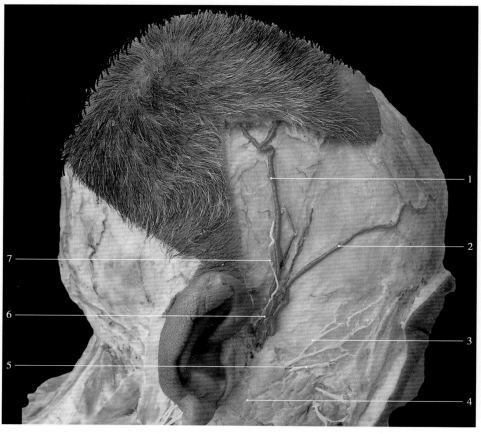

◀ 图 1-54　头皮血管神经右侧面观

Fig. 1-54　Right aspect of the vessel and nerve of the scalp

1. 颞浅动脉顶支 parietal branch of superficial temporal artery
2. 颞浅动脉额支 frontal branch of superficial temporal artery
3. 面神经颞支 temporal branch of facial nerve
4. 腮腺 parotid gland
5. 面神经颧支 zygomatic branch of facial nerve
6. 颞浅静脉 superficial temporal vein
7. 耳颞神经 auriculotemporal nerve

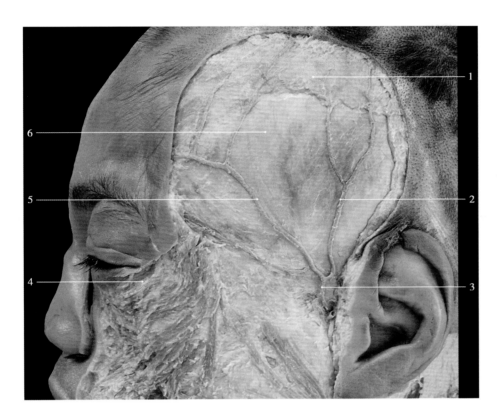

◀ 图 1-55 左侧颞浅动脉
Fig. 1-55 Left superficial temporal artery

1. 颞浅筋膜 superficial temporal fascia
2. 顶支 parietal branch
3. 颞浅动脉 superficial temporal artery
4. 眼轮匝肌 orbicularis oculi
5. 额支 frontal branch
6. 颞深筋膜 deep temporal fascia

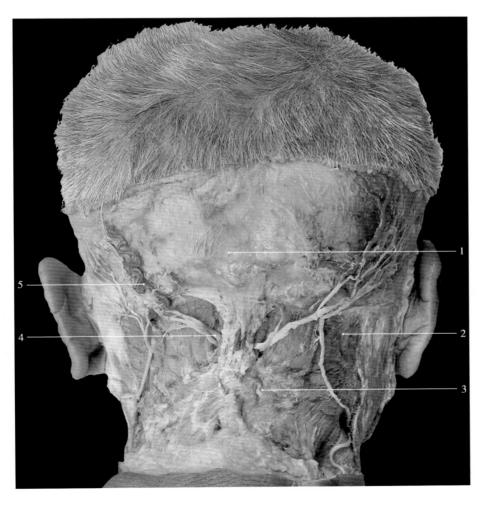

◀ 图 1-56 头皮血管神经后面观
Fig. 1-56 Posterior aspect of the vessel and nerve of the scalp

1. 枕外隆凸 external occipital protuberance
2. 头夹肌 splenius capitis
3. 斜方肌 trapezius
4. 枕大神经 greater occipital nerve
5. 枕动脉 occipital artery

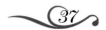

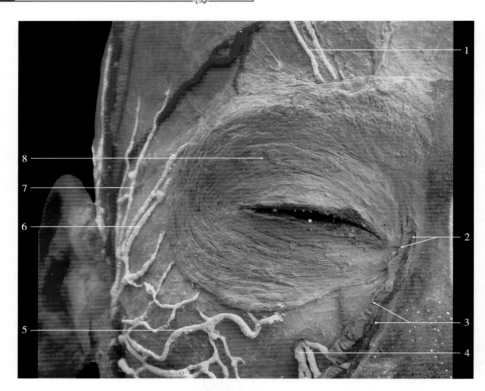

图 1-57　眶区浅层结构前面观

Fig. 1-57　Anterior aspect of the superficial structures of the orbital region

1. 眶上神经 supraorbital nerve
2. 内眦动脉、静脉 angular artery and vein
3. 面动脉、静脉 facial artery and vein
4. 眶下神经 infraorbital nerve
5. 面神经颊支 buccal branch of facial nerve
6. 面神经颧支 zygomatic branch of facial nerve
7. 面神经颞支 temporal branch of facial nerve
8. 眼轮匝肌 orbicularis oculi

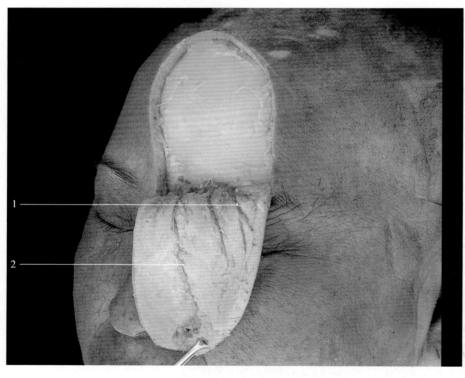

图 1-58　眶上皮瓣

Fig. 1-58　Supraorbital skin flap

1. 滑车上动脉 supratrochlear artery
2. 眶上动脉 supratrorbital artery

眶上皮瓣的应用解剖学要点

　　眶上皮瓣是带有眶上动脉、静脉、滑车上动脉、静脉的皮下组织蒂和额肌的复合组织瓣。该瓣可一次带蒂修复鼻背、鼻尖的组织缺损、畸形。因蒂部血管较粗大,血供丰富,皮下组织松软,通过鼻根、鼻背的皮下隧道而达鼻尖,鼻部皮肤不留瘢痕(图 1-52、图 1-58)。

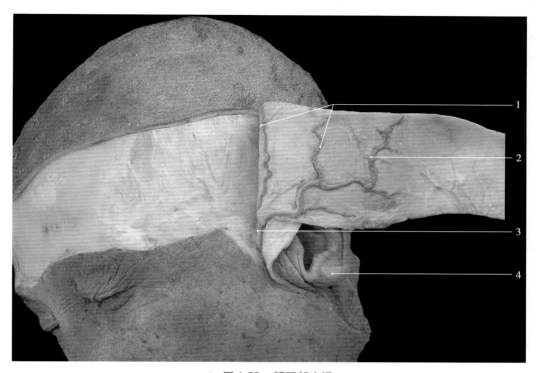

▲ 图 1-59　额颞部皮瓣
Fig. 1-59　Frontotemporal skin flap

1. 顶支 parietal branch　　3. 颞浅动脉 superficial temporal artery
2. 额支 frontal branch　　　4. 耳垂 auricular lobule

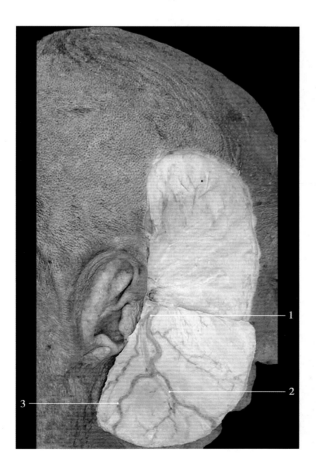

◀ 图 1-60　颞区皮瓣
Fig. 1-60　Temporal skin flap

1. 颞浅动脉 superficial temporal artery
2. 额支 frontal branch
3. 顶支 parietal branch

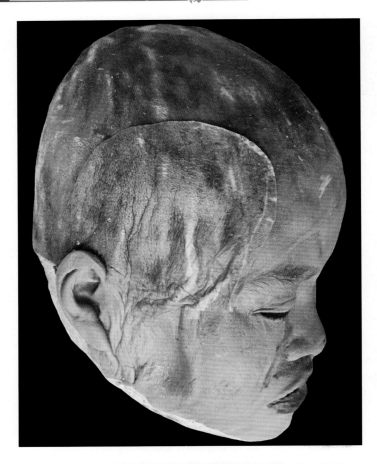

◀ 图 1-61　颞区手术入路切口（一）
Fig. 1-61　Incision of the temporal region（1）

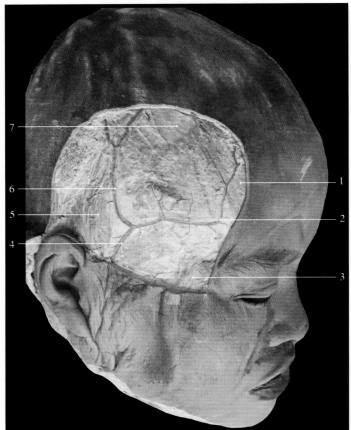

◀ 图 1-62　颞区手术入路切口（二）
Fig. 1-62　Incisions of the temporal region（2）

1. 额肌 frontal belly of occipitofrontalis
2. 额支 frontal branch
3. 眼轮匝肌 orbicularis oculi
4. 颞浅动脉 superficial temporal artery
5. 耳上肌 auricularis superior
6. 顶支 parietal branch
7. 帽状腱膜 epicranial aponeurosis

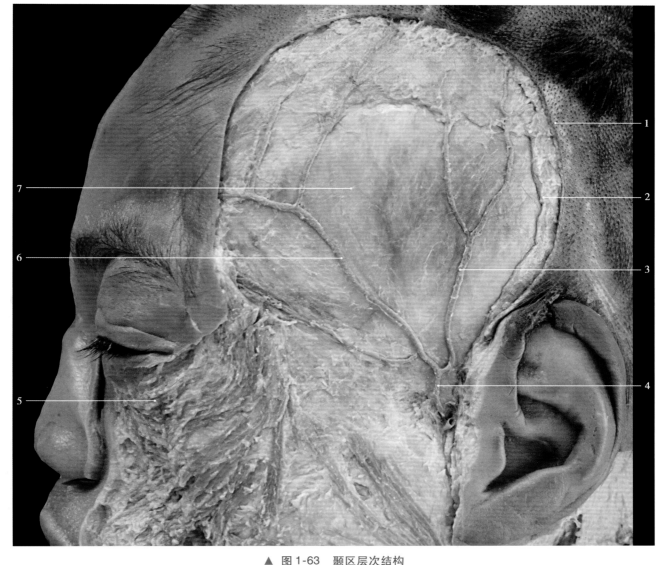

▲ 图 1-63　颞区层次结构

Fig. 1-63　Layered structures of the temporal region

1. 皮肤 skin
2. 颞浅筋膜 superficial temporal fascia
3. 顶支 parietal branch
4. 颞浅动脉 superficial temporal artery
5. 眼轮匝肌 orbicularis oculi
6. 额支 frontal branch
7. 颞深筋膜 deep temporal fascia

颞区皮瓣的应用解剖学要点

　　颞区皮瓣是以颞浅动脉主干或分支(顶支、额支)为蒂的皮瓣。该供区的优点是皮瓣区内有较粗的血管和感觉神经(耳颞神经),行程浅表,解剖位置恒定,血供丰富,供区接近面颊、额部,可形成的蒂较长,转移方便,是修复面颊部、额部缺损的理想供区之一(图 1-59、图 1-60)。

　　应用解剖要点:

　　颞区皮瓣主要动脉为颞浅动脉,该动脉起于颈外动脉,至颞区分为额支(向前内)和顶支(向上),可与对侧的同名动脉、后方的耳后动脉及前方的眶上动脉之间有丰富的吻合。颞区皮瓣切取后,供区需要再次植皮。

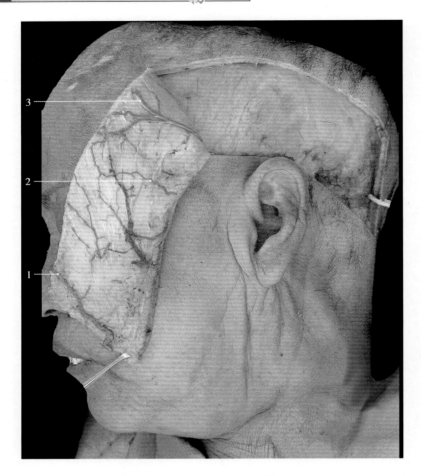

◀ 图 1-64　颞枕皮瓣
Fig. 1-64　Temporo-occipital skin flap

1. 枕支 occipital branch
2. 顶支 parietal branch
3. 额支 frontal branch

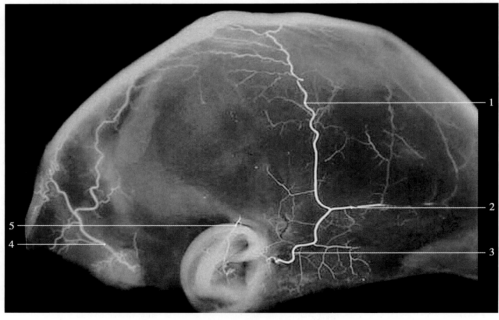

▲ 图 1-65　右侧颞枕皮瓣 X 光片
Fig. 1-65　X-ray of the right temporo-occipital skin flap

1. 顶支 parietal branch　　　　　4. 枕动脉 occipital artery
2. 额支 frontal branch　　　　　5. 耳后动脉 posterior auricular artery
3. 颞浅动脉 superficial temporal artery

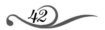

颞枕皮瓣的应用解剖学要点

颞枕皮瓣是以颞浅动脉及其分支和枕动脉为蒂的纵跨同侧颞枕区的长形皮瓣。枕动脉与颞浅动脉、耳后动脉之间有丰富的血管吻合,该皮瓣血供丰富,并有静脉和神经伴行。该皮瓣有毛发,是修复头皮与发际部位缺损的良好供区(图1-64、图1-65)。

应用解剖要点:

供区由颞枕部设计蒂位于发际缘,皮瓣宽(上→下)为5cm,蒂长(前→后)为24cm左右为宜,切口距耳后约3cm,枕部至项中线约4cm。供区内应含有耳后动脉与颞浅动脉在内。提起皮瓣,小心钝性分离皮瓣蒂部,注意供区内走行的血管免于损伤。

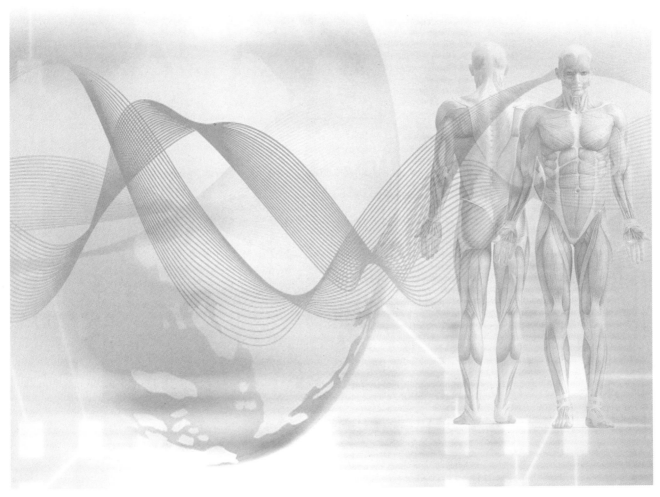

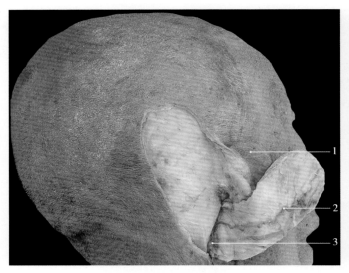

▲ 图 1-66　耳后皮瓣

Fig. 1-66　Posterior auricular skin flap

1. 耳郭 auricle
2. 耳后动脉 posterior auricular artery
3. 茎乳动脉 stylomastoid artery

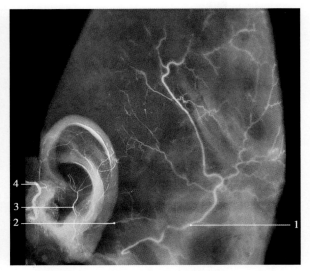

▲ 图 1-67　左侧耳后皮瓣 X 光片

Fig. 1-67　X ray of the left posterior auricular skin flap

1. 枕动脉 occipital artery
2. 乳突支 mastoid branch
3. 耳后动脉 posterior auricular artery
4. 颞浅动脉 superficial temporal artery

耳后皮瓣的应用解剖学要点

耳后区可形成以耳后动脉、静脉或以颞浅动脉、静脉为蒂的耳后皮瓣。该皮瓣具有皮肤薄、皮下脂肪少、皮肤的色质与面部接近、质地柔软、厚薄适宜，供区隐蔽等优点，是修复面部、耳郭的理想供区（图1-66、图1-67）。

应用解剖要点：

耳后动脉在下颌角平面上方两横指处起于颈外动脉，紧贴乳突与耳郭软骨之间的皮下组织内分为耳支和枕支，耳支发出后经耳后肌的深面上行，沿途发出数条小分支分布于耳郭背面和耳后区的皮肤，其分支与颞浅动脉和枕动脉的分支间有吻合。

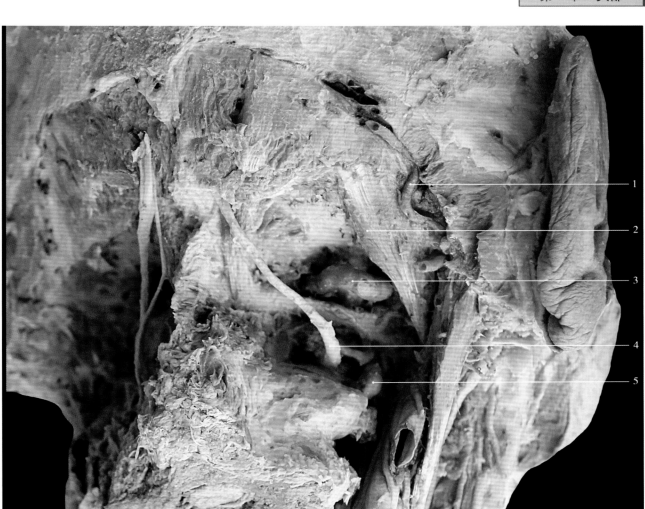

▲ 图 1-68　枕大神经

Fig. 1-68　Greater occipital nerve

1. 枕动脉 occipital artery
2. 头上斜肌 obliquus capitis superior
3. 椎动脉寰椎部 atlantic part of vertebral artery
4. 枕大神经 greater occipital nerve
5. 椎动脉横突部 transverse part of vertebral artery
6. 颈内动脉 internal carotid artery

枕大神经阻滞术的应用解剖学要点

枕大神经是第 2 颈神经的背侧支,在寰椎后弓与枢椎椎弓之间后行,于头下斜肌下方穿出并行于头下斜肌与头半棘肌之间,穿过头半棘肌和斜方肌枕部的附着处,分布于颅顶部皮肤(图 1-68)。

应用解剖要点：

枕大神经在枕部的阻滞术:进针点选在枕外隆凸外上方 2.5cm 或枕外隆凸与乳突尖连线的中点处。

穿刺层次为:皮肤→浅筋膜→斜方肌→枕大神经(患者有放射感)。

第四节 面深部结构

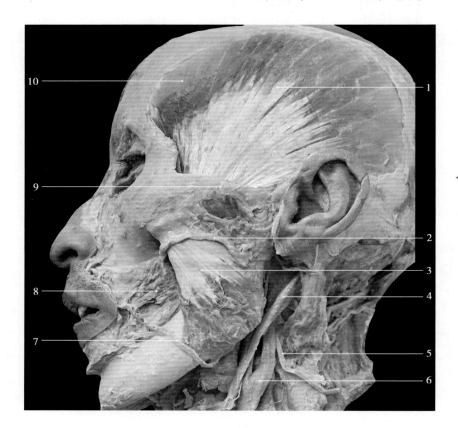

◀ 图 1-69 左侧颞肌和咬肌
Fig. 1-69 Left temporalis and masseter

1. 颞肌 temporalis
2. 腮腺管 parotid duct
3. 咬肌 masseter
4. 茎突 styloid process
5. 迷走神经 vagus nerve
6. 颈动脉窦 carotid artery
7. 面动脉 facial artery
8. 颊肌 buccinator
9. 颧弓 zygomatic arch
10. 颞筋膜 temporal fascia

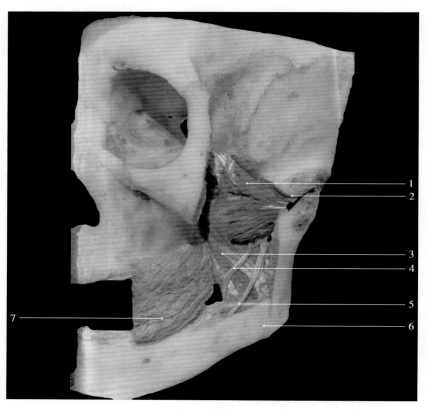

◀ 图 1-70 翼外肌、翼内肌和颊肌
Fig. 1-70 Lateral pterygoid, medial pterygoid and buccinator

1. 翼外肌 lateral pterygoid
2. 关节盘 articular disc
3. 翼内肌 medial pterygoid
4. 舌神经 lingual nerve
5. 下牙槽神经 inferior alveolar nerve
6. 下颌角 angle of mandible
7. 颊肌 buccinator

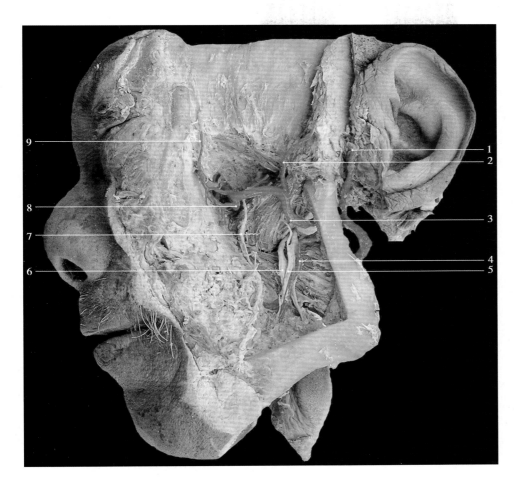

◀ 图 1-71　上颌动脉
Fig. 1-71　Maxillary artery

1. 颞浅动脉 superficial temporal artery
2. 颞深后动脉 posterior deep temporal artery
3. 上颌动脉 maxillary artery
4. 下牙槽动脉 inferior alveolar artery
5. 下牙槽神经 inferior alveolar nerve
6. 舌神经 lingual nerve
7. 颊神经 buccal nerve
8. 蝶腭动脉 sphenopalatine artery
9. 颞深前动脉 anterior deep temporal artery

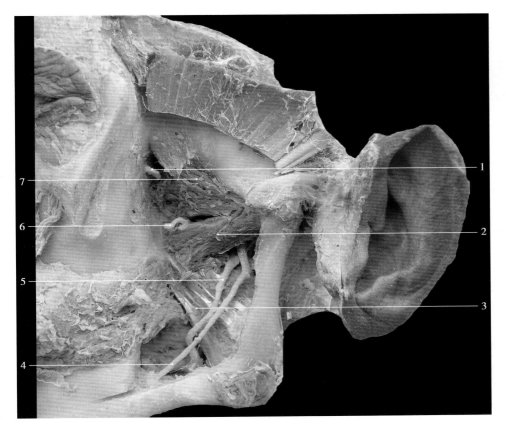

◀ 图 1-72　左侧舌神经和下牙槽神经外侧面观
Fig. 1-72　Lateral aspect of the left lingual nerve and inferior alveolar nerve

1. 眶下神经 infraorbital nerve
2. 翼外肌横头 transverse head of lateral pterygoid
3. 翼内肌 medial pterygoid
4. 下牙槽神经 inferior alveolar nerve
5. 舌神经 lingual nerve
6. 颊神经 buccal nerve
7. 翼外肌斜头 oblique head of lateral pterygoid

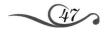

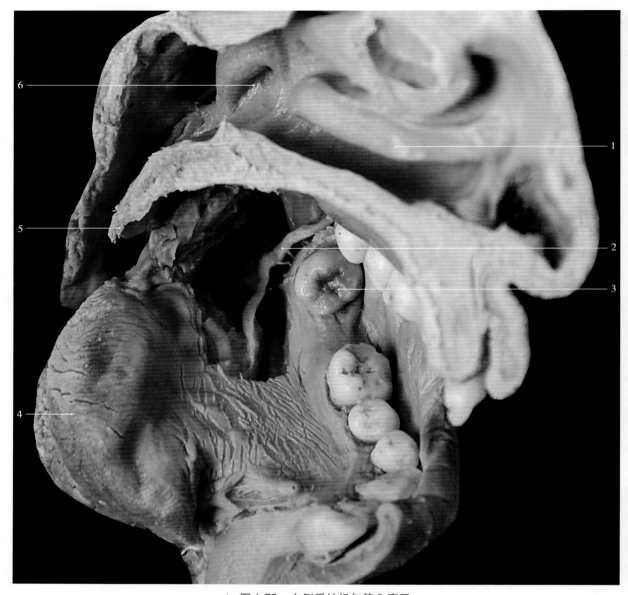

▲ 图 1-73　左侧舌神经与第 3 磨牙
Fig. 1-73　Left lingual nerve and the 3rd molar

1. 下鼻甲 inferior nasal concha
2. 舌神经 lingual nerve
3. 下颌第 3 磨牙 the 3rd molar of mandible
4. 舌（翻向外）tongue（turned laterally）
5. 腭垂 uvula
6. 咽鼓管咽口 pharyngeal opening of auditory tube

舌神经的应用解剖学要点

　　舌神经起于下颌神经的后干，起初行于腭帆张肌与翼外肌之间，在此处有鼓索支加入。从翼外肌下缘穿出后向前下行，位于翼内肌表面，逐渐与下颌支内侧相贴近，最后于下颌第 3 磨牙后根的相对侧，此处舌神经仅被牙龈黏膜、骨膜所覆盖。行下颌神经切除术时，可在此处切开黏膜，分离出舌神经，并沿舌神经向上向内分离至侧后方的下牙槽神经后，可一直分离至下颌神经本干。此点舌神经在下牙槽嵴下方 2～3mm，在下颌舌骨肌深面上方，舌神经向前下行于黏膜下层跨过舌沟，此处舌神经位于下颌下腺深部上面，继而在下颌下腺导管下方通过，向上、向前和向内进入舌。拔除下颌第 3 磨牙和切除下颌下腺时有伤及舌神经的危险（图 1-69～图 1-73）。

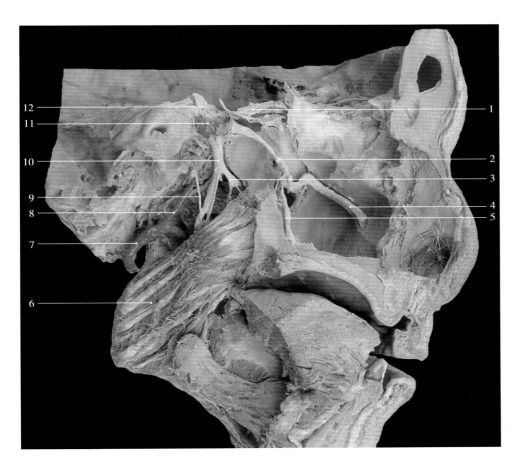

◀ 图 1-74　三叉神经内侧面观
Fig. 1-74　Medial aspect of the trigeminal nerve

1. 眼 神 经 ophthalmic nerve
2. 上 颌 神 经 maxillary nerve
3. 颊神经 buccal nerve
4. 眶下神经 infraorbital nerve
5. 腭大神经 greater palatine nerve
6. 翼内肌 medial pterygoid
7. 上 颌 动 脉 maxillary artery
8. 脑 膜 中 动 脉 middle meningeal artery
9. 鼓索 chorda tympanic
10. 下 颌 神 经 mandibular nerve
11. 三 叉 神 经 节 trigeminal ganglion
12. 三 叉 神 经 trigeminal nerve

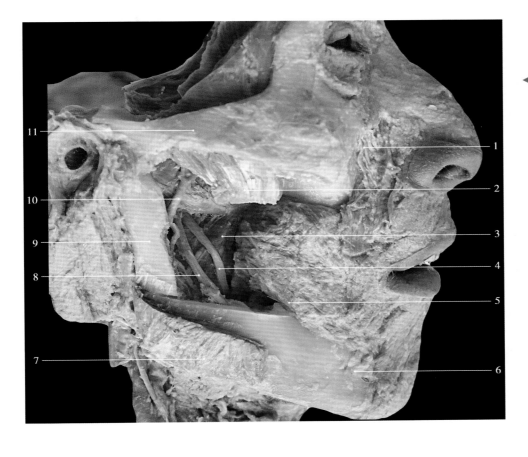

◀ 图 1-75　右侧下牙槽神经外侧面观
Fig. 1-75　Lateral aspect of the right inferior alveolar nerve

1. 眶下神经 infraorbital nerve
2. 颞肌 temporalis
3. 翼内肌 medial pterygoid
4. 舌神经 lingual nerve
5. 颊肌 buccinator
6. 颏神经 mental nerve
7. 咬肌 masseter
8. 下牙槽神经 inferior alveolar nerve
9. 下颌支 ramus of mandible
10. 上 颌 动 脉 maxillary artery
11. 颧弓 zygomatic arch

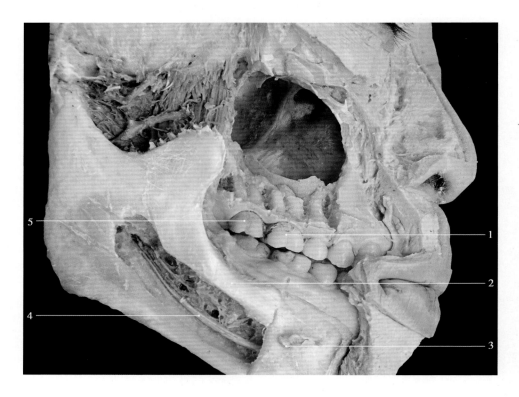

◀ 图 1-76 下牙槽神经管内段外侧面观
Fig. 1-76 Lateral aspect of the inferior alveolar nerve in the mandibular canal

1. 上颌第 1 磨牙 the 1st molar of maxilla
2. 下颌体 mandibular body
3. 颏孔 mental foramen
4. 下牙槽神经 inferior alveolar nerve
5. 上颌第 2 磨牙 the 2nd molar of maxilla

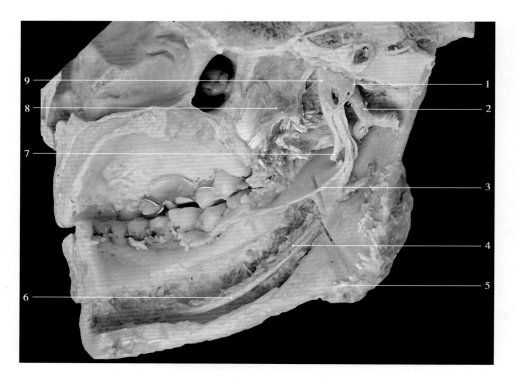

◀ 图 1-77 下牙槽神经管内段内侧面观
Fig. 1-77 Medial aspect of the inferior alveolar nerve in the mandibular canal

1. 鼓索 chorda tympanic
2. 上颌动脉 maxillary artery
3. 下颌舌骨肌支 mylohyoid branch
4. 下牙槽动脉 inferior alveolar artery
5. 下颌角 angle of mandible
6. 下牙槽神经管内段 inferior alveolar nerve in mandibular canal
7. 舌神经 lingual nerve
8. 腭帆张肌 circumflexus palati
9. 下颌神经 mandibular nerve

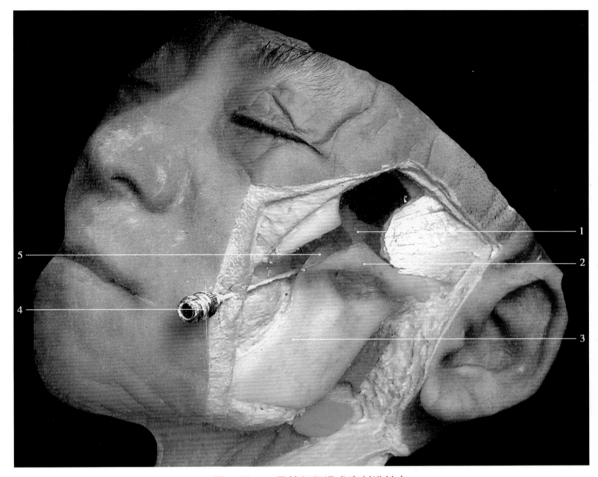

▲ 图1-78 三叉神经阻滞术穿刺进针点

Fig. 1-78 Needling point of the trigeminal nerve block

1. 三叉神经节 trigeminal ganglion
2. 颧弓 zygomatic arch
3. 下颌支 ramus of mandible
4. 穿刺针 transfixion pin
5. 冠突 coronoid process

三叉神经节阻滞术的应用解剖学要点

三叉神经是混合性脑神经,分布于头面部、黏膜、皮肌的一般感觉。三叉神经由感觉纤维、运动纤维组成,自脑桥腹外侧出脑,伸向前外侧经小脑幕与岩上窦下方至颞骨岩部前方终于三叉神经节,该节位于岩尖部三叉神经压迹处。小脑幕附着缘前端下方硬脑膜凹处形成三叉神经腔,蛛网膜与蛛网膜下隙也延伸入腔内包绕三叉神经根与三叉神经节的后部。硬脑膜及蛛网膜与神经节的结缔组织相融合,三叉神经节的内侧邻颈内动脉和海绵窦后部,节的下方靠近岩大神经。三叉神经节呈半月形,凸缘向前外。节的前缘由上向下分别连有眼神经、上颌神经和下颌神经(图1-78)。

应用解剖要点:

三叉神经节阻滞术的进针点常选在:颧弓后1/3下方,口角外侧2.5cm稍上方正对第2磨牙处进针,沿下颌支内侧面刺向后内侧至翼突基部达圆孔前方,在X线下证实针尖的位置后,改向后上刺入卵圆孔达三叉神经节。

穿刺层次:皮肤→皮下组织→口轮匝肌→翼外肌→卵圆孔→三叉神经节。

注意事项:三叉神经节阻滞术是经颅底达颅内的操作,是绝对无菌术的操作。因三叉神经节毗邻关系复杂,操作者一定要熟悉相关的应用解剖知识。

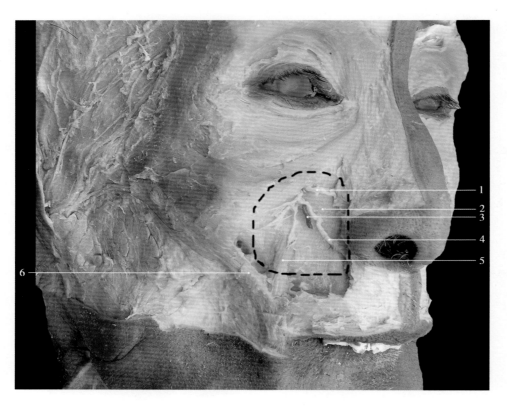

◀ 图 1-79　上颌窦前壁结构

Fig. 1-79　Structures of the anterior wall of the maxillary sinus

1. 眶下神经鼻外支 external nasal branch of infraorbital nerve
2. 上颌窦前壁 anterior wall of maxillary sinus
3. 眶下动脉 infraorbital artery
4. 眶下神经上唇支 superior labial branch of infraorbital nerve
5. 提口角肌 levator anguli oris
6. 颧大肌 zygomaticus major

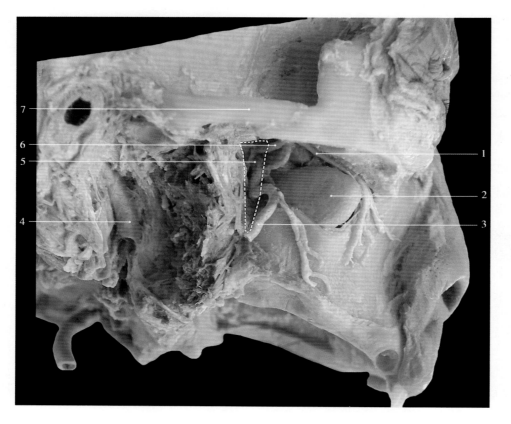

◀ 图 1-80　上颌窦黏膜外侧面观

Fig. 1-80　Lateral aspect of the mucous membrane of the maxillary sinus

1. 眶下神经 infraorbital nerve
2. 上颌窦黏膜 mucous membrane of maxillary sinus
3. 上颌动脉 maxillary artery
4. 颈内动脉 internal carotid artery
5. 翼腭窝 pterygopalatine fossa
6. 上颌神经 maxillary nerve
7. 颧弓 zygomatic arch

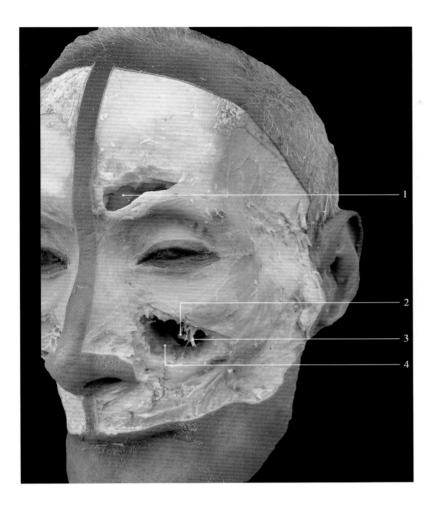

◀ 图 1-81 额窦和上颌窦（前壁已打开）
Fig. 1-81 Frontal and maxillary sinus (the anterior wall was opened)

1. 额窦 frontal sinus
2. 眶下动脉 infraorbital artery
3. 眶下神经 infraorbital nerve
4. 上颌窦 maxillary sinus

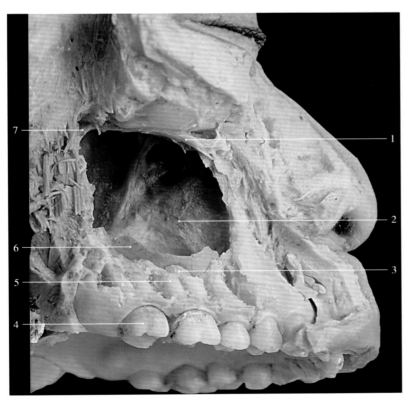

◀ 图 1-82 上颌窦底与上颌磨牙牙根
Fig. 1-82 Floor of the maxillary sinus and the roots of the maxillary molars

1. 眶下神经 infraorbital nerve
2. 上颌窦（已除去前外侧壁黏膜）maxillary sinus（the mucosa of the anterolateral wall was removed）
3. 上颌窦底骨质 bone of floor of maxillary sinus
4. 第 2 磨牙 the 2nd molar
5. 第 1 磨牙牙根 roots of the 1st molar
6. 上颌窦底黏膜 mucosa of floor of maxillary sinus
7. 上颌神经 maxillary nerve

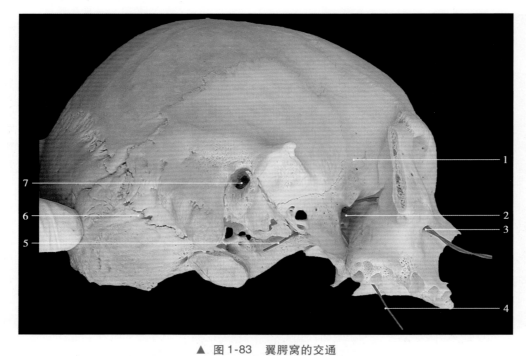

▲ 图1-83 翼腭窝的交通

Fig. 1-83 Communication of the pterygopalatine fossa

1. 翼点 pterion
2. 经圆孔至翼腭窝 through foramen rotundum to pterygopalatine fossa
3. 经眶下孔至翼腭窝 through infraorbital foramen to pterygopalatine fossa
4. 经翼腭管至翼腭窝 through pterygopalatine to pterygopalatine fossa
5. 经翼管至翼腭窝 through pterygoid canal to pterygopalatine fossa
6. 人字缝 lambdoid suture
7. 外耳门 external acoustic pore

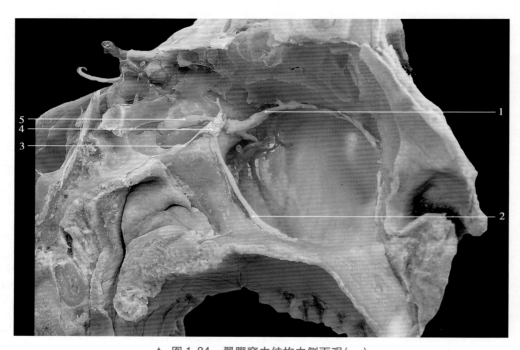

▲ 图1-84 翼腭窝内结构内侧面观（一）

Fig. 1-84 Medial aspect of the structures in the pterygopalatine fossa（1）

1. 眶下神经 infraorbital nerve
2. 腭大神经 greater palatine nerve
3. 翼管神经 nerve of pterygoid canal
4. 翼腭神经节 pterygopalatine ganglion
5. 上颌神经 maxillary nerve

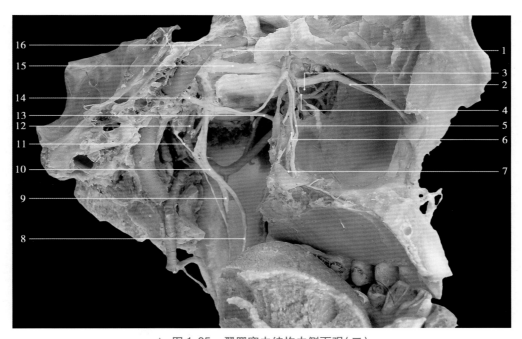

▲ 图 1-85　翼腭窝内结构内侧面观（二）
Fig. 1-85　Medial aspect of the structures in the pterygopalatine fossa（2）

1. 眼神经 ophthalmic nerve
2. 眶下神经 infraorbital nerve
3. 翼腭窝 pterygopalatine fossa
4. 蝶腭动脉 sphenopalatine artery
5. 腭大神经 greater palatine nerve
6. 腭小神经 lesser palatine nerve
7. 腭降动脉 descending palatine artery
8. 舌神经 lingual nerve
9. 下牙槽神经 inferior alveolar nerve
10. 下颌神经 mandibular nerve
11. 鼓索 chorda tympanic
12. 脑膜中动脉 middle meningeal artery
13. 颊神经 buccal nerve
14. 翼管神经 nerve of pterygoid canal
15. 上颌神经 maxillary nerve
16. 颈内动脉海绵窦部 cavernous part of internal carotid artery

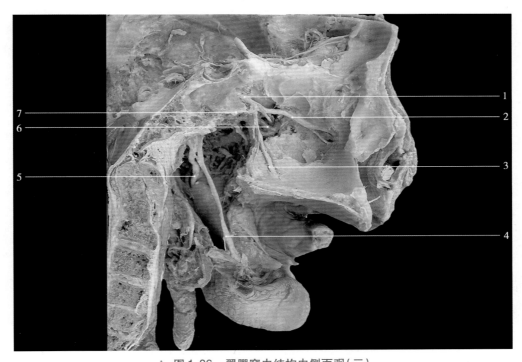

▲ 图 1-86　翼腭窝内结构内侧面观（三）
Fig. 1-86　Medial aspect of the structures in the pterygopalatine fossa（3）

1. 上颌神经 maxillary nerve
2. 眶下神经 infraorbital nerve
3. 腭大神经 greater palatine nerve
4. 舌神经 lingual nerve
5. 下牙槽神经 inferior alveolar nerve
6. 蝶腭动脉 sphenopalatine artery
7. 翼管神经 nerve of pterygoid canal

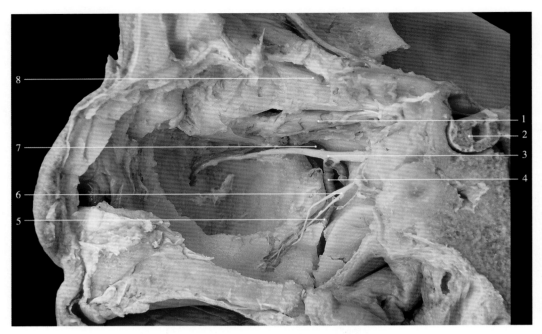

▲ 图 1-87 翼腭窝内结构内侧面观（四）
Fig. 1-87 Medial aspect of the structures in the pterygopalatine fossa（4）

1. 视神经 optic nerve
2. 垂体 hypophysis
3. 眶下神经 infraorbital nerve
4. 蝶腭动脉 sphenopalatine artery
5. 腭降动脉 descending palatine artery
6. 腭大神经 greater palatine nerve
7. 翼腭窝 pterygopalatine fossa
8. 内直肌 medial rectus

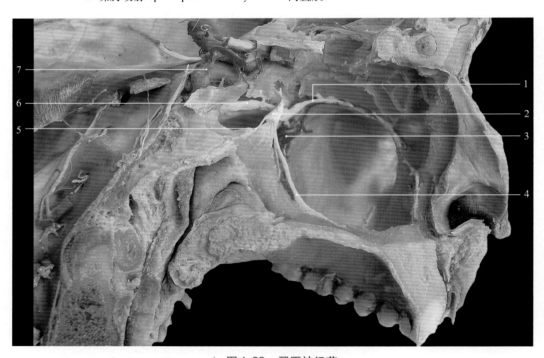

▲ 图 1-88 翼腭神经节
Fig. 1-88 Pterygopalatine ganglion

1. 眶下神经 infraorbital nerve
2. 翼腭神经节 pterygopalatine ganglion
3. 蝶腭动脉 sphenopalatine artery
4. 腭大神经 greater palatine nerve
5. 翼管神经 nerve of pterygoid canal
6. 上颌神经 maxillary nerve
7. 颈内动脉海绵窦部 cavernous part of internal carotid artery

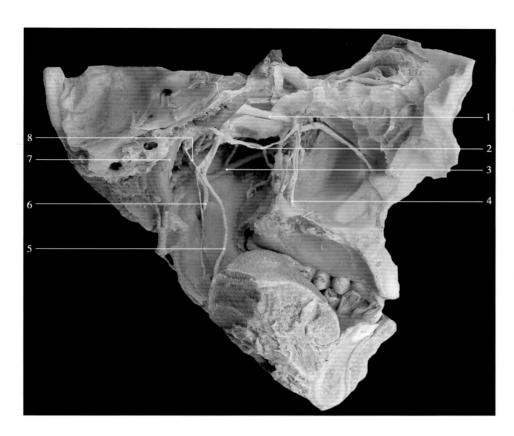

◀ 图 1-89 翼管神经
Fig. 1-89 Nerve of pterygoid canal

1. 上颌神经 maxillary nerve
2. 翼管神经 nerve of pterygoid canal
3. 上颌动脉 maxillary artery
4. 腭大神经 greater palatine nerve
5. 舌神经 lingual nerve
6. 下牙槽神经 inferior alveolar nerve
7. 颈内动脉岩部 petrosal part of internal carotid artery
8. 鼓索 chorda tympanic

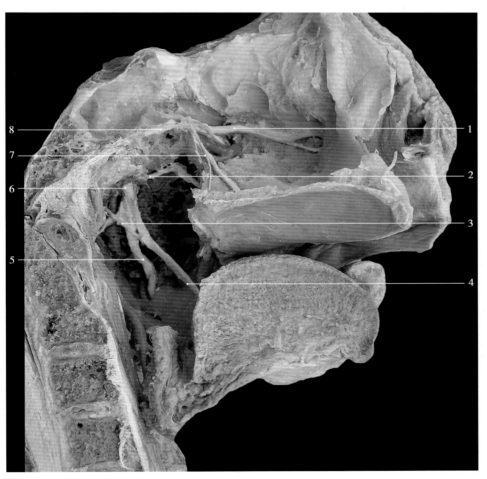

◀ 图 1-90 鼓索内侧面观
Fig. 1-90 Medial aspect of the chorda tympanic

1. 眶下神经 infraorbital nerve
2. 颊神经 buccal nerve
3. 鼓索 chorda tympanic
4. 舌神经 lingual nerve
5. 下牙槽神经 inferior alveolar nerve
6. 下颌神经 mandibular nerve
7. 腭大神经 greater palatine nerve
8. 上颌神经 maxillary nerve

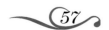

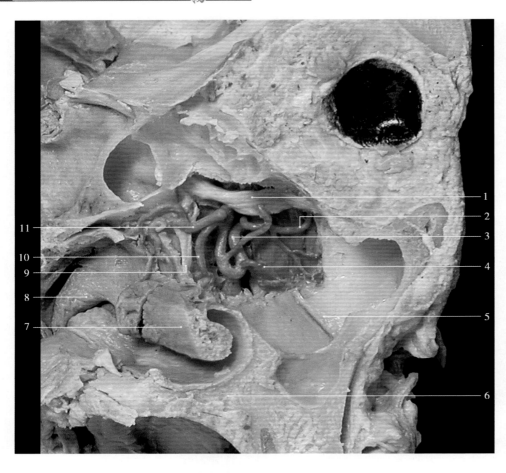

◀ 图 1-91 翼腭窝内侧面观 (示神经血管位置关系)
Fig. 1-91 Medial aspect of the pterygopalatine fossa (showing the positional relation of the nerves and vessels)

1. 上颌神经 maxillary nerve
2. 眶下动脉 infraorbital artery
3. 蝶腭动脉 sphenopalatine artery
4. 上牙槽中动脉 middle superior alveolar artery
5. 上颌窦 maxillary sinus
6. 硬腭 hard palate
7. 中鼻甲 middle nasal concha
8. 咽鼓管圆枕 tubal torus
9. 腭神经 palatine nerve
10. 腭降动脉 descending palatine artery
11. 鼻后外侧动脉 posterior lateral nasal artery

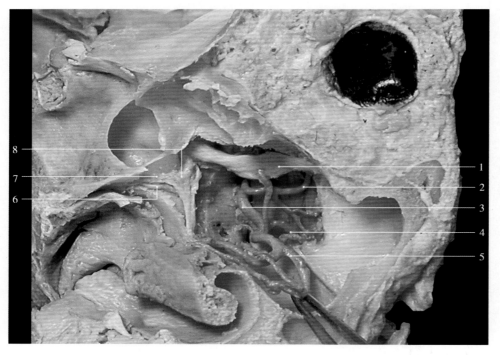

◀ 图 1-92 翼腭神经节和翼管神经内侧面观
Fig. 1-92 Medial aspect of the pterygopalatine ganglion and nerve of pterygoid canal

1. 眶下神经 infraorbital nerve
2. 眶下动脉 infraorbital artery
3. 蝶腭动脉 sphenopalatine artery
4. 上牙槽中动脉 middle superior alveolar artery
5. 鼻后外侧动脉 posterior lateral nasal arteries
6. 翼管动脉 artery of pterygoid canal
7. 翼管神经 nerve of pterygoid canal
8. 翼腭神经节 pterygopalatine ganglion

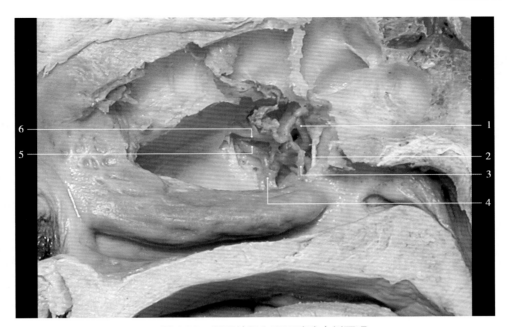

▲ 图 1-93 眶下神经和眶下动脉内侧面观

Fig. 1-93 Medial aspect of the infraorbital nerve and artery

1. 蝶腭动脉 sphenopalatine artery
2. 腭神经 palatine nerve
3. 腭降动脉 descending palatine artery
4. 鼻后外侧动脉 posterior lateral nasal arteries
5. 眶下动脉 infraorbital artery
6. 眶下神经 infraorbital nerve

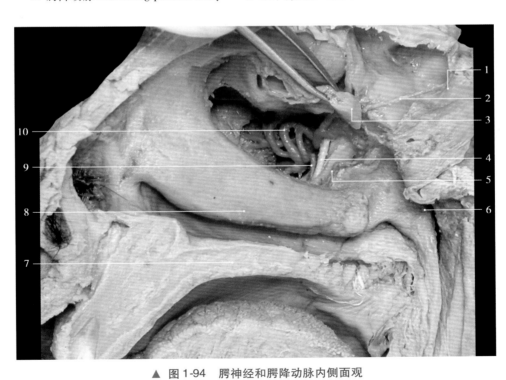

▲ 图 1-94 腭神经和腭降动脉内侧面观

Fig. 1-94 Medial aspect of the palatine nerve and descending palatine artery

1. 鼻中隔（翻向上）nasal septum（turned up）
2. 鼻中隔后动脉 posterior nasal septal artery
3. 上鼻甲（翻向上）superior nasal concha（turned up）
4. 腭神经 palatine nerve
5. 鼻后外侧动脉 posterior lateral nasal artery
6. 咽隐窝 pharyngeal recess
7. 硬腭 hard palate
8. 下鼻甲 inferior nasal concha
9. 腭降动脉 descending palatine artery
10. 蝶腭动脉 sphenopalatine artery

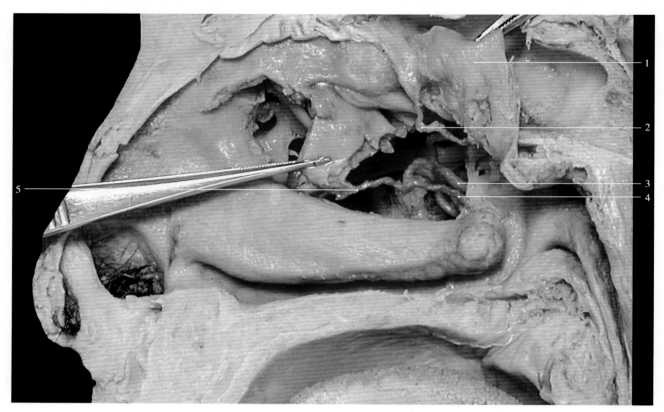

▲ 图 1-95　鼻后外侧动脉内侧面观

Fig. 1-95　Medial aspect of the posterior lateral nasal artery

1. 鼻中隔（翻向上）nasal septum（turned up）
2. 鼻中隔支 nasal septal branch
3. 鼻后外侧动脉 posterior lateral nasal artery
4. 中鼻甲支 middle nasoturbinal branch
5. 上鼻甲支 superior nasoturbinal branch

翼腭窝内神经血管的应用解剖学要点

翼腭窝是位于上颌骨体、蝶骨翼突、腭骨之间的狭小锥体形间隙。外侧借翼上颌裂与颞下窝相邻，其前壁为上颌窦后壁，内侧壁为腭骨垂直板，后壁为蝶骨翼突根部及大翼前部的下面，顶壁为蝶骨体的下面，下面移行为翼腭管。翼腭窝内有上颌神经、翼腭神经节、上颌动脉及其分支，窝内充满疏松的脂肪组织。

翼腭窝是许多手术操作涉及的区域，如颅底肿瘤切除术、翼管神经切除术等。其中口内入路经上颌窦在翼腭窝内行上颌神经经圆孔外高位切断加末梢神经撕脱术，用于对药物治疗无效的三叉神经上颌支痛是有效的（图 1-83～图 1-95）。

应用解剖要点：

1. 上颌神经出圆孔后随即分为两支，一支在上颌窦上壁与后壁交界的中点处进入眶下管，另一支在上颌窦后壁与内侧壁交界处下行，两者走行方向垂直。

2. 上颌动脉在翼腭窝内盘曲走行，其分支位于上颌窦后壁平行的平面内，在翼腭窝外侧部，动脉位于上颌神经主干的下方；在翼腭窝上部，动脉位于翼腭神经节的前方；在翼腭窝内侧部，动脉恒定地位于腭降神经的外侧。

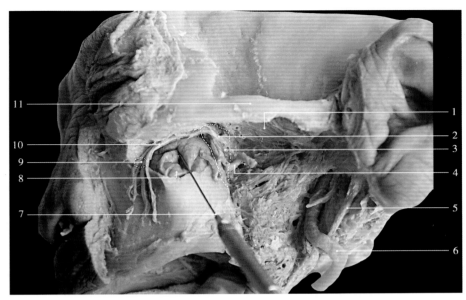

▲ 图 1-96 经上颌窦至翼腭窝上颌神经切除术手术入路外侧面观（左）

Fig. 1-96 Lateral aspect of excision of the maxillary nerve from the maxillary sinus to the pterygopalatine fossa (left)

1. 翼外肌 lateral pterygoid
2. 上颌神经 maxillary nerve
3. 翼腭窝 pterygopalatine fossa
4. 上颌动脉 maxillary artery
5. 茎突 styloid process
6. 颈内动脉 internal carotid artery
7. 探针 probe
8. 上颌窦黏膜 mucous membrane of maxillary sinus
9. 眶下孔 infraorbital foramen
10. 眶下神经 infraorbital nerve
11. 颧弓 zygomatic arch

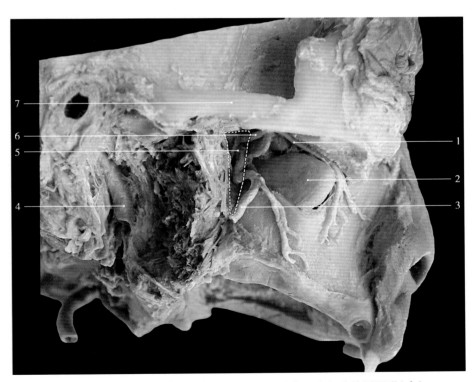

▲ 图 1-97 经上颌窦至翼腭窝上颌神经切除术手术入路外侧面观（右）

Fig. 1-97 Lateral aspect of excision of the maxillary nerve from the maxillary sinus to the pterygopalatine fossa (right)

1. 眶下神经 infraorbital nerve
2. 上颌窦黏膜 mucous membrane of maxillary sinus
3. 上颌动脉 maxillary artery
4. 颈内动脉 internal carotid artery
5. 翼腭窝 pterygopalatine fossa
6. 上颌神经 maxillary nerve
7. 颧弓 zygomatic arch

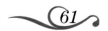

上颌神经的应用解剖学要点

上颌神经为感觉性神经,发自三叉神经节的凸侧,贴硬脑膜下、海绵窦外侧壁下部前行,经圆孔至翼腭窝,向前外侧经眶下裂入眶后称眶下神经。上颌神经分布于眼裂与口裂之间的皮肤、鼻、腭部黏膜和上颌牙、牙龈的一般感觉(图1-96、图1-97)。

应用解剖要点:

1. 上颌神经阻滞术的进针点常选在颧弓中点下缘处　穿刺层次为:皮肤→浅筋膜→深筋膜→咬肌筋膜→咬肌→翼内肌→翼外肌→翼腭窝→上颌神经。

2. 经上颌窦上颌神经切除术　在上唇与上颌牙龈交界处切开黏膜后沿上颌骨前面钝性分离上唇与上颌骨至眶下孔处,在眶下孔下方将上颌骨凿开2.5cm×2.5cm,经上颌窦前壁至后壁,凿开后壁至翼腭窝,沿上颌神经本干分离至圆孔,将上颌神经在圆孔处切断。

此手术入路的优点为:

1. 切断包括上牙槽后神经在内的上颌神经颅外段全部,可有效降低上颌神经切除后的复发率。

2. 经唇切至眶下孔其切口隐蔽,有效保护了患者的面容而且手术方法易被患者接受。

3. 注意事项

(1) 在翼腭窝内分离上颌神经时要注意窝内的上颌动脉,动脉位于神经的外侧。

(2) 撕拽上颌神经时,要防止脑脊液漏。

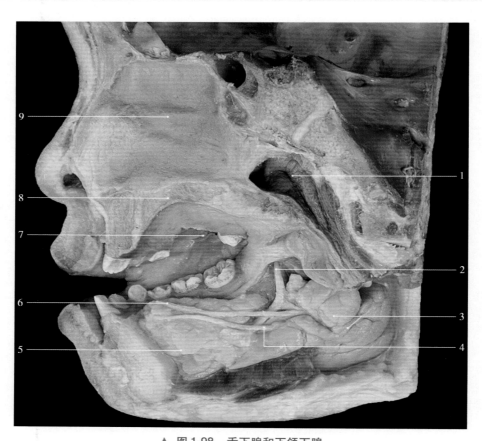

▲ 图1-98　舌下腺和下颌下腺
Fig. 1-98　Sublingual gland and submandibular gland

1. 咽鼓管圆枕 tubal torus
2. 舌神经 lingual nerve
3. 下颌下腺 submandibular gland
4. 舌下腺导管 sublingual duct
5. 舌下腺 sublingual gland
6. 下颌下腺导管 submandibular gland duct
7. 腮腺乳头 parotid papilla
8. 硬腭 hard palate
9. 鼻中隔 nasal septum

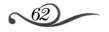

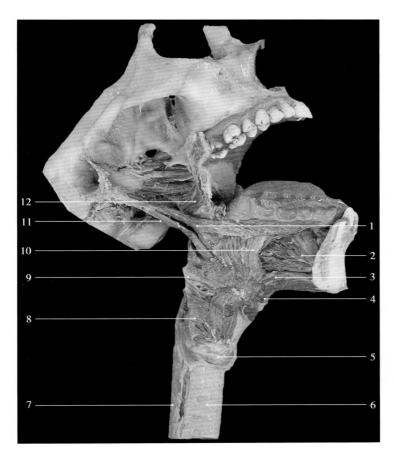

◀ 图 1-99 舌肌外侧面观
Fig. 1-99 Lateral aspect of the muscle of the tongue

1. 茎突舌肌 styloglossus
2. 颏舌肌 genioglossus
3. 颏舌骨肌 geniohyoid
4. 下颌舌骨肌 mylohyoid
5. 环状软骨 cricoid cartilage
6. 气管 trachea
7. 食管 esophagus
8. 咽中缩肌 middle constrictor of pharynx
9. 舌骨大角 greater cornu of hyoid bone
10. 舌骨舌肌 hyoglossus
11. 茎突舌肌 styloglossus
12. 咽上缩肌 superior constrictor of pharynx

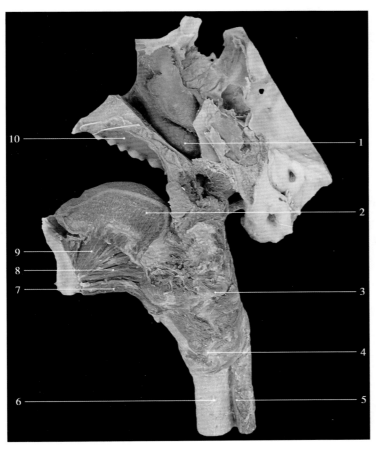

◀ 图 1-100 舌肌正中矢状切面
Fig. 1-100 Medial sagittal section of the muscle of the tongue

1. 下鼻甲 inferior nasal concha
2. 舌 tongue
3. 舌骨 hyoid bone
4. 环甲肌 cricothyroid
5. 食管 esophagus
6. 气管 trachea
7. 下颌舌骨肌 mylohyoid
8. 颏舌骨肌 geniohyoid
9. 颏舌肌 genioglossus
10. 硬腭 hard palate

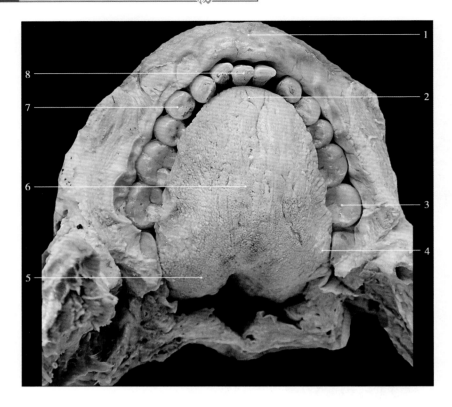

◀ 图 1-101 舌
Fig. 1-101　Tongue

1. 下唇 lower lip
2. 舌尖 apex of tongue
3. 第 2 磨牙 the 2nd molar
4. 舌缘 border of tongue
5. 舌根 root of tongue
6. 舌体 body of tongue
7. 第 1 前磨牙 the 1st premolar
8. 切牙 incisor

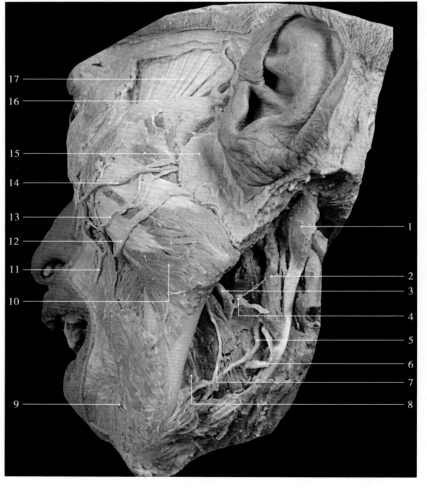

◀ 图 1-102　左侧下颌下神经节
Fig. 1-102　Left submandibular ganglion

1. 二腹肌后腹 posterior belly of digastric
2. 茎突舌骨肌 stylohyoid
3. 舌神经 lingual nerve
4. 下颌下神经节 submandibular ganglion
5. 舌动脉 lingual artery
6. 舌下神经 hypoglossal nerve
7. 下颌舌骨肌支 mylohyoid branch
8. 下颌舌骨肌 mylohyoid
9. 降口角肌 depressor anguli oris
10. 咬肌 masseter
11. 面动脉 facial artery
12. 腮腺管 parotid duct
13. 面神经颊支 buccal branches
14. 面横动脉 transverse facial artery
15. 腮腺 parotid gland
16. 颧弓 zygomatic arch
17. 颞肌 temporalis

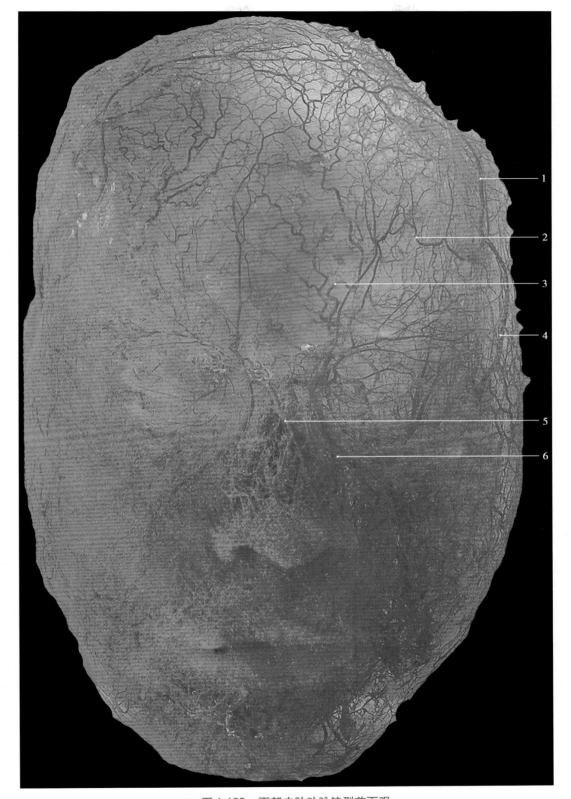

▲ 图 1-103　面部皮肤动脉铸型前面观

Fig. 1-103　Anterior aspect of the arterial cast of the facial skin

1. 颞浅动脉顶支 parietal branch of superficial temporal artery
2. 颞浅动脉额支 frontal branch of superficial temporal artery
3. 眶上动脉 supraorbital artery
4. 颞浅动脉 superficial temporal artery
5. 鼻背动脉 dorsal nasal artery
6. 面动脉 facial artery

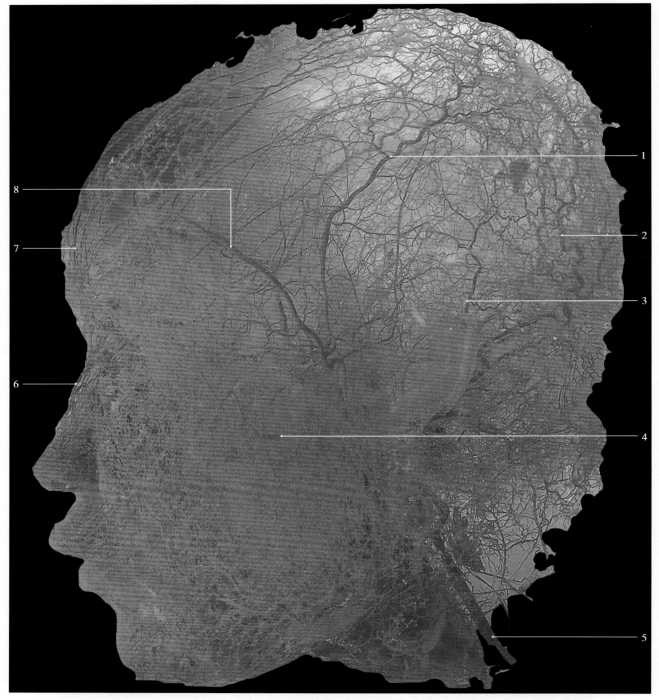

▲ 图 1-104 顶颞部皮肤动脉铸型左侧面观

Fig. 1-104 Left aspect of the arterial cast of the parietal-temporal skin

1. 颞浅动脉顶支 parietal branch of superficial temporal artery
2. 枕动脉 occipital artery
3. 耳后动脉 posterior auricular artery
4. 面横动脉 transverse facial artery
5. 颈外动脉 external carotid artery
6. 鼻背动脉 dorsal nasal artery
7. 眶上动脉 supraorbital artery
8. 颞浅动脉额支 frontal branch of superficial temporal artery

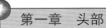

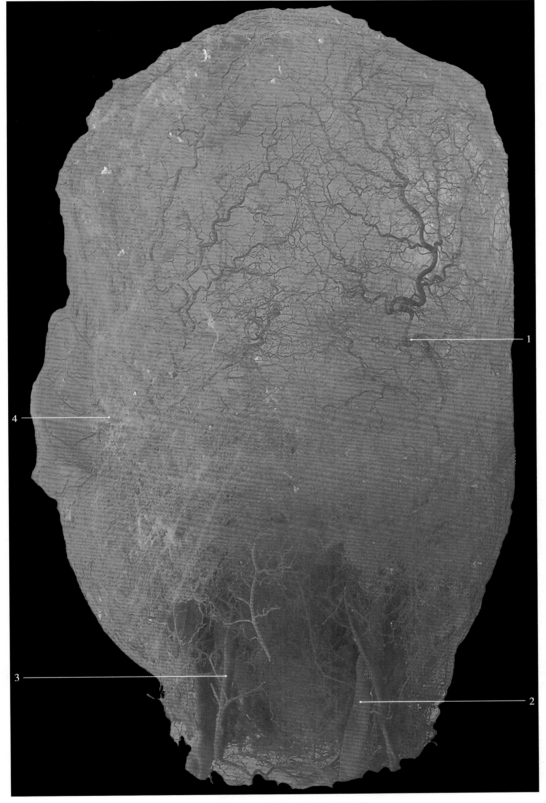

▲ 图 1-105 顶枕部皮肤动脉铸型
Fig. 1-105 Arterial cast of the parietal-occipital skin

1. 枕动脉 occipital artery   3. 椎动脉 vertebral artery
2. 颈内动脉 internal carotid artery   4. 耳后动脉 posterior auricular artery

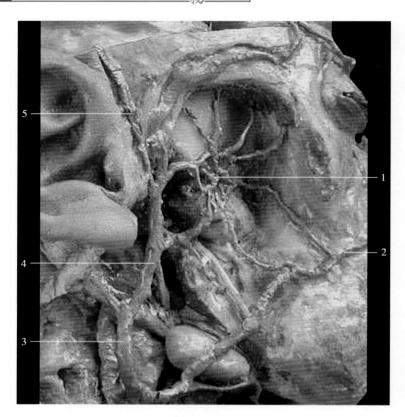

◀ 图 1-106　翼静脉丛
Fig. 1-106　Pterygoid venous plexus

1. 翼静脉丛 pterygoid venous plexus
2. 面静脉 facial vein
3. 下颌后静脉 retromandibular vein
4. 上颌静脉 maxillary vein
5. 颞浅静脉 superficial temporal vein

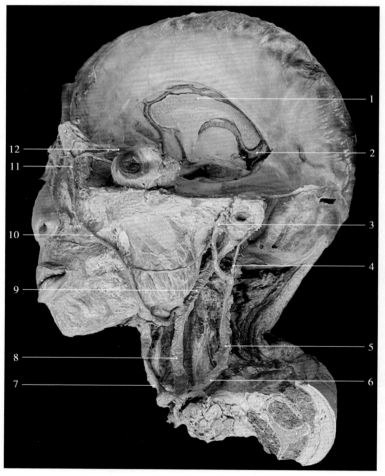

◀ 图 1-107　头颈部静脉
Fig. 1-107　Vein of the head and neck

1. 胼胝体 corpus callosum
2. 大脑大静脉 great cerebral vein
3. 颞浅静脉 superficial temporal vein
4. 耳后静脉 posterior auricular vein
5. 颈外静脉 external jugular vein
6. 锁骨下静脉 subclavian vein
7. 颈前静脉 anterior jugular vein
8. 颈内静脉 internal jugular vein
9. 下颌后静脉 retromandibular vein
10. 面静脉 facial vein
11. 内眦静脉 angular vein
12. 眼静脉 ophthalmic vein

第五节 眶腔结构

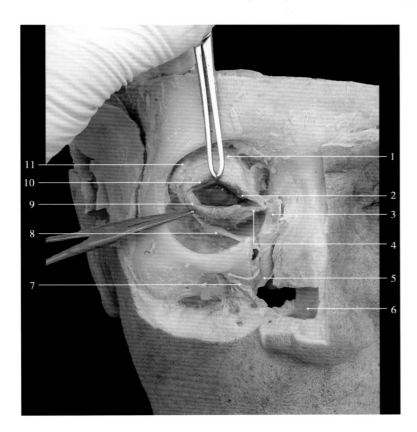

◀ 图 1-108 泪器
Fig. 1-108 Lacrimal apparatus

1. 上睑板 superior tarsus
2. 上泪点 superior lacrimal punctum
3. 泪囊 lacrimal sac
4. 下泪小管 inferior lacrimal ductule
5. 鼻泪管 nasolacrimal duct
6. 下鼻道 inferior nasal meatus
7. 眶下神经 infraorbital nerve
8. 下斜肌 inferior obliquus
9. 下睑缘 inferior palpebral edge
10. 上睑缘 superior palpebral edge
11. 泪腺 lacrimal gland

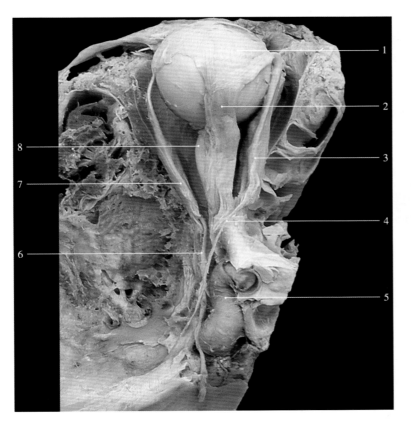

◀ 图 1-109 眶内结构上面观
Fig. 1-109 Superior aspect of the structures in the orbit

1. 眼球 eyeball
2. 上直肌 superior rectus
3. 上斜肌 superior obliquus
4. 滑车神经 trochlear nerve
5. 颈内动脉海绵窦部 cavernous part of internal carotid artery
6. 展神经 abducent nerve
7. 外直肌 lateral rectus
8. 视神经 optic nerve

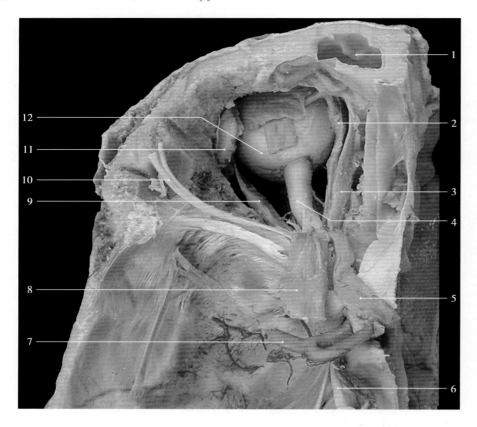

◀ 图 1-110　眼球外肌上面观
Fig. 1-110　Superior aspect of the ocular muscles

1. 额窦 frontal sinus
2. 内直肌 medial rectus
3. 上斜肌 superior obliquus
4. 视神经 optic nerve
5. 上睑提肌 levator palpebrae superioris
6. 动眼神经 oculomotor nerve
7. 大脑中动脉 middle cerebral artery
8. 上直肌 superior rectus
9. 外直肌 lateral rectus
10. 额神经 frontal nerve
11. 泪腺 lacrimal gland
12. 眼球 eyeball

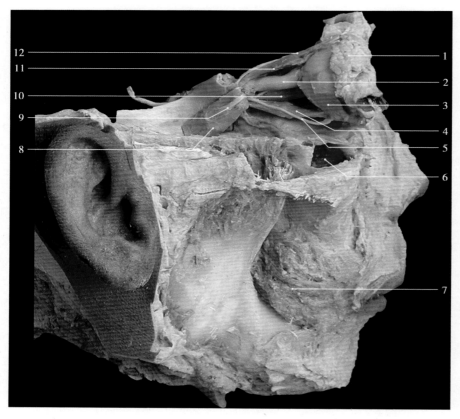

◀ 图 1-111　眼球外肌外侧面观
Fig. 1-111　Lateral aspect of the ocular muscles

1. 泪腺 lacrimal gland
2. 视神经 optic nerve
3. 下斜肌 inferior obliquus
4. 下直肌 inferior rectus
5. 动眼神经下支 inferior branch of culomotor nerve
6. 上颌窦 maxillary sinus
7. 颊肌 buccinator
8. 外直肌（向后翻）lateral rectus（turned posteriorly）
9. 展神经 abducent nerve
10. 内直肌 medial rectus
11. 上直肌 superior rectus
12. 上睑提肌 levator palpebrae superioris

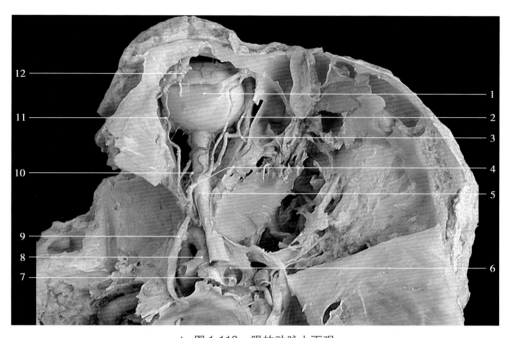

▲ 图 1-112　眼的动脉上面观

Fig. 1-112　Superior aspect of the arteries of the eye

1. 眼球 eyeball
2. 筛前动脉 anterior ethmoidal artery
3. 筛后动脉 posterior ethmoidal artery
4. 眼动脉 ophthalmic artery
5. 视神经 optic nerve
6. 鞍膈 diaphragma sellae

7. 漏斗 infundibulum
8. 颈内动脉 internal carotid artery
9. 动眼神经 oculomotor nerve
10. 睫后长动脉 long posterior ciliary artery
11. 泪腺动脉 lacrimal artery
12. 泪腺 lacrimal gland

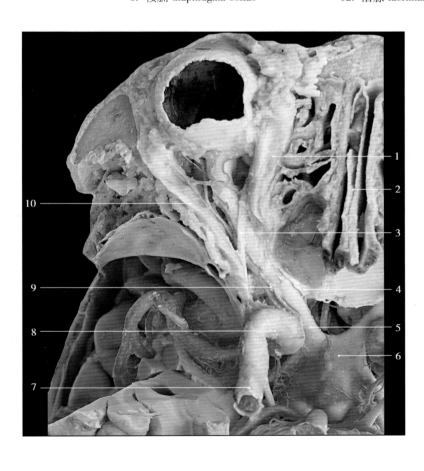

◀ 图 1-113　眼的动脉下面观

Fig. 1-113　Inferior aspect of the arteries of the eye

1. 内直肌 medial rectus
2. 鼻中隔 nasal septum
3. 动眼神经下支 inferior branch of oculo-motor nerve
4. 视神经管 optic canal
5. 视神经 optic nerve
6. 视交叉 optic chiasma
7. 颈内动脉 internal carotid artery
8. 床突上段 supraclinoid part
9. 眼动脉 ophthalmic artery
10. 外直肌 lateral rectus

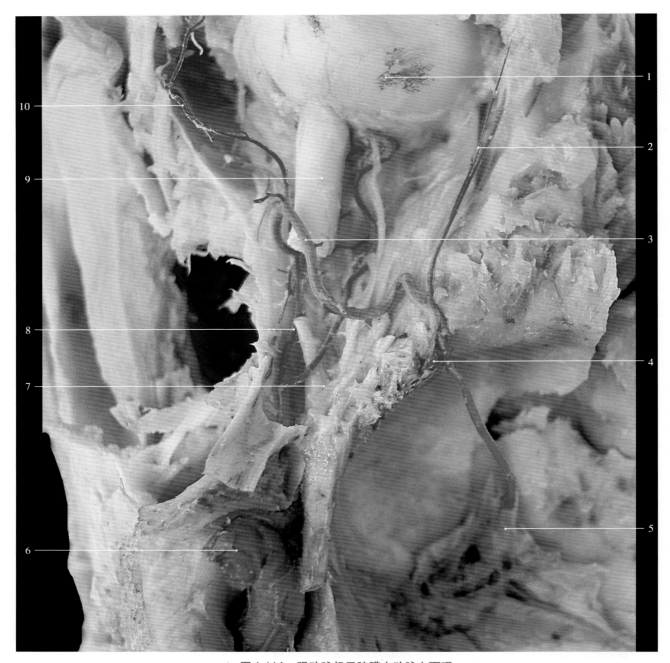

▲ 图 1-114 眼动脉起于脑膜中动脉上面观

Fig. 1-114 Superior aspect of the ophthalmic artery coming from the middle meningeal artery

1. 眼球 eyeball
2. 泪腺动脉 lacrimal artery
3. 眼动脉 ophthalmic artery
4. 脑膜中动脉吻合支 anastomosing branch of middle meningeal artery
5. 脑膜中动脉 middle meningeal artery
6. 颈内动脉 internal carotid artery
7. 动眼神经 oculomotor nerve
8. 筛后动脉 posterior ethmoidal artery
9. 视神经 optic nerve
10. 筛前动脉 anterior ethmoidal artery

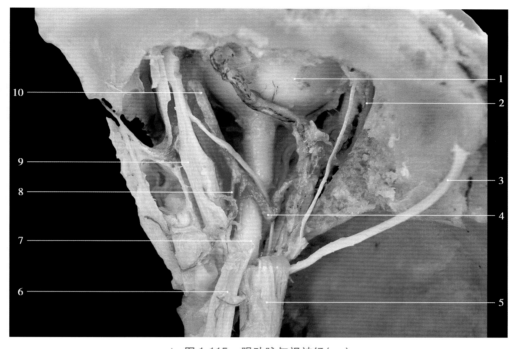

▲ 图 1-115　眼动脉与视神经（一）

Fig. 1-115　Ophthalmic artery and optic nerve（1）

1. 眼球 eyeball
2. 泪腺动脉 lacrimal artery
3. 额神经 frontal nerve
4. 眼动脉 ophthalmic artery
5. 上睑提肌（翻向后）levator palpebrae superioris（turned posteriorly）
6. 上直肌（翻向后）superior rectus（turned posteriorly）
7. 视神经 optic nerve
8. 眼肌动脉 muscular artery
9. 上斜肌 superior obliquus
10. 筛前动脉 anterior ethmoidal artery

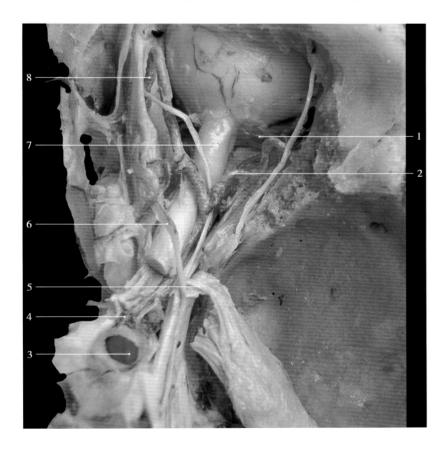

◀ 图 1-116　眼动脉与视神经（二）

Fig. 1-116　Ophthalmic artery and optic nerve（2）

1. 睫后短动脉 short posterior ciliary artery
2. 泪腺动脉 lacrimal artery
3. 颈内动脉 internal carotid artery
4. 眼动脉 ophthalmic artery
5. 展神经（翻向后）abducent nerve（turned posteriorly）
6. 滑车神经 trochlear nerve
7. 视神经 optic nerve
8. 筛前动脉 anterior ethmoidal artery

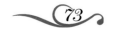

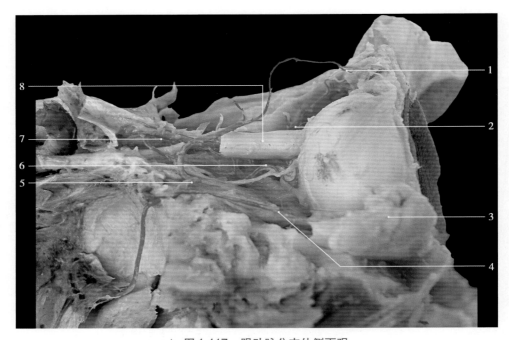

▲ 图 1-117　眼动脉分支外侧面观
Fig. 1-117　Lateral aspect of the branches of the ophthalmic artery

1. 筛前动脉 anterior ethmoidal artery
2. 睫后长动脉 long posterior ciliary artery
3. 泪腺 lacrimal gland
4. 泪腺动脉 lacrimal artery
5. 眼动脉 ophthalmic artery
6. 睫后短动脉 short posterior ciliary artery
7. 筛后动脉 posterior ethmoidal artery
8. 视神经 optic nerve

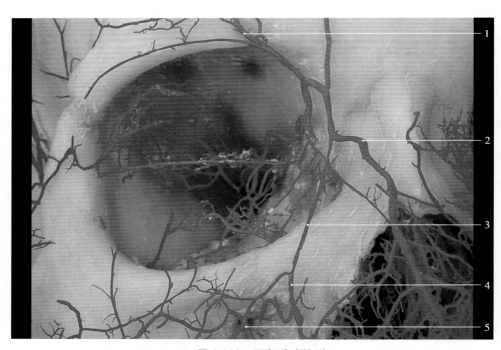

▲ 图 1-118　眶部动脉铸型
Fig. 1-118　Cast of the arteries around the orbit

1. 眶上动脉 supraorbital artery
2. 鼻外侧支 lateral nasal branch
3. 内眦动脉 angular artery
4. 面动脉 facial artery
5. 眶下动脉 infraorbital artery

第六节 脑

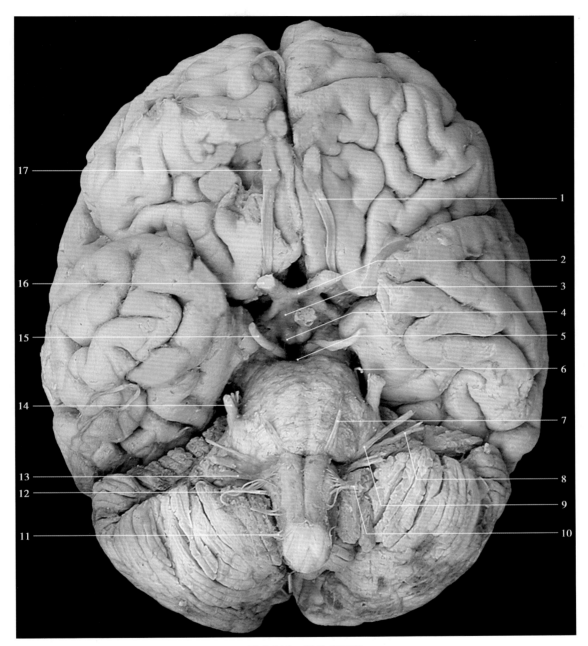

▲ 图 1-119 脑的底面观
Fig. 1-119 Basal aspect of the brain

1. 嗅束 olfactory tract
2. 视交叉 optic chiasma
3. 灰结节 tuber cinereum
4. 乳头体 mamillary body
5. 脚间窝 interpeduncular fossa
6. 滑车神经 trochlear nerve
7. 展神经 abducent nerve
8. 前庭蜗神经 vestibulocochlear nerve
9. 面神经 facial nerve
10. 舌下神经 hypoglossal nerve
11. 副神经 accessory nerve
12. 迷走神经 vagus nerve
13. 舌咽神经 glossopharyngeal nerve
14. 三叉神经 trigeminal nerve
15. 动眼神经 oculomotor nerve
16. 视神经 optic nerve
17. 嗅球 olfactory bulb

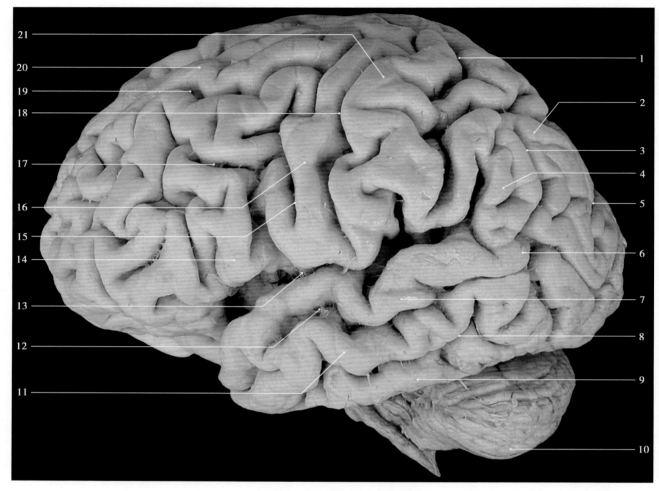

▲ 图 1-120　脑的背外侧面观
Fig. 1-120　Dorso-lateral aspect of the brain

1. 中央后沟 postcentral sulcus
2. 顶上小叶 superior parietal lobule
3. 顶内沟 intraparietal sulcus
4. 缘上回 supramarginal gyrus
5. 顶枕沟 parietooccipital sulcus
6. 角回 angular gyrus
7. 颞上回 superior temporal gyrus
8. 颞下沟 inferior temporal sulcus
9. 颞下回 inferior temporal gyrus
10. 小脑 cerebellum
11. 颞中回 middle temporal gyrus
12. 颞上沟 superior temporal sulcus
13. 外侧沟 lateral sulcus
14. 额下回 inferior frontal gyrus
15. 中央前沟 precentral sulcus
16. 中央前回 precentral gyrus
17. 额下沟 inferior frontal sulcus
18. 中央沟 central sulcus
19. 额上沟 superior frontal sulcus
20. 额上回 superior frontal gyrus
21. 中央后回 postcentral gyrus

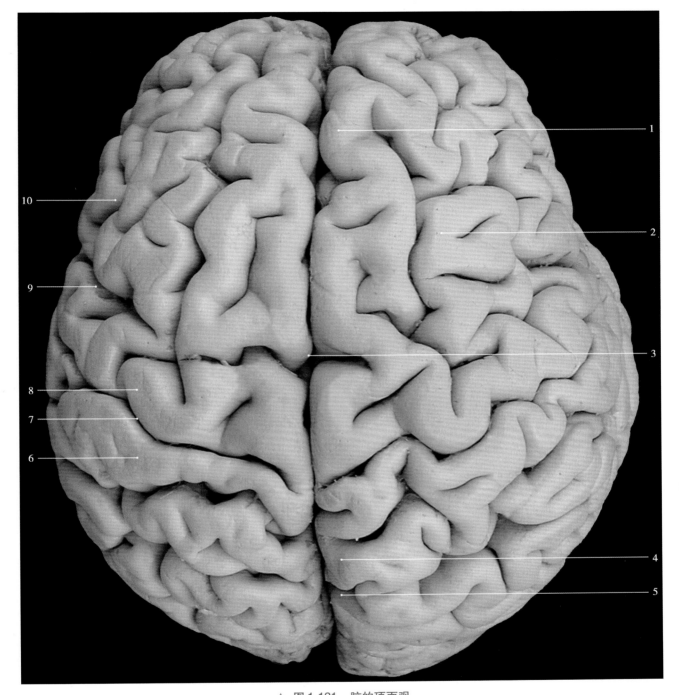

▲ 图 1-121 脑的顶面观
Fig. 1-121 Parietal aspect of the brain

1. 额上回 superior frontal gyrus
2. 额中回 middle frontal gyrus
3. 大脑纵裂 cerebral longitudinal fissure
4. 顶上小叶 superior parietal lobule
5. 顶枕沟 parietooccipital sulcus

6. 中央后回 postcentral gyrus
7. 中央沟 central sulcus
8. 中央前回 precentral gyrus
9. 外侧沟 lateral sulcus
10. 额下回 inferior frontal gyrus

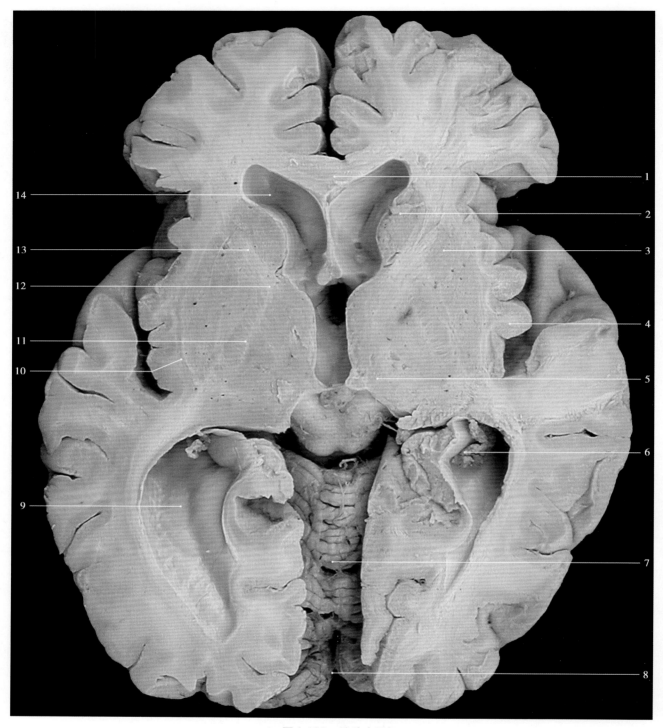

▲ 图 1-122 端脑水平切

Fig. 1-122 Horizontal section of the brain

1. 胼胝体 corpus callosum
2. 尾状核头 head of caudate nucleus
3. 豆状核 lentiform nucleus
4. 脑岛 insula
5. 背侧丘脑 dorsal thalamus
6. 侧脑室脉络丛 choroid plexus of lateral ventricle
7. 小脑蚓 vermis

8. 小脑后切迹 posterior cerebellar notch
9. 后角 posterior horn
10. 屏状核 claustrum
11. 内囊后肢 posterior limb of internal capsule
12. 内囊膝 genu of internal capsule
13. 内囊前肢 anterior limb of internal capsule
14. 前角 anterior horn

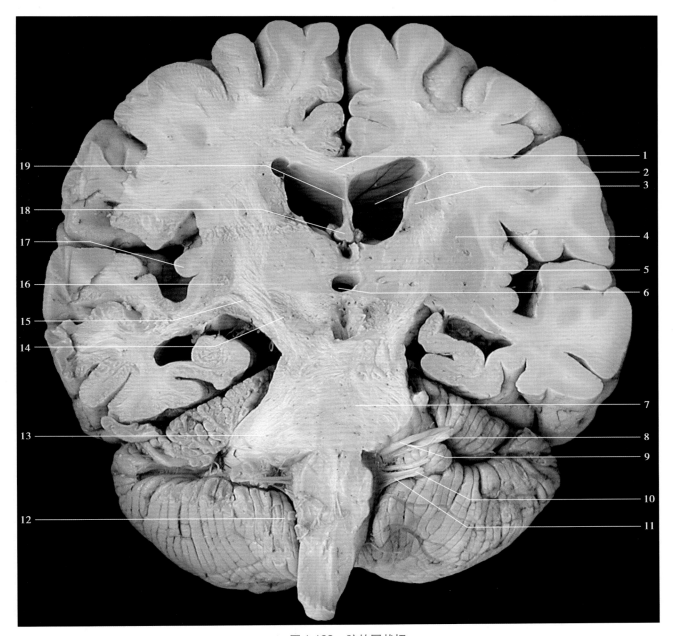

▲ 图1-123 脑的冠状切
Fig. 1-123 Coronary section of the brain

1. 胼胝体 corpus callosum
2. 侧脑室 lateral ventricle
3. 尾状核 caudate nucleus
4. 豆状核 lentiform nucleus
5. 背侧丘脑 dorsal thalamus
6. 第三脑室 third ventricle
7. 脑桥 pons
8. 前庭蜗神经 vestibulocochlear nerve
9. 面神经 facial nerve
10. 舌咽神经 glossopharyngeal nerve

11. 迷走神经 vagus nerve
12. 小脑扁桃体 tonsil of cerebellum
13. 小脑中脚 middle cerebellar peduncle
14. 黑质 substantia nigra
15. 内囊 internal capsule
16. 豆状核壳 putamen of lentiform nucleus
17. 脑岛 insula
18. 穹隆 fornix
19. 透明隔 septum pellucidum

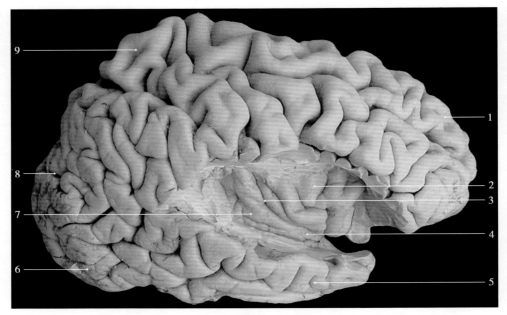

▲ 图 1-124 脑岛
Fig. 1-124 Insula

1. 额叶 frontal lobe
2. 岛短回 short gyri of insula
3. 岛中央沟 central sulcus of insula
4. 岛阈 limen insulae
5. 颞叶 temporal lobe
6. 枕叶 occipital lobe
7. 岛长回 long gyrus of insula
8. 顶枕沟 parietooccipital sulcus
9. 顶叶 parietal lobe

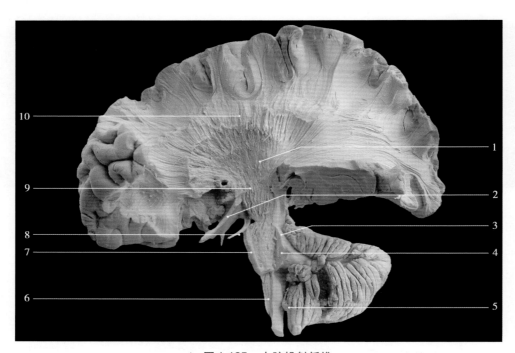

▲ 图 1-125 大脑投射纤维
Fig. 1-125 Projective fiber of the cerebrum

1. 内囊 internal capsule
2. 视束 optic tract
3. 上髓帆 superior medullary velum
4. 小脑中脚 middle cerebellar peduncle
5. 小脑扁桃体 tonsil of cerebellum
6. 延髓 medulla oblongata
7. 脑桥 pons
8. 动眼神经 oculomotor nerve
9. 锥体束 pyramidal tract
10. 辐射冠 corona radiate

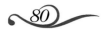

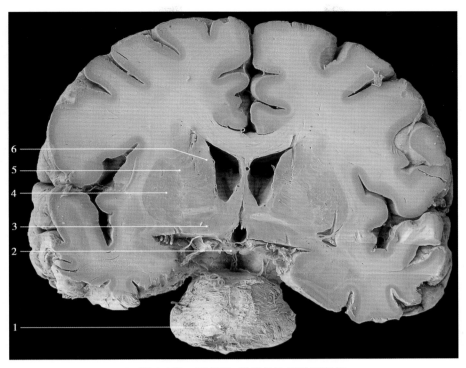

▲ 图 1-126　豆状核、尾状核和丘脑冠状切
Fig. 1-126　Coronary section of the lentiform nucleus，caudate nucleus and thalamus

1. 脑桥 pons　　　　　3. 丘脑 thalamus　　　　　5. 内囊 internal capsule
2. 乳头体 mamillary body　　4. 豆状核 lentiform nucleus　　6. 尾状核头 head of caudate nucleus

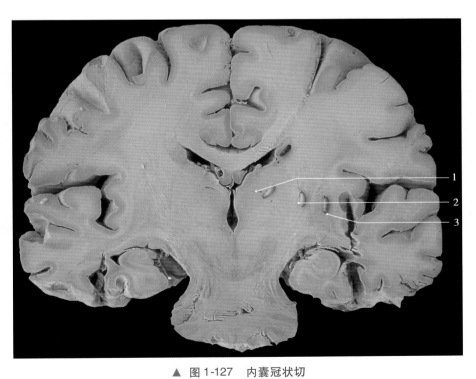

▲ 图 1-127　内囊冠状切
Fig. 1-127　Coronary section of the internal capsule

1. 尾状核头 head of caudate nucleus　　　2. 内囊 internal capsule　　　3. 豆状核 lentiform nucleus

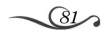

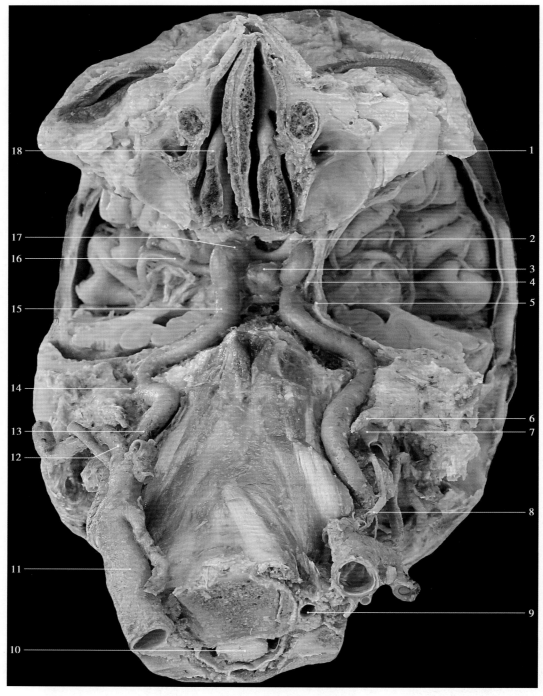

▲ 图 1-128　垂体下面观

Fig. 1-128　Inferior aspect of the hypophysis

1. 上颌窦口 ostium of maxillary sinus
2. 视神经 optic nerve
3. 垂体 hypophysis
4. 动眼神经 oculomotor nerve
5. 海绵窦外侧壁 lateral wall of cavernous sinus
6. 茎突 styloid process
7. 颈内静脉 internal jugular vein
8. 迷走神经 vagus nerve
9. 椎动脉 vertebral artery

10. 颈髓 cervical spinal cord
11. 颈总动脉 common carotid artery
12. 颈外动脉 external carotid artery
13. 颈内动脉 internal carotid artery
14. 颈动脉管外口 external aperture of carotid canal
15. 破裂孔段 lacerum part
16. 大脑中动脉 middle cerebral artery
17. 床突上段 supraclinoid part
18. 中鼻甲 middle nasal concha

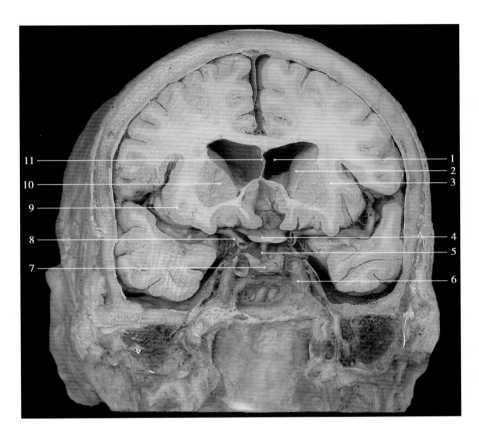

◀ 图 1-129 垂体冠状切
Fig. 1-129 Coronary section of the hypophysis

1. 侧脑室 lateral ventricle
2. 尾状核头 head of caudate nucleus
3. 内囊 internal capsule
4. 视交叉 optic chiasma
5. 垂体柄 hypophysial stalk
6. 颈内动脉海绵窦部 cavernous part of internal carotid artery
7. 垂体 hypophysis
8. 颈内动脉 internal carotid artery
9. 豆状核 lentiform nucleus
10. 丘脑 thalamus
11. 透明隔 septum pellucidum

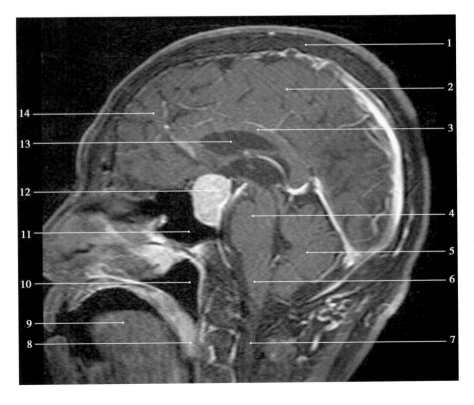

◀ 图 1-130 垂体瘤
Fig. 1-130 Hypophysoma

1. 颅骨 skull
2. 顶叶 parietal lobe
3. 胼胝体 corpus callosum
4. 脑桥 pons
5. 小脑 cerebellum
6. 延髓 medulla oblongata
7. 颈髓 cervical spinal cord
8. 腭垂 uvula
9. 舌 tongue
10. 鼻咽部 nasopharynx
11. 蝶窦 sphenoid sinus
12. 垂体瘤 hypophysoma
13. 侧脑室 lateral ventricle
14. 额叶 frontal lobe

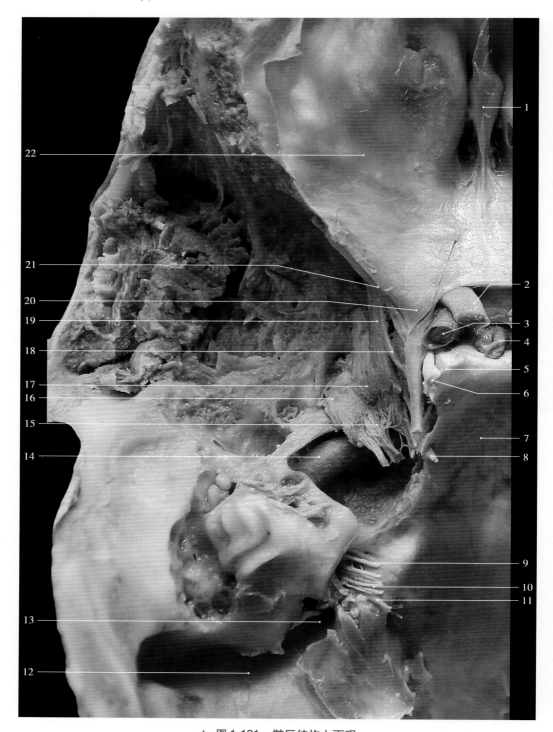

▲ 图 1-131 鞍区结构上面观

Fig. 1-131 Superior aspect of the structures of the sellar region

1. 鸡冠 crista galli
2. 视神经 optic nerve
3. 颈内动脉 internal carotid artery
4. 垂体柄 hypophysial stalk
5. 后床突 posterior clinoid process
6. 动眼神经 oculomotor nerve
7. 斜坡 clivus
8. 展神经 abducent nerve

9. 舌咽神经 glossopharyngeal nerve
10. 迷走神经 vagus nerve
11. 副神经 accessory nerve
12. 横窦 transverse sinus
13. 乙状窦 sigmoid sinus
14. 颈内动脉岩部 petrosal part of internal carotid artery
15. 三叉神经 trigeminal nerve

16. 下颌神经 mandibular nerve
17. 三叉神经节 trigeminal ganglion
18. 滑车神经 trochlear nerve
19. 眼神经 ophthalmic nerve
20. 前床突 anterior clinoid process
21. 眶上裂 superior orbital fissure
22. 颅前窝 anterior cranial fossa

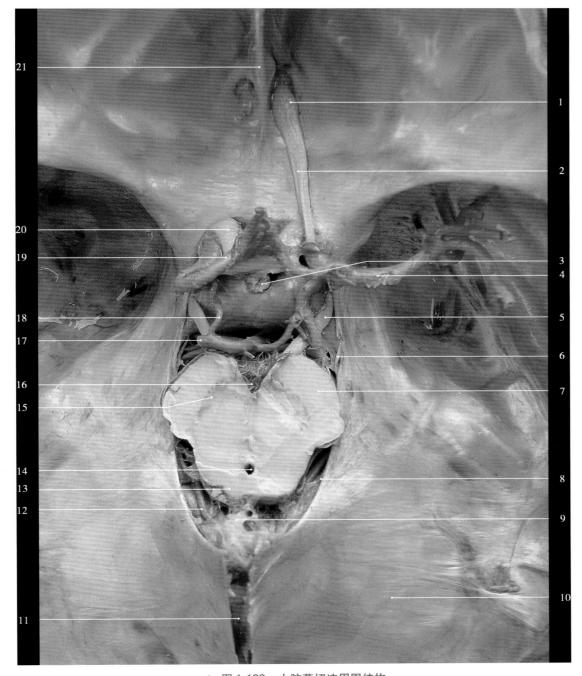

▲ 图 1-132 小脑幕切迹周围结构

Fig. 1-132 Structures around the tentorial notch

1. 嗅球 olfactory bulb
2. 嗅束 olfactory tract
3. 垂体柄 hypophysial stalk
4. 大脑中动脉 middle cerebral artery
5. 动眼神经 oculomotor nerve
6. 滑车神经 trochlear nerve
7. 大脑脚 cerebral peduncle
8. 小脑幕切迹 tentorial notch
9. 大脑深静脉 deep cerebral vein
10. 小脑幕 tentorium of cerebellum
11. 直窦 straight sinus
12. 小脑上动脉 superior cerebellar artery
13. 上丘 superior colliculus
14. 中脑导水管 mesencephalic aqueduct
15. 黑质 substantia nigra
16. 脚间窝 interpeduncular fossa
17. 大脑后动脉 posterior cerebral artery
18. 后交通动脉 posterior communicating artery
19. 大脑前动脉 anterior cerebral artery
20. 视神经 optic nerve
21. 鸡冠 crista galli

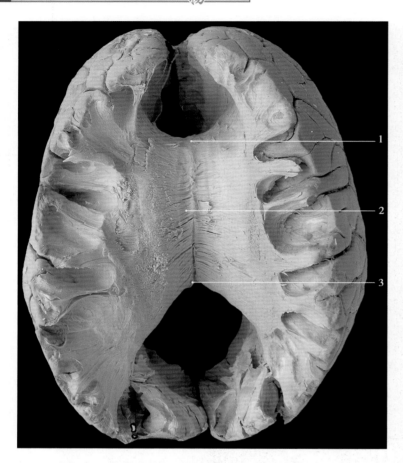

◀ 图 1-133 胼胝体上面观
Fig. 1-133 Superior aspect of the corpus callosum

1. 前钳 frontal forceps
2. 胼胝体干 trunk of corpus callosum
3. 后钳 occipital forceps

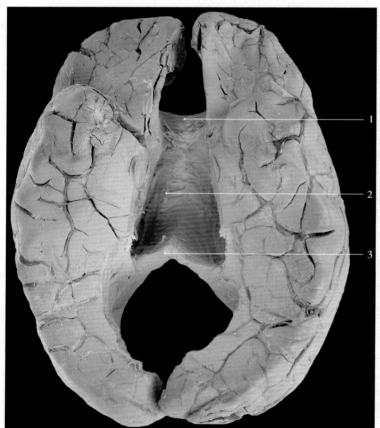

◀ 图 1-134 胼胝体下面观
Fig. 1-134 Inferior aspect of the corpus
callosum

1. 胼胝体膝 genu of corpus callosum
2. 胼胝体 corpus callosum
3. 胼胝体压部 splenium of corpus callosum

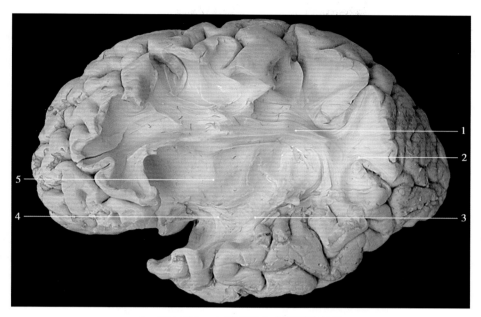

▲ 图 1-135　大脑半球内主要联络纤维
Fig. 1-135　Principle association fibers in the cerebral hemisphere

1. 上纵束 superior longitudinal fascicus
2. 大脑弓状纤维 cerebral arcuate fibers
3. 下纵束 inferior longitudinal fascicus
4. 钩束 uncinate fasciculus
5. 豆状核 lentiform nucleus

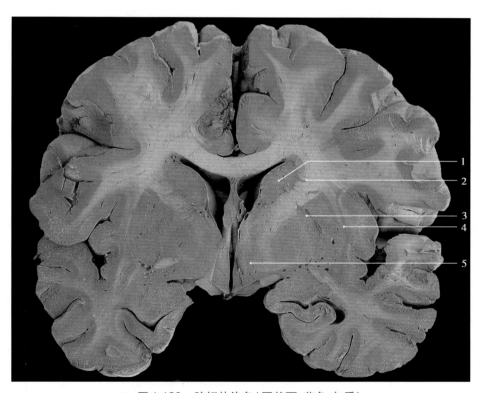

▲ 图 1-136　脑切片染色(冠状面,蓝色-灰质)
Fig. 1-136　Cerebral section-staining (coronary plane，blue-gray matter)

1. 尾状核头 head of caudate nucleus
2. 内囊前肢 anterior limb of internal capsule
3. 豆状核 lentiform nucleus
4. 屏状核 claustrum
5. 丘脑 thalamus

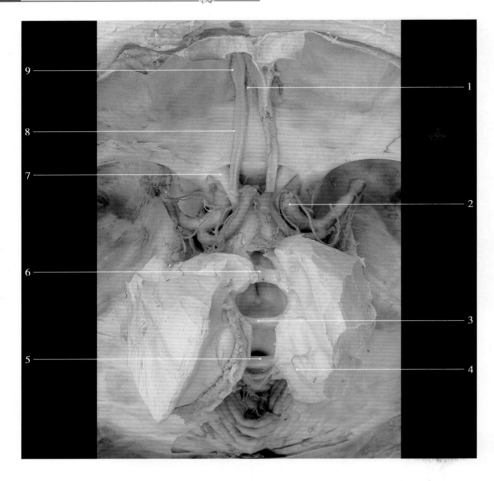

◀ 图 1-137　间脑间连合
Fig. 1-137　Commissure between the diencephalon

1. 鸡冠 crista galli
2. 颈内动脉 internal carotid artery
3. 丘脑间粘合 interthalamic adhesion
4. 丘脑 thalamus
5. 后连合 posterior commissure
6. 前连合 anterior commissure
7. 视神经 optic nerve
8. 嗅束 olfactory tract
9. 嗅球 olfactory bulb

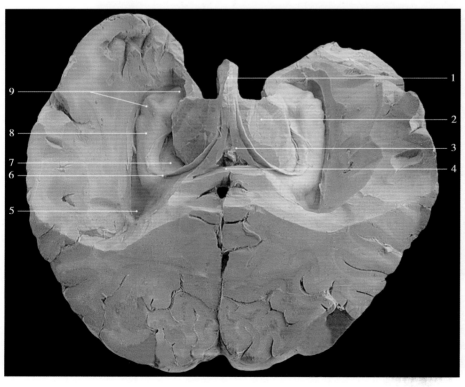

◀ 图 1-138　海马
Fig. 1-138　Hippocampus

1. 穹隆连合 commissure of fornix
2. 豆状核 lentiform nucleus
3. 穹隆脚 crus of fornix
4. 胼胝体 corpus callosum
5. 侧副三角 collateral trigone
6. 海马伞 fimbria of hippocampus
7. 海马旁回 parahippocampal gyrus
8. 海马 hippocampus
9. 海马足 pes hippocampi

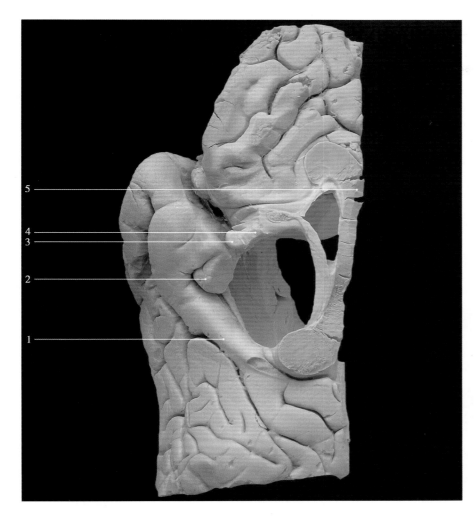

◀ 图 1-139 穹隆柱和乳头体
Fig. 1-139 Column of fornix and mamillary body

1. 海马旁回 parahippocampal gyrus
2. （海马旁回）钩 uncus of parahippocampal gyrus
3. 乳头体 mamillary body
4. 穹隆柱 column of fornix
5. 胼胝体 corpus callosum

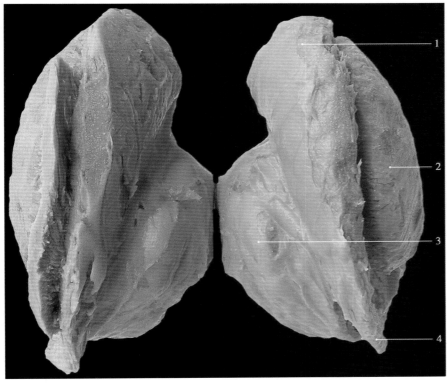

◀ 图 1-140 基底核上面观
Fig. 1-140 Superior aspect of the basal nuclei

1. 尾状核头 head of caudate nucleus
2. 豆状核 lentiform nucleus
3. 丘脑 thalamus
4. 尾状核尾 tail of caudate nucleus

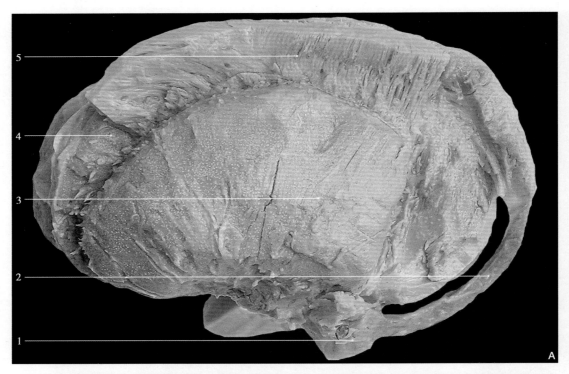

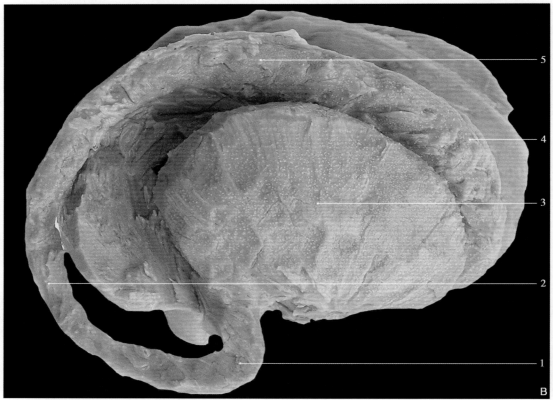

▲ 图 1-141　基底核外侧面观
Fig. 1-141　Lateral aspect of the basal nuclei

A：左侧　B：右侧

1. 杏仁核 amygdala
2. 尾状核尾 tail of caudate nucleus
3. 豆状核 lentiform nucleus
4. 尾状核头 head of caudate nucleus
5. 尾状核体 body of caudate nucleus

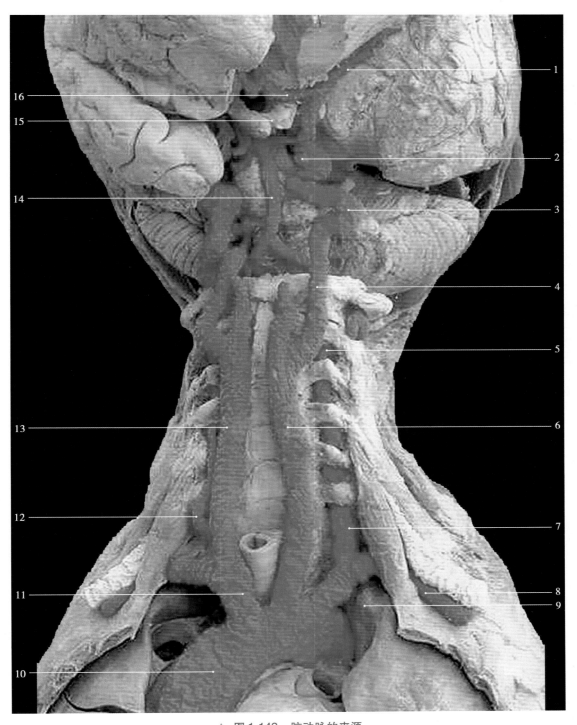

▲ 图 1-142　脑动脉的来源
Fig. 1-142　Source of the cerebral artery

1. 大脑中动脉 middle cerebral artery
2. 颈内动脉海绵窦部 cavernous part of internal carotid artery
3. 颈内动脉岩部 petrosal part of internal carotid artery
4. 左颈内动脉 left internal carotid artery
5. 左椎动脉横突部 transverse part of left vertebral artery
6. 左颈总动脉 left common carotid artery
7. 左椎动脉椎前部 prevertebral part of left vertebral artery
8. 左锁骨下动脉 left subclavian artery

9. 肺尖 apex of lung
10. 升主动脉 ascending aorta
11. 头臂干 brachiocephalic trunk
12. 右椎动脉 right vertebral artery
13. 右颈总动脉 right common carotid artery
14. 基底动脉 basilar artery
15. 视交叉 optic chiasma
16. 大脑前动脉 anterior cerebral artery

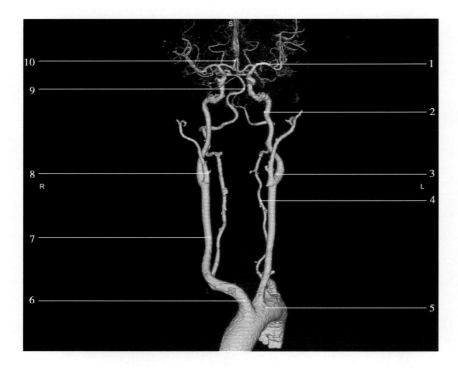

◀ 图 1-143 脑血管起源
Fig. 1-143 Origin of the cerebral vessels

1. 大脑中动脉 middle cerebral artery
2. 颈内动脉 internal carotid artery
3. 颈动脉窦 carotid sinus
4. 椎动脉 vertebral artery
5. 主动脉弓 aortic arch
6. 头臂干 brachiocephalic trunk
7. 颈总动脉 common carotid artery
8. 颈外动脉 external carotid artery
9. 基底动脉 basilar artery
10. 大脑前动脉 anterior cerebral artery

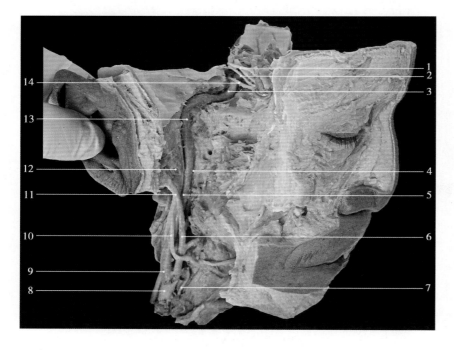

◀ 图 1-144 颈内动脉岩部右侧面观
Fig. 1-144 Right aspect of the petrosal part of internal carotid artery

1. 眼神经 ophthalmic nerve
2. 滑车神经 trochlear nerve
3. 颈内动脉破裂孔段 lacerum part of internal carotid artery
4. 颈动脉管外口 external aperture of carotid canal
5. 颈内动脉 internal carotid artery
6. 颈外动脉 external carotid artery
7. 甲状腺上动脉 superior thyroid artery
8. 颈总动脉 common carotid artery
9. 颈动脉窦 carotid sinus
10. 舌下神经 hypoglossal nerve
11. 枕动脉 occipital artery
12. 茎突根部 base of styloid process
13. 颈内动脉岩部 petrosal part of internal carotid artery
14. 展神经 abducent nerve

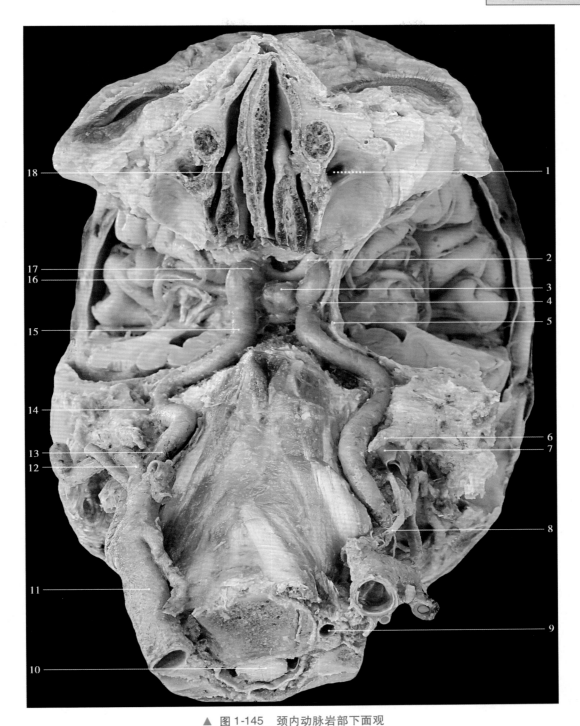

▲ 图 1-145 颈内动脉岩部下面观

Fig. 1-145 Inferior aspect of the petrosal part of internal carotid artery

1. 上颌窦口 ostium of maxillary sinus
2. 视神经 optic nerve
3. 垂体 pituitary
4. 动眼神经 oculomotor nerve
5. 海绵窦外侧壁 lateral wall of the cavernous sinus
6. 茎突 styloid process
7. 颈内静脉 internal jugular vein
8. 迷走神经 vagus nerve
9. 椎动脉 vertebral artery
10. 颈髓 cervical spinal cord
11. 颈总动脉 common carotid artery
12. 颈外动脉 external carotid artery
13. 颈内动脉 internal carotid artery
14. 颈动脉管外口 external aperture of carotid canal
15. 破裂孔段 lacerum part of internal carotid artery
16. 大脑中动脉 middle cerebral artery
17. 床突上段 supraclinoid part of internal carotid artery
18. 中鼻甲 middle nasal concha

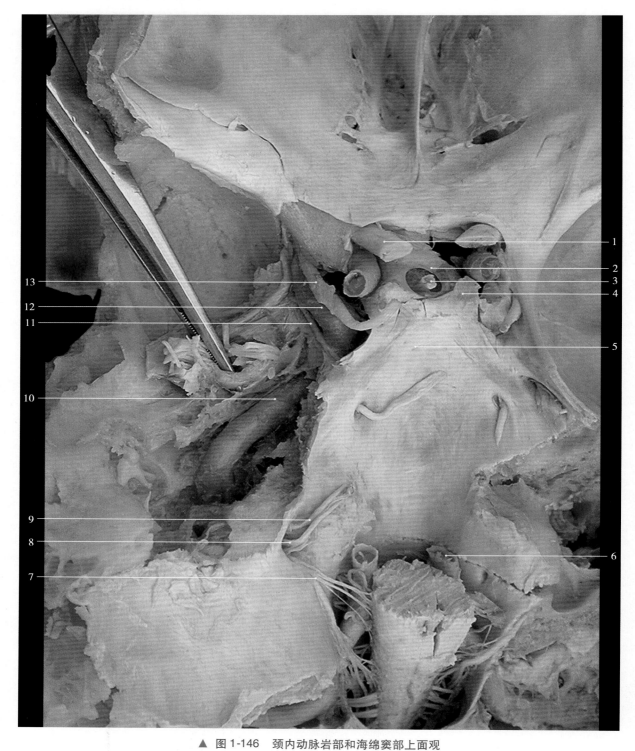

▲ 图 1-146　颈内动脉岩部和海绵窦部上面观

Fig. 1-146　Superior aspect of the petrosal and cavernous part of internal carotid artery

1. 视神经 optic nerve
2. 鞍膈 diaphragma sellae
3. 垂体柄 hypophysial stalk
4. 后床突 posterior clinoid process
5. 斜坡 clivus
6. 椎动脉 vertebral artery
7. 副神经 accessory nerve
8. 迷走神经 vagus nerve
9. 舌咽神经 glossopharyngeal nerve
10. 颈内动脉岩部 petrosal part of internal carotid artery
11. 展神经 abducent nerve
12. 颈内动脉海绵窦部 cavernous part of internal carotid artery
13. 动眼神经 oculomotor nerve

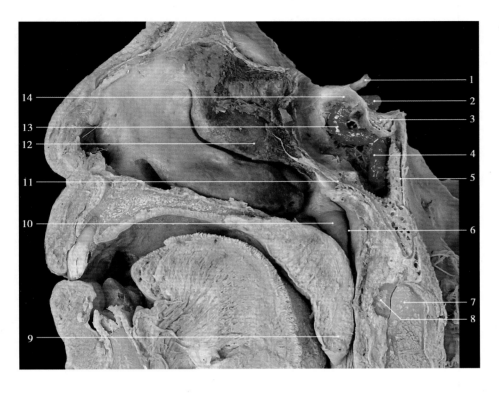

◀ 图1-147 颈内动脉海绵窦部内侧面观(一)
Fig. 1-147 Medial aspect of the cavernous part of internal carotid artery(1)

1. 视神经 optic nerve
2. 床突上段 supraclinoid part of internal carotid artery
3. 垂体 hypophysis
4. 破裂孔段 lacerum part of internal carotid artery
5. 斜坡 clivus
6. 咽隐窝 pharyngeal recess
7. 齿突 odontoid process of axis
8. 寰椎前弓 anterior arch of atlas
9. 腭垂 uvula
10. 咽鼓管圆枕 tubal torus
11. 咽结节 pharyngeal tubercle
12. 上鼻甲 superior nasal concha
13. 颈内动脉海绵窦部 cavernous part of internal carotid artery
14. 前床突 anterior clinoid process

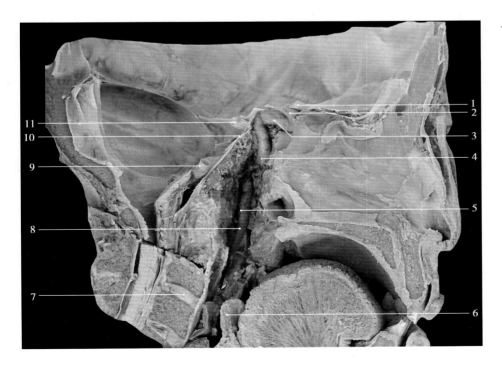

◀ 图1-148 颈内动脉海绵窦部内侧面观(二)
Fig. 1-148 Medial aspect of the cavernous part of internal carotid artery(2)

1. 视神经 optic nerve
2. 床突上段 supraclinoid part of internal carotid artery
3. 颈内动脉海绵窦部 cavernous part of internal carotid artery
4. 破裂孔段 lacerum part of internal carotid artery
5. 颈内动脉岩部 petrosal part of internal carotid artery
6. 会厌 epiglottis
7. 椎间盘 intervertebral disc
8. 颈内动脉 internal carotid artery
9. 椎动脉 vertebral artery
10. 斜坡 clivus
11. 三叉神经 trigeminal nerve

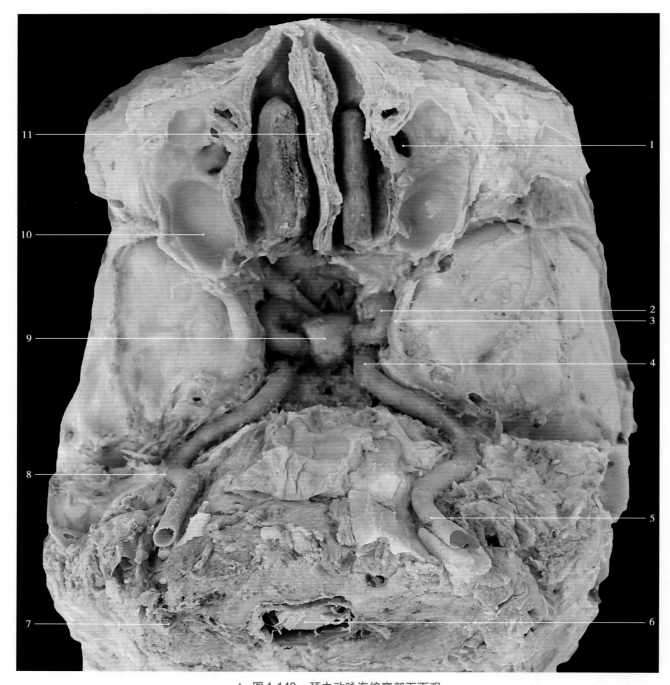

▲ 图 1-149　颈内动脉海绵窦部下面观

Fig. 1-149　Inferior aspect of the cavernous part of internal carotid artery

1. 上颌窦开口 ostium of maxillary sinus
2. 海绵窦部 cavernous part of internal carotid artery
3. 海绵窦外侧壁 lateral wall of cavernous sinus
4. 破裂孔段 lacerum part of internal carotid artery
5. 颈内动脉 internal carotid artery
6. 颈髓 cervical spinal cord
7. 椎动脉 vertebral artery
8. 颈动脉管外口 external aperture of carotid canal
9. 垂体 hypophysis
10. 上颌窦顶 roof of maxillary sinus
11. 鼻中隔 nasal septum

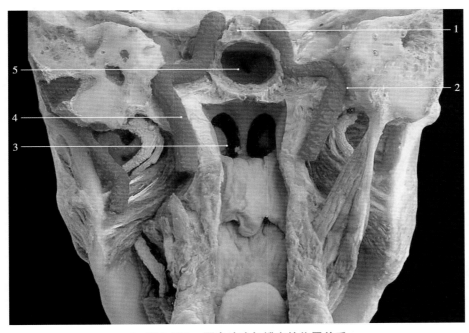

▲ 图 1-150 颈内动脉与蝶窦的位置关系

Fig. 1-150 Positional relation of the internal carotid artery and sphenoidal sinus

1. 鞍背 dorsum sellae   4. 颈内动脉 internal carotid artery
2. 颈动脉管 carotid canal   5. 蝶窦 sphenoidal sinus
3. 鼻后孔 posterior nare

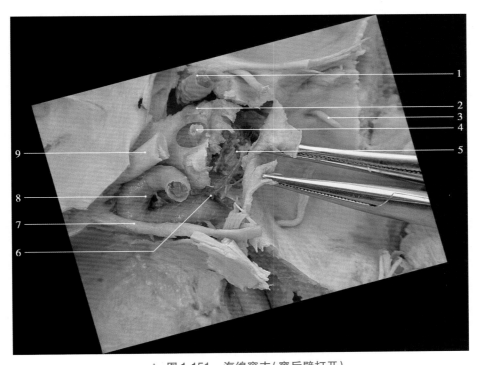

▲ 图 1-151 海绵窦支(窦后壁打开)

Fig. 1-151 Branch of the cavernous sinus (the posterior wall of sinus was opened)

1. 颈内动脉 internal carotid artery   6. 海绵窦支 branch of cavernous sinus
2. 鞍膈 diaphragma sellae   7. 动眼神经 oculomotor nerve
3. 展神经 abducent nerve   8. 颈内动脉海绵窦部 cavernous part of internal carotid artery
4. 垂体柄 hypophysial stalk   9. 视神经 optic nerver
5. 海绵窦 cavernous sinus

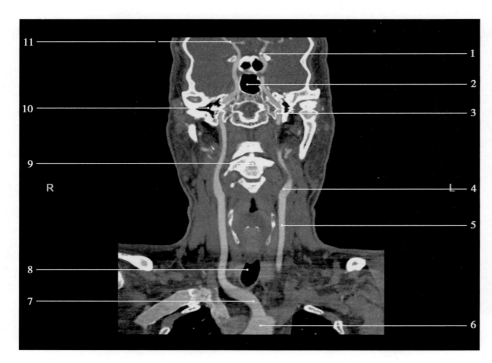

◀ 图 1-152 颈内动脉 CTA 前面观
Fig. 1-152 Anterior aspect of the internal carotid artery by CTA

1. 颈内动脉海绵窦部 cavernous part of internal carotid artery
2. 鼻咽 nasopharynx
3. 颈内动脉岩部 petrosal part of internal carotid artery
4. 颈总动脉分叉部 furcation of common carotid artery
5. 颈总动脉 common carotid artery
6. 主动脉弓 aortic arch
7. 头臂干 brachiocephalic trunk
8. 气管 trachea
9. 寰椎椎体 vertebral body of atlas
10. 中耳 middle ear
11. 大脑中动脉 middle cerebral artery

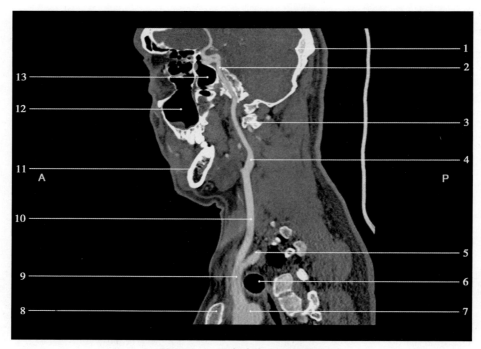

▲ 图 1-153 颈内动脉 CTA 左侧面观
Fig. 1-153 Left aspect of the internal carotid artery by CTA

1. 枕内隆起 internal occipital protuberance
2. 颈内动脉海绵窦部 cavernous part of internal carotid artery
3. 寰椎侧块 lateral mass of atlas
4. 颈动脉窦 carotid sinus
5. 锁骨下动脉 subclavian artery
6. 气管 trachea
7. 主动脉弓 aortic arch
8. 胸骨 sternum
9. 头臂干 brachiocephalic trunk
10. 颈总动脉 common carotid artery
11. 下颌骨 mandible
12. 上颌窦 maxillary sinus
13. 蝶窦 sphenoidal sinus

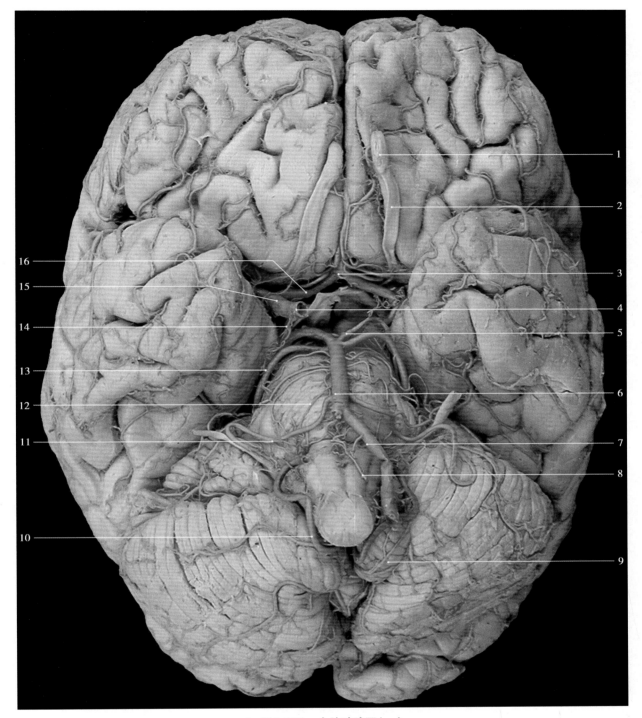

▲ 图 1-154 大脑动脉环（一）
Fig. 1-154 Cerebral arterial circle（1）

1. 嗅球 olfactory bulb
2. 嗅束 olfactory tract
3. 前交通动脉 anterior communicating artery
4. 颈内动脉 internal carotid artery
5. 大脑后动脉 posterior cerebral artery
6. 基底动脉 basilar artery
7. 左椎动脉 left vertebral artery
8. 脊髓前动脉 anterior spinal artery
9. 小脑扁桃体 tonsil of cerebellum
10. 小脑下后动脉 posterior inferior cerebellar artery
11. 小脑下前动脉 anterior inferior cerebellar artery
12. 脑桥动脉 pontine artery
13. 小脑上动脉 superior cerebellar artery
14. 后交通动脉 posterior communicating artery
15. 大脑中动脉 middle cerebral artery
16. 大脑前动脉 anterior cerebral artery

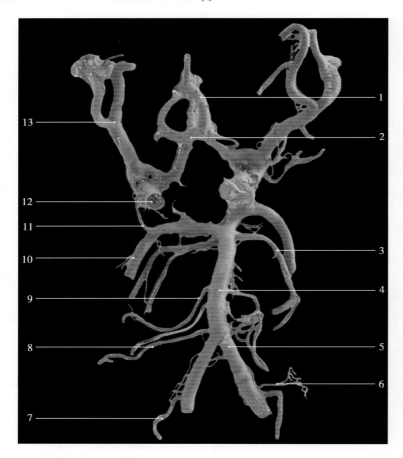

◀ 图 1-155　大脑动脉环（二）
Fig. 1-155　Cerebral arterial circle（2）

1. 大脑前动脉 anterior cerebral artery
2. 前交通动脉 anterior communicating artery
3. 小脑上动脉 superior cerebellar artery
4. 基底动脉 basilar artery
5. 左椎动脉 left vertebral artery
6. 小脑下后动脉 posterior inferior cerebellar artery
7. 脊髓前动脉 anterior spinal artery
8. 小脑下前动脉 anterior inferior cerebellar artery
9. 脑桥动脉 pontine artery
10. 大脑后动脉 posterior cerebral artery
11. 后交通动脉 posterior communicating artery
12. 颈内动脉 internal carotid artery
13. 大脑中动脉 middle cerebral artery

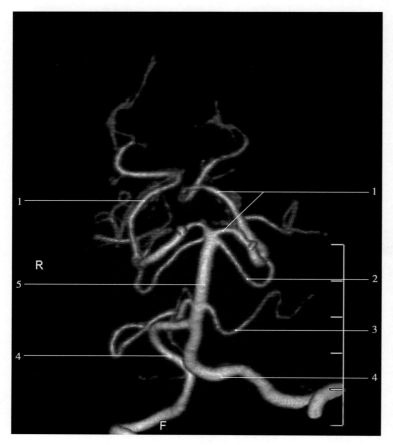

◀ 图 1-156　椎-基底动脉系
Fig. 1-156　Vertebrobasilar artery system

1. 大脑后动脉 posterior cerebral artery
2. 小脑上动脉 superior cerebellar artery
3. 小脑下前动脉 anterior inferior cerebellar artery
4. 椎动脉 vertebral artery
5. 基底动脉 basilar artery

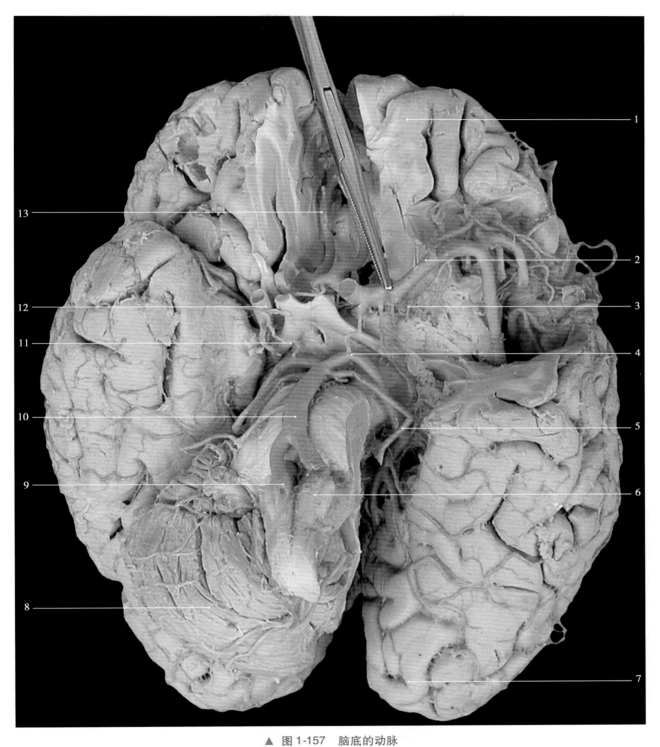

▲ 图 1-157　脑底的动脉
Fig. 1-157　Arteries at the base of the brain

1. 眶回 orbital gyri
2. 大脑中动脉 middle cerebral artery
3. 前外侧中央动脉 anterolateral central artery
4. 大脑后动脉 posterior cerebral artery
5. 小脑上动脉 superior cerebellar artery
6. 锥体 pyramid
7. 枕叶 occipital lobe
8. 小脑 cerebellum
9. 椎动脉 vertebral artery
10. 基底动脉 basilar artery
11. 后交通动脉 posterior communicating artery
12. 颈内动脉 internal carotid artery
13. 大脑前动脉 anterior cerebral artery

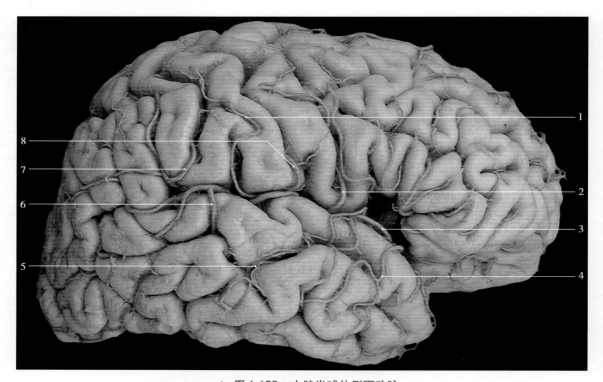

▲ 图 1-158　大脑半球外侧面动脉
Fig. 1-158　Arteries on the lateral surface of the cerebral hemisphere

1. 中央后沟动脉 artery of postcentral sulcus
2. 中央前沟动脉 artery of precentral sulcus
3. 前外侧中央动脉 anterolateral central artery
4. 颞叶前动脉 anterior temporal artery
5. 颞叶中动脉 middle temporal artery
6. 颞叶后动脉 posterior temporal artery
7. 角回动脉 artery of angular gyrus
8. 中央沟动脉 artery of central sulcus

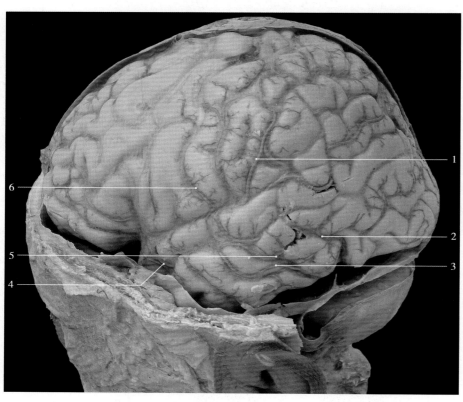

◀ 图 1-159　脑血管背外侧面观
Fig. 1-159　Dorsal lateral aspect of the cerebral vessels

1. 中央后沟动脉 artery of postcentral sulcus
2. 颞叶后动脉 posterior temporal artery
3. 颞叶底外侧动脉 lateral basilar temporal artery
4. 颞叶前动脉 anterior temporal artery
5. 颞叶中动脉 middle temporal artery
6. 中央前沟动脉 artery of precentral sulcus

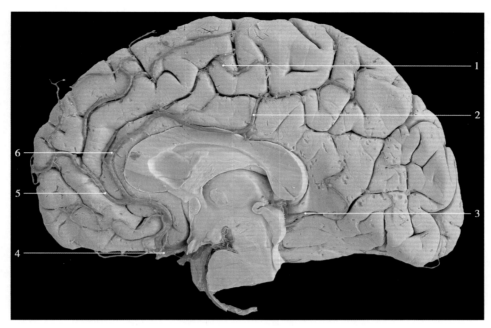

▲ 图 1-160 右侧大脑前动脉(一)
Fig. 1-160 Right anterior cerebral artery (1)

1. 额叶中内侧支 mediomedial frontal branch
2. 额叶后内侧支 posteromedial frontal branch
3. 大脑后动脉 posterior cerebral artery
4. 大脑前动脉 anterior cerebral artery
5. 额叶前内侧支 anteromedial frontal branch
6. 扣带支 cingular branch

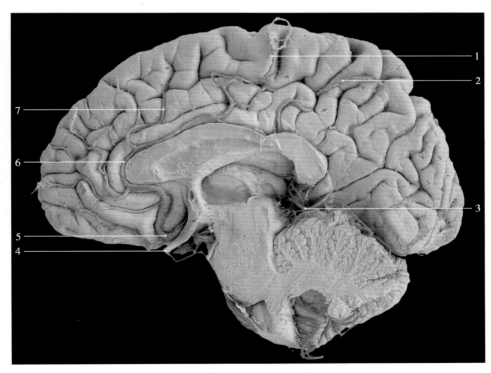

▲ 图 1-161 右侧大脑前动脉(二)
Fig. 1-161 Right anterior cerebral artery (2)

1. 额叶后内侧支 posteromedial frontal branch
2. 顶枕动脉 parietooccipital artery
3. 大脑后动脉 posterior cerebral artery
4. 视神经 optic nerve
5. 大脑前动脉 anterior cerebral artery
6. 扣带支 cingular branch
7. 额叶中内侧支 mediomedial frontal branch

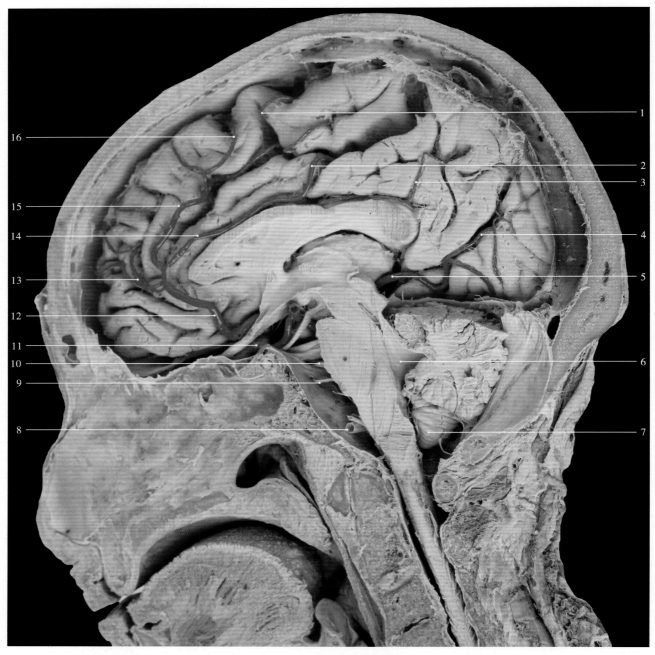

▲ 图 1-162　右侧大脑前动脉（三）
Fig. 1-162　Right anterior cerebral artery（3）

1. 额中内侧动脉 mediomedial frontal artery　　　9. 展神经 abducent nerve
2. 额后内侧动脉 posteromedial frontal artery　　10. 三叉神经 trigeminal nerve
3. 楔前动脉 precuneal artery　　　　　　　　　11. 颈内动脉 internal carotid artery
4. 顶枕动脉 parietooccipital artery　　　　　　12. 大脑前动脉 anterior cerebral artery
5. 大脑后动脉 posterior cerebral artery　　　　13. 额极动脉 frontopolar artery
6. 第四脑室 fourth ventricle　　　　　　　　　14. 胼周动脉 paricallosal artery
7. 小脑扁桃体 tonsil of cerebellum　　　　　　15. 胼胝体缘动脉 callosomarginal artery
8. 椎动脉 vertebral artery　　　　　　　　　　16. 额前内侧动脉 anteromedial frontal artery

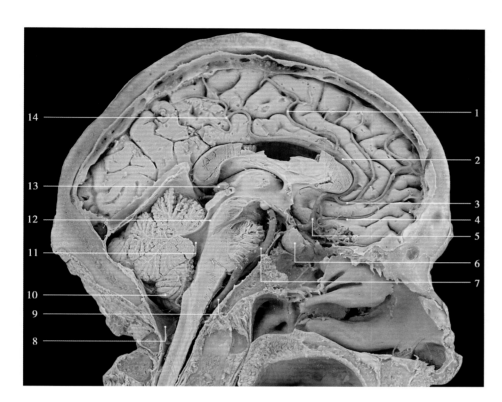

◀ 图 1-163 左侧大脑前动脉（一）
Fig. 1-163 Left anterior cerebral artery（1）

1. 额中内侧动脉 medio-medial frontal artery
2. 胼周动脉 pericallosal artery
3. 额前内侧动脉 antero-medial frontal artery
4. 眶动脉 orbital artery
5. 大脑前动脉 anterior cerebral artery
6. 垂体 hypophysis
7. 基底动脉 basilar artery
8. 小脑延髓池 cerebello-medullary cistern
9. 椎动脉 vertebral artery
10. 小脑扁桃体 tonsil of cerebellum
11. 第四脑室 fourth ventricle
12. 中脑导水管 mesence-phalic aqueduct
13. 松果体 pineal body
14. 额后内侧动脉 postero-medial frontal artery

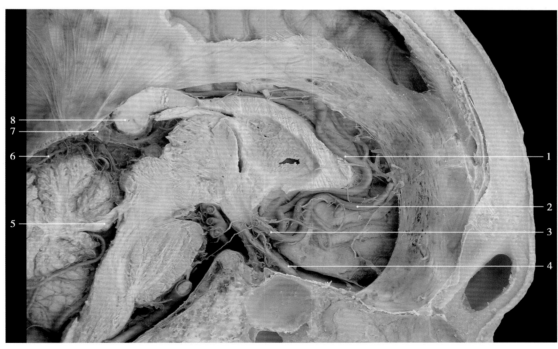

▲ 图 1-164 左侧大脑前动脉（二）
Fig. 1-164 Left anterior cerebral artery（2）

1. 胼胝体缘动脉 callosomarginal artery
2. 额叶前内侧支 anteromedial frontal branch
3. 大脑前动脉 anterior cerebral artery
4. 视神经 optic nerve
5. 上髓帆 superior medullary velum
6. 蚓支 vermian branch
7. 大脑深静脉 deep cerebral vein
8. 胼胝体压部 splenium of corpus callosum

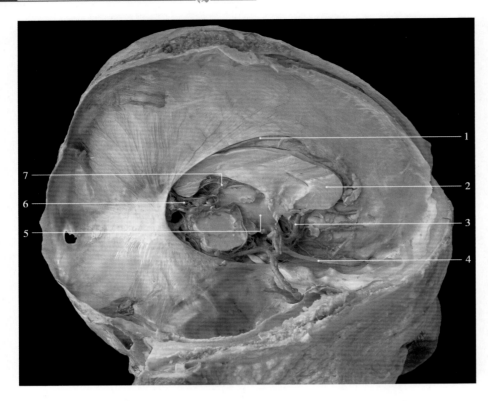

◀ 图 1-165 大脑前动脉与嗅束
Fig. 1-165 Anterior cerebral artery and olfactory tract

1. 胼胝体缘动脉 callosomarginal artery
2. 胼胝体膝 genu of corpus callosum
3. 大脑前动脉 anterior cerebral artery
4. 嗅束 olfactory tract
5. 第三脑室 third ventricle
6. 大脑深静脉 deep cerebral vein
7. 脉络丛前动脉 anterior choroidal artery

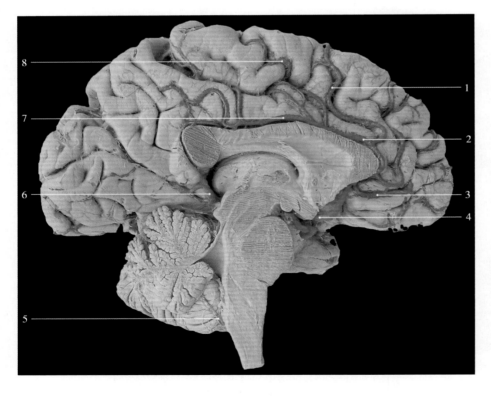

◀ 图 1-166 胼胝体缘动脉
Fig. 1-166 Callosomarginal artery

1. 额叶中内侧支 mediomedial frontal branch
2. 胼胝体缘动脉 callosomarginal artery
3. 额叶前内侧支 anteromedial frontal branch
4. 大脑前动脉 anterior cerebral artery
5. 小脑扁桃体支 cerebellar tonsillar branch
6. 大脑后动脉 posterior cerebral artery
7. 扣带支 cingular branch
8. 额叶后内侧支 posteromedial frontal branch

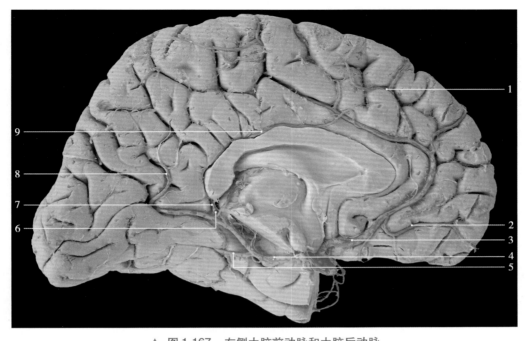

▲ 图 1-167 左侧大脑前动脉和大脑后动脉

Fig. 1-167 Left anterior cerebral artery and posterior cerebral artery

1. 额叶中内侧支 mediomedial frontal branch
2. 额叶前内侧支 anteromedial frontal branch
3. 大脑前动脉 anterior cerebral artery
4. 大脑后动脉 posterior cerebral artery
5. 颞叶中动脉 middle temporal artery
6. 脉络丛后内侧支 posterior medial choroidal branch
7. 脉络丛后外侧支 posterior lateral choroidal branch
8. 顶叶支 parietal branch
9. 扣带支 cingular branch

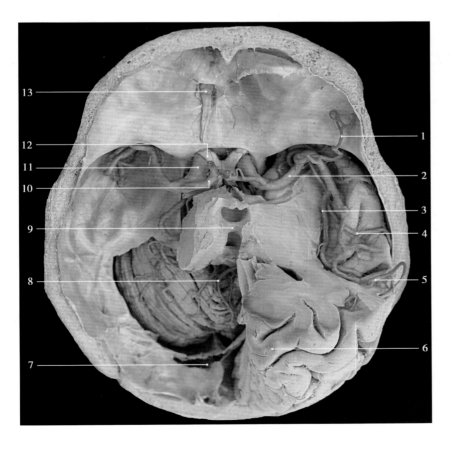

◀ 图 1-168 大脑中动脉（一）
Fig. 1-168 Middle cerebral artery（1）

1. 外侧眶额动脉 lateral orbitofrontal artery
2. 大脑中动脉 middle cerebral artery
3. 大脑中动脉上干 superior trunk of middle cerebral artery
4. 大脑中动脉下干 inferior trunk of middle cerebral artery
5. 顶后动脉 posterior parietal artery
6. 顶叶 parietal lobe
7. 横窦 transverse sinus
8. 小脑上动脉 superior cerebellar artery
9. 丘脑间粘合 interthalamic adhesion
10. 大脑前动脉 anterior cerebral artery
11. 颈内动脉 internal carotid artery
12. 视神经 optic nerve
13. 嗅球 olfactory bulb

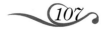

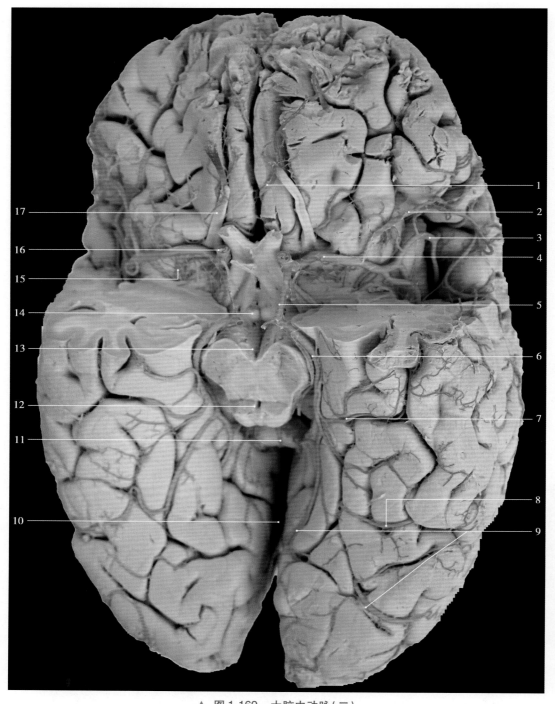

▲ 图 1-169 大脑中动脉(二)
Fig. 1-169 Middle cerebral artery(2)

1. 眶额内侧动脉 medial orbitofrontal artery
2. 颞极动脉 temporal polarartery
3. 大脑中动脉上干 anterior trunk middle cerebral artery
4. 大脑中动脉 middle cerebral artery
5. 后交通动脉 posterior communicating artery
6. 大脑后动脉 posterior cerebral artery
7. 颞下中动脉 middle inferior temporal artery
8. 颞下后动脉 posterior inferior temporal artery
9. 颞枕动脉 occipitotemporal artery
10. 大脑纵裂 cerebral longitudinal fissure
11. 胼胝体动脉 artery of corpus callosum
12. 中脑导水管 mesencephalic aqueduct
13. 脚间窝 interpeduncal fossa
14. 乳头体 mammillary body
15. 豆纹动脉外侧组 lateral group of lenticulostriate artery
16. 颈内动脉 internal carotid artery
17. 嗅束 olfactory tract

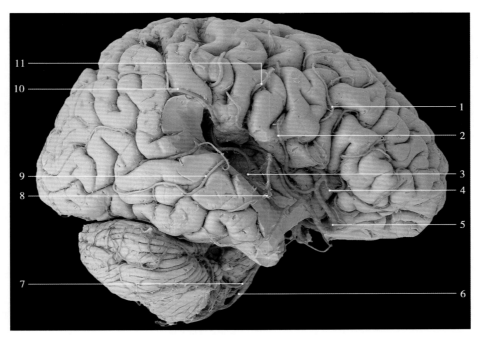

▲ 图 1-170 右大脑中动脉（一）

Fig. 1-170 Right middle cerebral artery（1）

1. 中央前沟动脉 artery of precentral sulcus
2. 颞叶中央沟动脉 temporal artery of central sulcus
3. 岛动脉 insular artery
4. 颞前动脉 anterior temporal artery
5. 大脑中动脉 middle cerebral artery
6. 基底动脉 basilar artery
7. 小脑上动脉 superior cerebellar artery
8. 颞叶中动脉 middle temporal artery
9. 颞叶后动脉 posterior temporal artery
10. 顶叶前动脉 anterior parietal artery
11. 中央后沟动脉 artery of postcentral sulcus

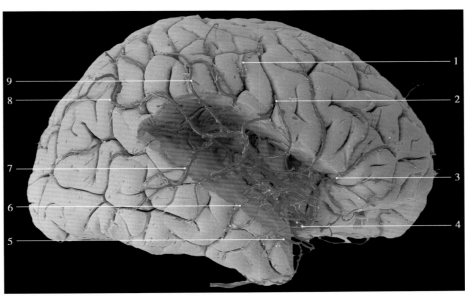

▲ 图 1-171 右大脑中动脉（二）

Fig. 1-171 Right middle cerebral artery（2）

1. 中央前沟动脉 artery of precentral sulcus
2. 中央沟动脉 artery of central sulcus
3. 额叶前外侧支 anterolateral frontal branch
4. 大脑中动脉 middle cerebral artery
5. 颞叶前动脉 anterior temporal artery
6. 颞叶中动脉 middle temporal artery
7. 颞叶后动脉 posterior temporal artery
8. 顶叶后动脉 posterior parietal artery
9. 中央后沟动脉 artery of postcentral sulcus

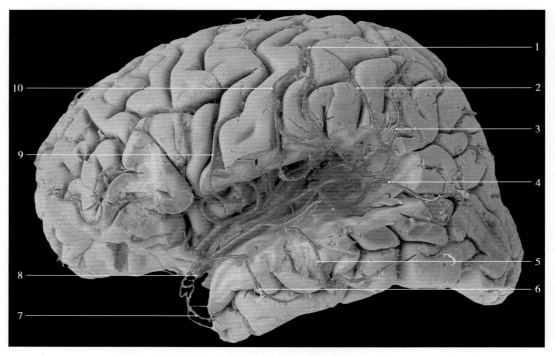

▲ 图 1-172　左大脑中动脉
Fig. 1-172　Left middle cerebral artery

1. 中央后沟动脉 artery of postcentral sulcus
2. 顶叶前动脉 anterior parietal artery
3. 顶叶后动脉 posterior parietal artery
4. 颞叶后动脉 posterior temporal artery
5. 颞叶中动脉 middle temporal artery
6. 颞叶前动脉 anterior temporal artery
7. 额叶底外侧动脉 lateral frontobasal artery
8. 大脑中动脉 middle cerebral artery
9. 中央前沟动脉 artery of precentral sulcus
10. 中央沟动脉 artery of central sulcus

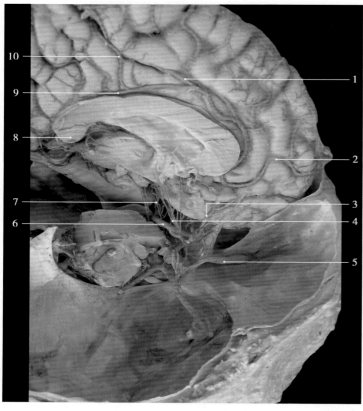

◀ 图 1-173　大脑中动脉及其分支（一）
Fig. 1-173　Middle cerebral artery and its branches（1）

1. 额叶中内侧支 mediomedial frontal branch
2. 额叶前内侧支 anteromedial frontal branch
3. 额叶底外侧动脉 lateral frontobasal artery
4. 内侧支 medial branch
5. 嗅束 olfactory tract
6. 大脑中动脉 middle cerebral artery
7. 前外侧中央动脉 anterolateral central artery
8. 胼胝体压部 splenium of corpus callosum
9. 胼胝体缘动脉 callosomarginal artery
10. 额叶后内侧支 posteromedial frontal branch

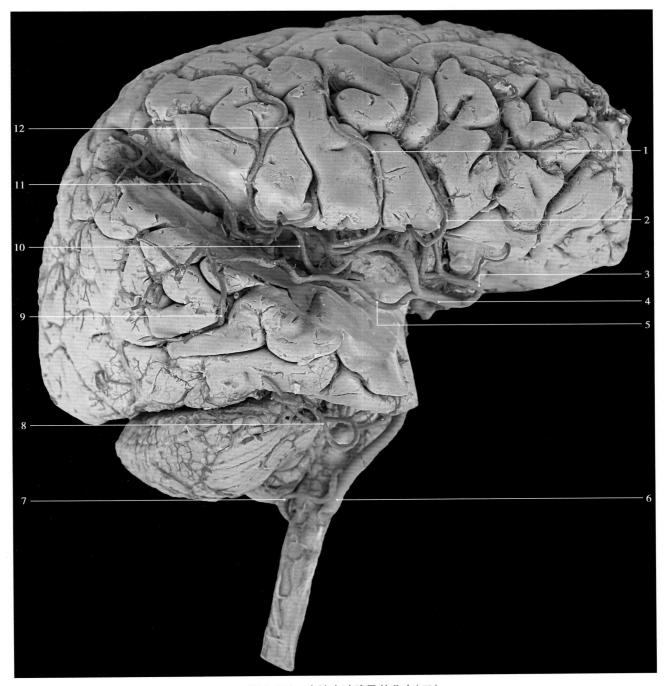

▲ 图 1-174　大脑中动脉及其分支(二)
Fig. 1-174　Middle cerebral artery and its branches (2)

1. 中央沟动脉 artery of central sulcus
2. 中央前沟动脉 artery of precentral sulcus
3. 眶额动脉 orbitofrontal artery
4. 大脑中动脉 middle cerebral artery
5. 大脑中动脉下干 inferior trunk of middle cerebral artery
6. 基底动脉 basilar artery
7. 小脑后下动脉 posterior inferior cerebellar artery
8. 小脑上动脉 superior cerebellar artery
9. 颞中动脉 middle temporal artery
10. 大脑中动脉上干 superior trunk of middle cerebral artery
11. 顶叶后动脉 posterior parietal artery
12. 中央后沟动脉 artery of postcentral sulcus

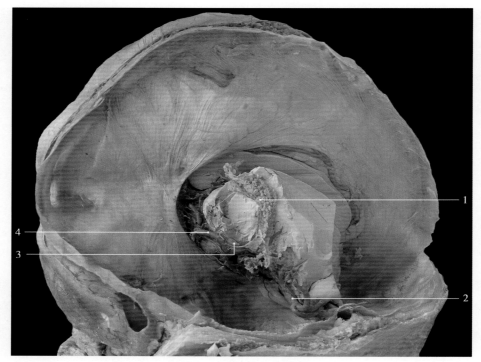

▲ 图 1-175 脉络丛动脉
Fig. 1-175 Choroidal artery

1. 侧脑室内脉络丛 choroids plexus in lateral ventricle
2. 大脑中动脉 middle cerebral artery
3. 脉络丛动脉 choroidal artery
4. 大脑后动脉 posterior cerebral artery

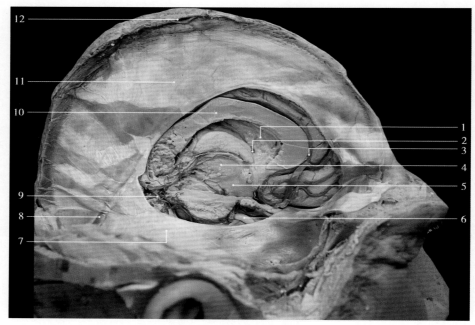

▲ 图 1-176 脉络丛后动脉
Fig. 1-176 Posterior choroidal artery

1. 透明隔 septum pellucidum
2. 室间孔 interventricular foramen
3. 胼胝体缘动脉 callosomarginal artery
4. 丘脑 thalamus
5. 第三脑室 third ventricle
6. 动眼神经 oculomotor nerve
7. 小脑幕 tentorium of cerebellum
8. 直窦 straight sinus
9. 脉络丛后动脉 posterior choroidal artery
10. 胼胝体 corpus callosum
11. 大脑镰 cerebral falx
12. 上矢状窦 superior sagittal sinus

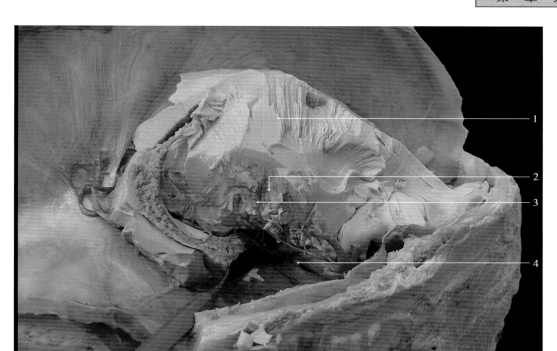

▲ 图 1-177 豆纹动脉
Fig. 1-177 Artery of cerebral hemorrhage

1. 内囊 internal capsule
2. 豆状核 lentiform nucleus
3. 豆纹动脉 artery of cerebral hemorrhage
4. 大脑中动脉 middle cerebral artery

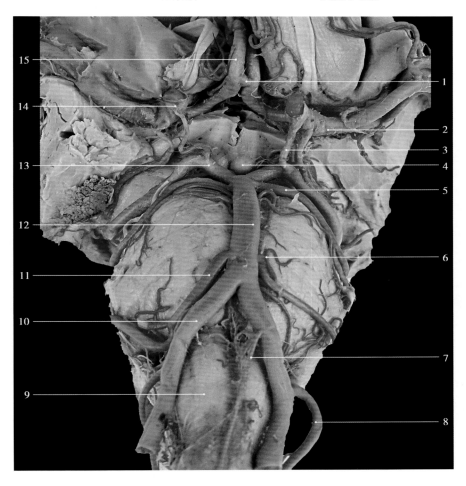

◀ 图 1-178 大脑后动脉
Fig. 1-178 Posterior cerebral artery

1. 前交通动脉 anterior communicating artery
2. 大脑中动脉 middle cerebral artery
3. 后交通动脉 posterior communicating artery
4. 乳头体 mamillary body
5. 小脑上动脉 superior cerebellar artery
6. 桥支 pontine branch
7. 脊髓前动脉 anterior spinal artery
8. 小脑下后动脉 posterior inferior cerebellar artery
9. 锥体 pyramid
10. 椎动脉 vertebral artery
11. 小脑下前动脉 anterior inferior cerebellar artery
12. 基底动脉 basilar artery
13. 大脑后动脉 posterior cerebral artery
14. 颈内动脉 internal carotid artery
15. 大脑前动脉 anterior cerebral artery

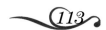
113

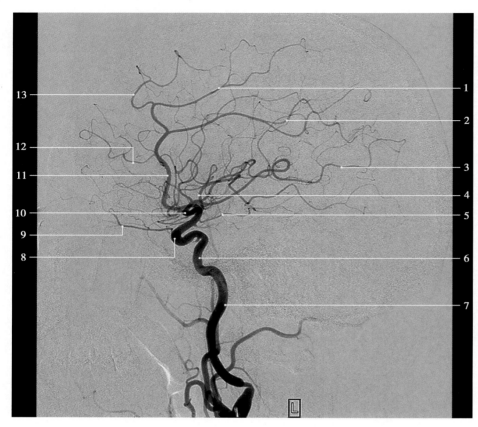

◀ 图 1-179 左颈内动脉侧位
动脉期
Fig. 1-179 Lateral position
of the left internal carotid artery in the arterial phase

1. 额中内侧动脉 mediomedial
frontal artery
2. 额后内侧动脉 posteromedi-
al frontal artery
3. 角回动脉 artery of angular
gyrus
4. 大脑中动脉 middle cere-
bral artery
5. 脉络丛前动脉 anterior cho-
roidal artery
6. 颈内动脉岩部 petrosal part
of internal carotid artery
7. 颈内动脉颈部 cervical part
of internal carotid artery
8. 颈内动脉海绵窦部 cavern-
ous part of internal carotid
artery
9. 眼动脉 ophthalmic artery
10. 床突上段 superior part of
clinoid process
11. 大脑前动脉 anterior cere-
bral artery
12. 额极动脉 frontopolar ar-
tery
13. 额内侧动脉 medial frontal
artery

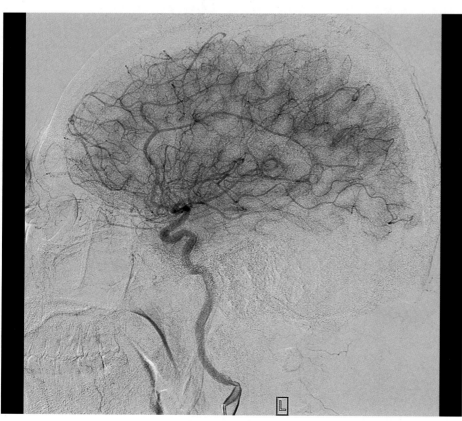

◀ 图 1-180 颈内动脉侧位实
质期
Fig. 1-180 Lateral position
of the internal carotid artery
in the parenchymal phase

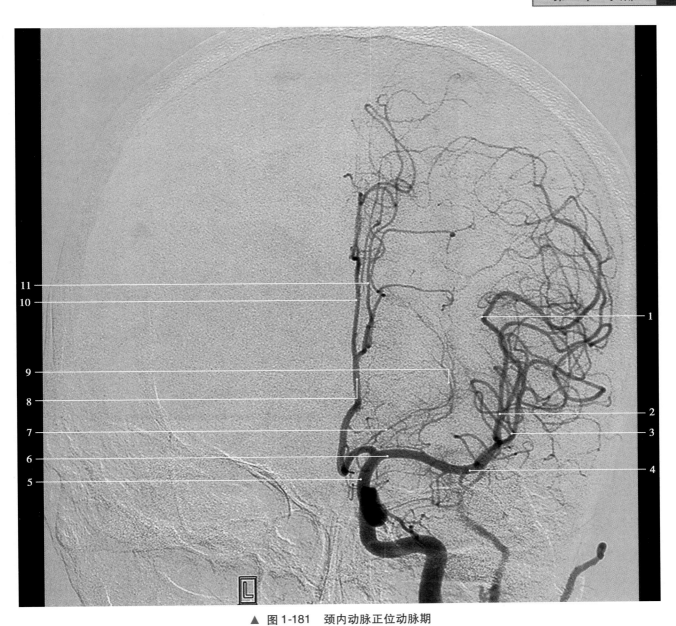

▲ 图 1-181 颈内动脉正位动脉期

Fig. 1-181 Normotopia of the internal carotid artery in the arterial phase

1. 侧裂点 sylvian point
2. 大脑中动脉内侧支 medial branch of middle cerebral artery
3. 大脑中动脉外侧支 lateral branch of middle cerebral artery
4. 大脑中动脉 middle cerebral artery
5. 颈内动脉 internal carotid artery
6. 大脑中动脉 middle cerebral artery
7. 中央短动脉 short central artery
8. 大脑前动脉 anterior cerebral artery
9. 豆纹动脉 artery of cerebral hemorrhage
10. 胼周动脉 pericallosal artery
11. 胼胝体缘动脉 callosomarginal artery

脑复苏的应用解剖学基础

在心肺复苏后,应及时对患者的脑组织缺血、缺氧性损害程度作出初步的估计,对昏迷的深度和脑功能结果作出判断。患者瞳孔对光反射的存在和自主呼吸相继的出现是脑组织获得供血供氧的有力指征,医生应熟知脑组织血管的来源、走行和特点。脑的血液供应均起于颈根部,向上行至颅底:

1. 颈内动脉经颈动脉管外口→颈动脉管→颈动脉管内口→海绵窦→颅内。

2. 椎动脉发自锁骨下动脉经→C6~C1颈椎横突孔→寰椎上面的椎动脉沟→枕骨大孔→两侧椎动脉在延髓上端汇合为基底动脉→基底动脉的终末支为两条大脑后动脉。

颈内动脉发出的前交通动脉、两侧大脑前动脉的起始段、两条后交通动脉和大脑后动脉在脑底下方、蝶鞍上方,环绕视交叉、灰结节和乳头体构成大脑动脉环。大脑动脉环是颈内动脉与椎-基底动脉之间的相互交通。当构成此环中的某一动脉的血流减少或被阻塞时,可通过大脑动脉环在一定程度上使血流重新分配和代偿,以维持脑的营养供应和功能活动。

由于供应脑组织的血管均经颈部至颅底入脑,从解剖学角度讲在抢救患者时一定要将颈部置于正常的位置,即颈部处于正中位且不宜过度后伸或头屈向一侧,以保证经颈部上升供应脑组织的血管不受挤压或扭曲(图1-154~图1-181)。

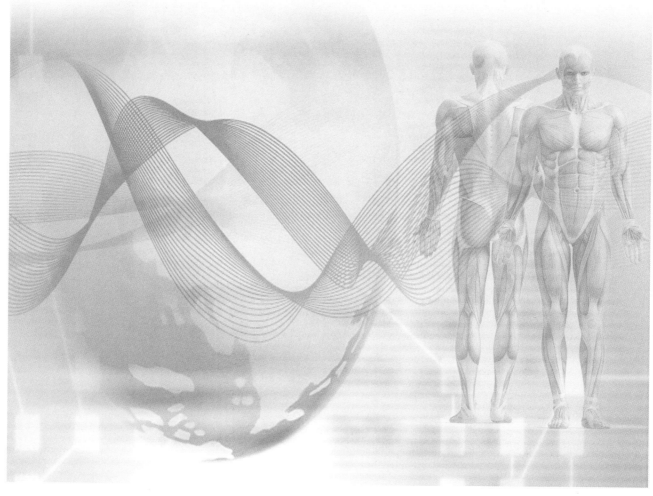

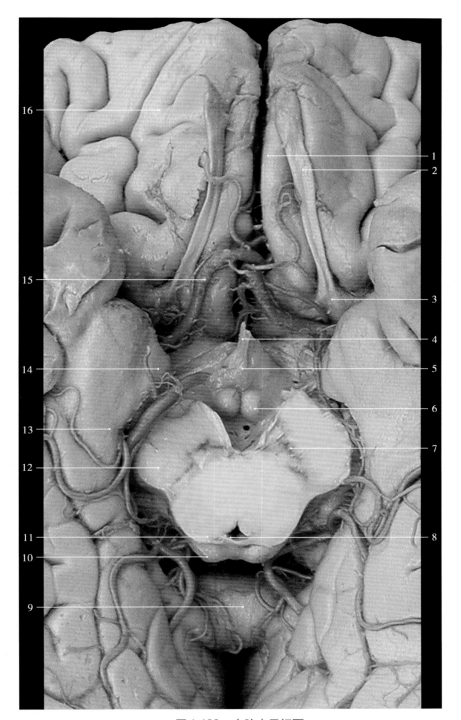

▲ 图 1-182　中脑水平切面

Fig. 1-182　Horizontal section of the midbrain

1. 直回 gyrus rectus
2. 嗅束 olfactory tract
3. 嗅三角 olfactory trigone
4. 漏斗 infundibulum
5. 灰结节 tuber cinereum
6. 乳头体 mamillary body
7. 黑质 substantia nigra
8. 中脑导水管 mesencephalic aqueduct

9. 胼胝体压部 splenium of corpus callosum
10. 上丘 superior colliculus
11. 顶盖 tectum
12. 大脑脚 cerebral peduncle
13. 海马旁回 parahippocampal gyrus
14. 钩 uncus
15. 大脑前动脉 anterior cerebral artery
16. 眶回 orbital gyrus

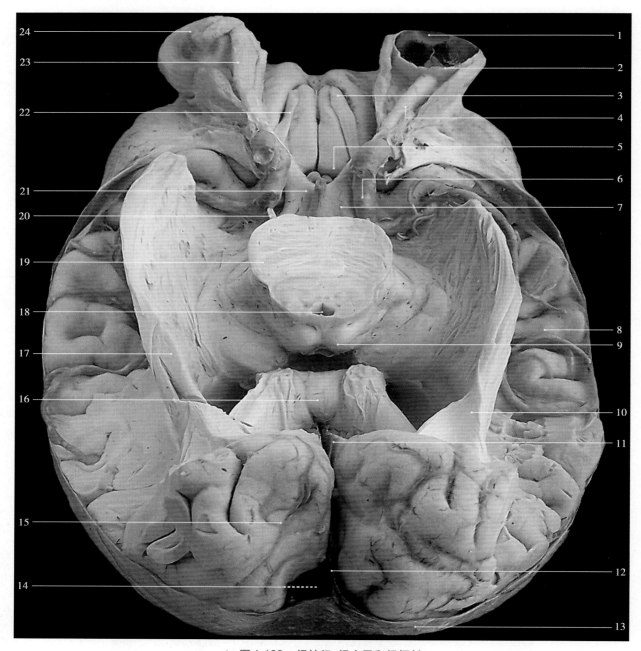

▲ 图 1-183　视神经、视交叉和视辐射
Fig. 1-183　Optic nerve, optic chiasma and optic radiation

1. 角膜 cornea
2. 巩膜 sclera
3. 嗅球 olfactory bulb
4. 视神经 optic nerve
5. 直回 gyrus rectus
6. 大脑中动脉 middle cerebral artery
7. 视束 optic tract
8. 颞叶 temporal lobe
9. 上丘 superior colliculus
10. 视辐射 optic radiation
11. 连合纤维 commissural fiber
12. 大脑镰 cerebral falx

13. 硬脑膜 cerebral dura mater
14. 上矢状窦 superior sagittal sinus
15. 枕叶 occipital lobe
16. 胼胝体压部 splenium of corpus callosum
17. 视辐射 optic radiation
18. 中脑导水管 mesencephalic aqueduct
19. 脑桥 pons
20. 动眼神经 oculomotor nerve
21. 视交叉 optic chiasma
22. 嗅束 olfactory tract
23. 内直肌 medial rectus
24. 眼球壁 wall of eyeball

角膜对光反射的应用解剖学要点

当一侧角膜受刺激时,引起双侧眼轮匝肌收缩而出现急速闭眼,这种现象叫作角膜反射。受刺激侧的角膜反射叫作直接角膜反射,另一侧的角膜反射称作间接角膜反射。角膜反射是防御性反射的一种,通过反射保护角膜以免受到伤害。临床上检查角膜反射是判断意识障碍程度的重要标志之一。

角膜反射的反射弧为:角膜受到刺激→眼神经→三叉神经节→三叉神经→三叉神经感觉主核和三叉神经脊束核→脑干网状结构→两侧面神经核→两侧面神经颞支和面神经颧支→两侧眼轮匝肌→引起双侧闭眼(图1-183)。

应用解剖要点:

角膜反射是一种比较恒定的可靠的反射,其减弱或消失可能有以下几种因素造成。

1. 麻醉(全麻)过深、醉酒可出现角膜反射减弱或消失。此种症状出现时已显示麻醉水平深达脑桥,应及时调整药量,否则可出现严重后果。

2. 反射弧受到损伤

(1)传入神经病变:如角膜病变、眼神经及三叉神经损伤、颈动脉瘤及颞叶肿瘤压迫三叉神经节等,均可出现病变侧直接角膜反射减弱或消失,健侧间接反射也出现减弱或消失。

(2)传出神经病变:如面神经颞支、颧支的损伤,面神经麻痹及脑桥小脑角肿瘤等均可出现患侧角膜反射减弱或消失,健侧间接角膜反射依然存在。

(3)脑桥病变:如脑桥肿瘤、脑疝等致反射中枢受损而致两侧角膜的直接反射和间接反射均消失。

(4)高级中枢病变:如内囊出血、脑水肿等造成意识障碍时,两侧的直接、间接角膜反射均消失。

3. 意识障碍 造成意识障碍的任何中枢神经疾病均可出现角膜反射减弱或消失。角膜反射存在为患者意识基本正常或为轻度昏迷。角膜反射减弱或消失为中度昏迷。角膜反射消失伴有瞳孔对光反射消失,肌肉松弛等症状时,可定为重度昏迷。

瞳孔对光反射的应用解剖学要点

瞳孔对光反射是医生在抢救、检查患者,特别是对患者实施全身麻醉时最常用的一种检查术。瞳孔对光反射是用强光照射一侧瞳孔,引起两眼瞳孔缩小,光线移开后,瞳孔随即散大。瞳孔对光反射的传入途径为:光线→角膜→房水→晶状体→玻璃体→视锥细胞/视杆细胞→双极细胞→神经节细胞→视神经→视交叉→视束→上丘臂→顶盖前区→双侧的动眼神经副核→动眼神经→睫状神经节→睫状短神经→瞳孔括约肌→两眼瞳孔缩小。由于视神经在视交叉处有部分纤维(来自视网膜的鼻侧纤维)交叉和顶盖前区发出的纤维终止于两侧的动眼神经副核,所以光线照射一侧瞳孔时能引起两侧瞳孔同时缩小。直接被光照射侧的瞳孔缩小现象称为直接对光反射,而对侧瞳孔缩小的现象称为间接对光反射(图1-183)。

应用解剖要点:

瞳孔对光反射障碍时有以下几种因素:

1. 传入神经损伤或病变 当一侧视神经完全损伤时,传入信息中断,光照患侧眼时,两眼瞳孔均不发生缩小,但光照健侧眼时,两眼瞳孔均能缩小,即双眼对光反射均存在(此时患侧直接对光反射消失,间接对光反射存在)。

2. 瞳孔对光反射中枢病变(中脑的顶盖前区) 两侧对光反射均消失,特别是在给患者实施全麻时,对患者瞳孔的观察是了解麻醉深度一个十分重要的指标,如瞳孔对光反射迟缓或消失,说明麻醉平面已达中脑,是一个很危险的信号。

3. 传出神经病变 一侧动眼神经损伤时,由于反射弧的传出神经中断,无论光照哪一侧的眼,患侧瞳孔均无反应,直接和间接对光反射均消失。

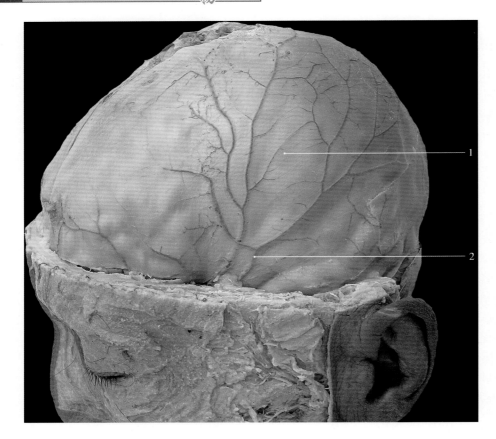

◀ 图 1-184　左侧硬脑膜的动脉

Fig. 1-184　Arteries of the left cerebral dura mater

1. 硬脑膜 cerebral dura mater
2. 脑膜中动脉 middle meningeal artery

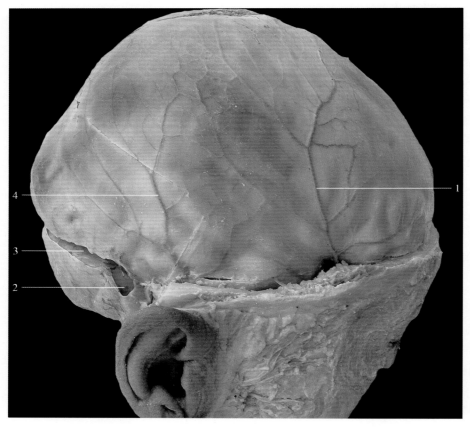

◀ 图 1-185　右侧硬脑膜的动脉

Fig. 1-185　Arteries of the right cerebral dura mater

1. 脑膜中动脉前支 anterior branch of middle meningeal artery
2. 乙状窦 sigmoid sinus
3. 横窦 transverse sinus
4. 脑膜中动脉后支 posterior branch of middle meningeal artery

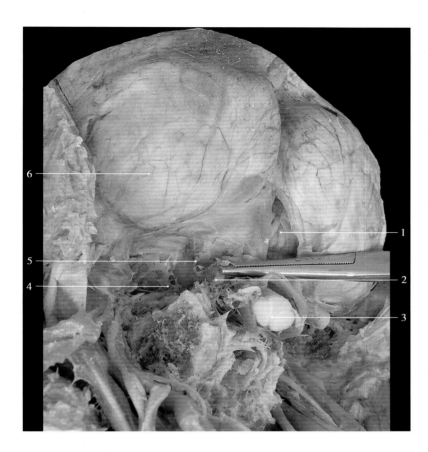

◀ 图 1-186　左脑膜后动脉
Fig. 1-186　Left posterior meningeal artery

1. 小脑延髓池 cerebellomedullary cistern
2. 椎动脉 vertebral artery
3. 脊髓 spinal cord
4. 枕骨大孔 foramen magnum of occipital bone
5. 脑膜后动脉 posterior meningeal artery
6. 颅后窝硬脑膜 cerebral dura mate of posterior cranial fossa

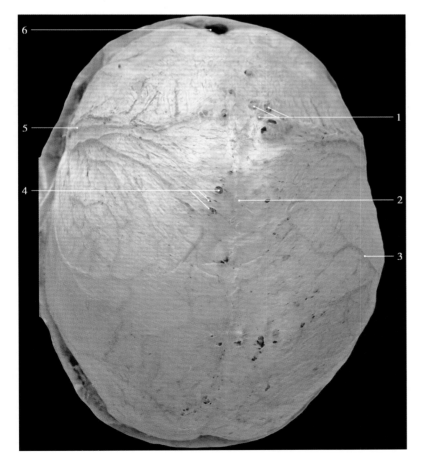

◀ 图 1-187　硬脑膜血管
Fig. 1-187　Artery of the cerebral dura mater

1. 蛛网膜粒 arachnoid granulations
2. 上矢状窦 superior sagittal sinus
3. 脑膜中动脉后支 posterior branch of middle meningeal artery
4. 蛛网膜粒 arachnoid granulations
5. 脑膜中动脉前支 anterior branch of middle meningeal artery
6. 额窦 frontal sinus

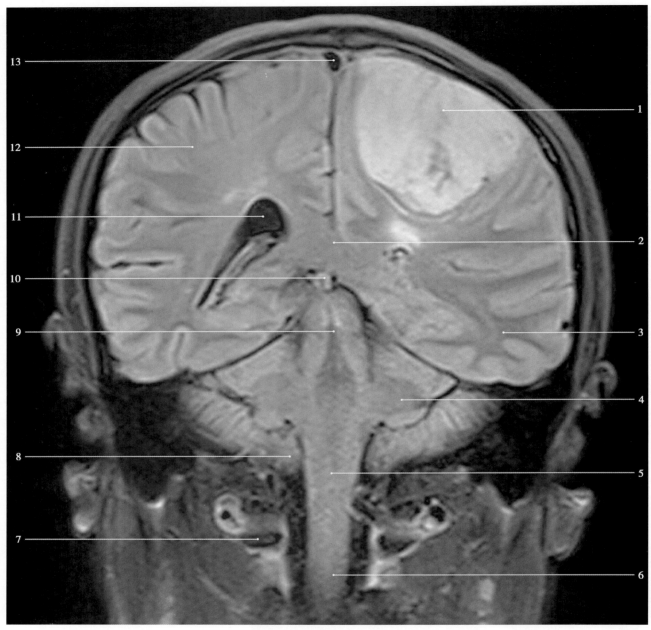

▲ 图 1-188　脑膜瘤
Fig. 1-188　Meningeoma

1. 脑膜瘤 meningeoma
2. 胼胝体压部 splenium of corpus callosum
3. 颞叶 temporal lobe
4. 小脑中脚 middle cerebellar peduncle
5. 颈髓 cervical spinal cord
6. 延髓 medulla oblongata
7. 颈内静脉 internal carotid vein

8. 小脑扁桃体 tonsil of cerebellum
9. 中脑导水管 mesencephalic aqueduct
10. 大脑大静脉 great cerebral vein
11. 侧脑室 lateral ventricle
12. 顶叶 parietal lobe
13. 上矢状窦 superior sagittal sinus

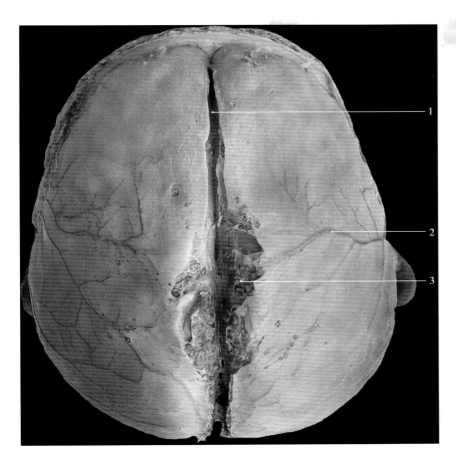

◀ 图 1-189 上矢状窦上面观
Fig. 1-189 Superior aspect of the superior sagittal sinus

1. 上矢状窦 superior sagittal sinus
2. 脑膜中动脉 middle meningeal artery
3. 蛛网膜粒 arachnoid granulations

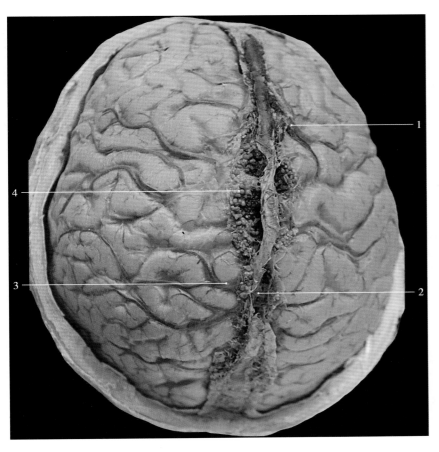

◀ 图 1-190 蛛网膜粒上面观
Fig. 1-190 Superior aspect of the arachnoid granulations

1. 大脑浅静脉上前组 anterior upper group of superficial cerebral vein
2. 上矢状窦 superior sagittal sinus
3. 大脑浅静脉上后组 posterior upper group of superficial cerebral vein
4. 蛛网膜粒 arachnoid granulations

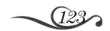

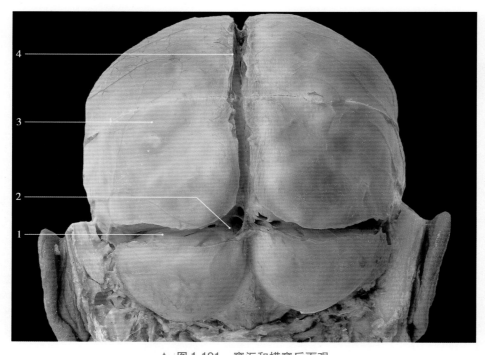

▲ 图 1-191　窦汇和横窦后面观

Fig. 1-191　Posterior aspect of the confluence of sinus and transverse sinus

1. 横窦 transverse sinus
2. 直窦开口 debouch of straight sinus
3. 硬脑膜 cerebral dura mater
4. 上矢状窦 superior sagittal sinus

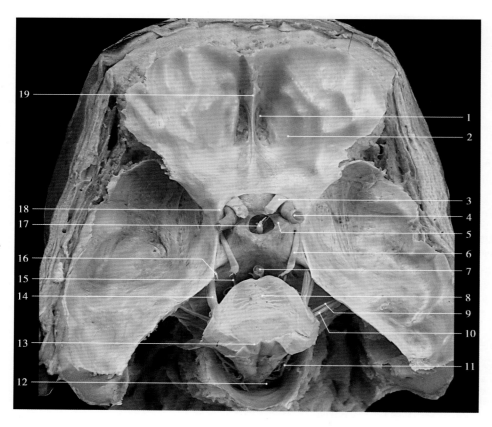

◀ 图 1-192　海绵窦

Fig. 1-192　Cavernous sinus

1. 筛孔 cribriform foramina
2. 颅前窝 anterior cranial fossa
3. 视神经 optic nerve
4. 颈内动脉 internal carotid artery
5. 鞍膈 diaphragma sellae
6. 动眼神经 oculomotor nerve
7. 基底动脉 basilar artery
8. 脑桥 pons
9. 面神经 facial nerve
10. 前庭蜗神经 vestibulo-cochlear nerve
11. 副神经 accessory nerve
12. 枕骨大孔 foramen magnum of occipital bone
13. 内侧隆起 medial eminence
14. 三叉神经 trigeminal nerve
15. 展神经 abducent nerve
16. 滑车神经 trochlear nerve
17. 垂体柄 hypophysial stalk
18. 前床突 anterior clinoid process
19. 鸡冠 crista galli

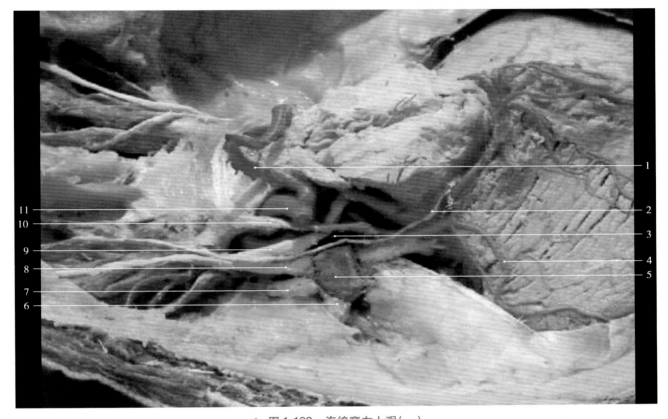

▲ 图 1-193　海绵窦左上观（一）

Fig. 1-193　Left superior aspect of the cavernous sinus（1）

1. 大脑前动脉 anterior cerebral artery
2. 滑车神经 trochlear nerve
3. 海绵窦外侧壁上三角 superior triangle in lateral wall of cavernous sinus
4. 小脑上动脉 superior cerebellar artery
5. 三叉神经节 trigeminal ganglion
6. 下颌神经 mandibular nerve
7. 上颌神经 maxillary nerve
8. 眼神经 ophthalmic nerve
9. 动眼神经 oculomotor nerve
10. 前床突 anterior clinoid process
11. 颈内动脉 internal carotid artery

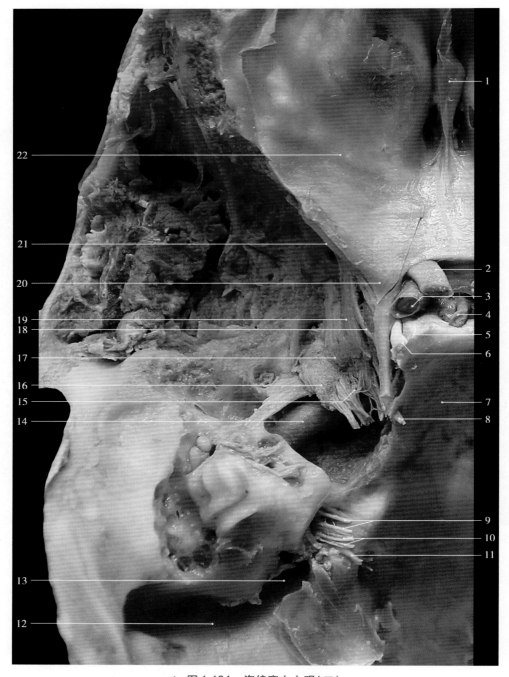

▲ 图 1-194　海绵窦左上观（二）

Fig. 1-194　Left superior aspect of the cavernous sinus（2）

1. 鸡冠 crista galli
2. 视神经 optic nerve
3. 颈内动脉 internal carotid artry
4. 垂体柄 hypophysial stalk
5. 后床突 posterior clinoid process
6. 动眼神经 oculomotor nerve
7. 斜坡 clivus
8. 展神经 abducent nerve
9. 舌咽神经 glossopharyngeal nerve
10. 迷走神经 vagus nerve
11. 副神经 accessory nerve

12. 横窦 transverse sinus
13. 乙状窦 sigmoid sinus
14. 颈内动脉岩部 petrosal part of internal carotid artery
15. 三叉神经 trigeminal nerve
16. 下颌神经 mandibular nerve
17. 三叉神经节 trigeminal ganglion
18. 滑车神经 trochlear nerve
19. 眼神经 ophthalmic nerve
20. 前床突 anterior clinoid process
21. 眶上裂 superior orbital fissure
22. 颅前窝 anterior cranial fossa

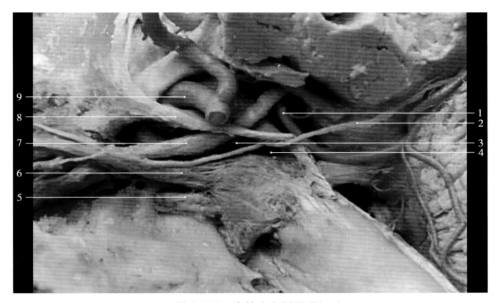

▲ 图 1-195　海绵窦左侧面观（一）

Fig. 1-195　Left aspect of the cavernous sinus（1）

1. 小脑上动脉 superior cerebellar artery
2. 滑车神经 trochlear nerve
3. 海绵窦外侧壁上三角 superior triangle in lateral wall of cavernous sinus
4. 海绵窦外侧壁下三角 inferior triangle in lateral wall of cavernous sinus （Parkinson triangle）
5. 上颌神经 maxillary nerve
6. 眼神经 ophthalmic nerve
7. 动眼神经 oculomotor nerve
8. 前床突 anterior clinoid process
9. 颈内动脉 internal carotid artery

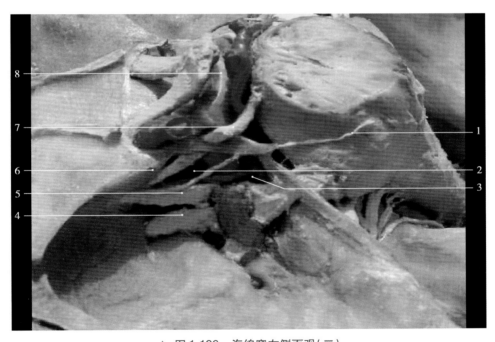

▲ 图 1-196　海绵窦左侧面观（二）

Fig. 1-196　Left aspect of the cavernous sinus（2）

1. 滑车神经 trochlear nerve
2. 海绵窦外侧壁上三角 superior triangle in lateral wall of cavernous sinus
3. 海绵窦外侧壁下三角 inferior triangle in lateral wall of cavernous sinus （Parkinson triangle）
4. 上颌神经 maxillary nerve
5. 眼神经 ophthalmic nerve
6. 前床突 anterior clinoid process
7. 动眼神经 oculomotor nerve
8. 后床突 posterior clinoid process

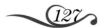

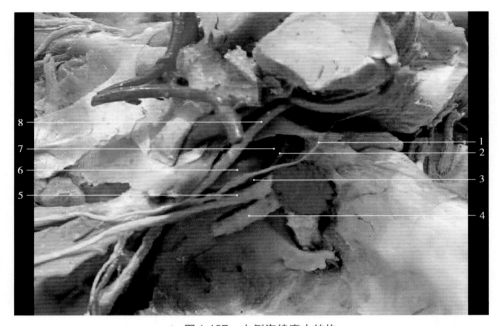

▲ 图 1-197　左侧海绵窦内结构
Fig. 1-197　Structures in the left cavernous sinus

1. 滑车神经 trochlear nerve
2. 展神经 abducent nerve
3. 海绵窦外侧壁下三角 inferior triangle in lateral wall of cavernous sinus（Parkinson triangle）
4. 上颌神经 maxillary nerve
5. 眼神经 ophthalmic nerve
6. 颈内动脉 internal carotid artery
7. 海绵窦外侧壁上三角 superior triangle in lateral wall of cavernous sinus
8. 动眼神经 oculomotor nerve

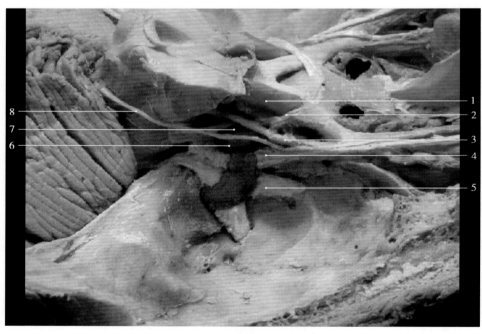

▲ 图 1-198　海绵窦右侧面观（一）
Fig. 1-198　Right aspect of the cavernous sinus（1）

1. 颈内动脉 internal carotid artery
2. 前床突 anterior clinoid process
3. 动眼神经 oculomotor nerve
4. 眼神经 ophthalmic nerve
5. 上颌神经 maxillary nerve
6. 海绵窦外侧壁下三角 inferior triangle in lateral wall of cavernous sinus（Parkinson triangle）
7. 海绵窦外侧壁上三角 superior triangle in lateral wall of cavernous sinus
8. 滑车神经 trochlear nerve

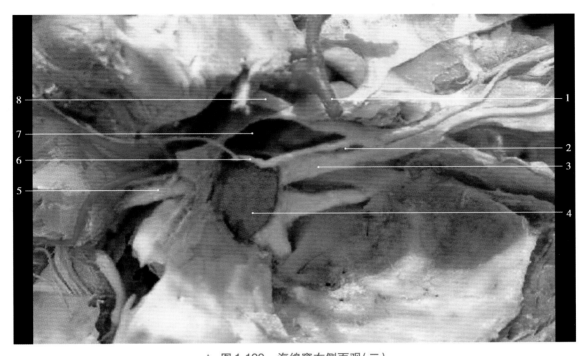

▲ 图 1-199 海绵窦右侧面观（二）
Fig. 1-199 Right aspect of the cavernous sinus（2）

1. 大脑中动脉 middle cerebral artery
2. 海绵窦外侧壁下三角 inferior triangle in lateral wall of cavernous sinus（Parkinson triangle）
3. 眼神经 ophthalmic nerve
4. 三叉神经节 trigeminal ganglion

5. 三叉神经 trigeminal nerve
6. 滑车神经 trochlear nerve
7. 海绵窦外侧壁上三角 superior triangle in lateral wall of cavernous sinus
8. 动眼神经 oculomotor nerve

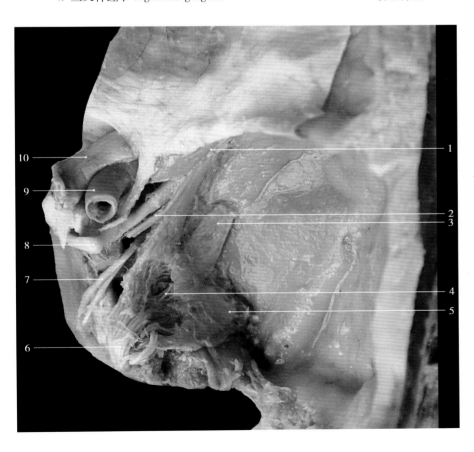

◀ 图 1-200 海绵窦右上观
Fig. 1-200 Right superior aspect of the cavernous sinus

1. 眶上裂 superior orbital fissure
2. 滑车神经 trochlear nerve
3. 上颌神经 maxillary nerve
4. 三叉神经节 trigeminal ganglion
5. 下颌神经 mandibular nerve
6. 三叉神经 trigeminal nerve
7. 展神经 abducent nerve
8. 动眼神经 oculomotor nerve
9. 颈内动脉 internal carotid artery
10. 视神经 optic nerve

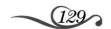

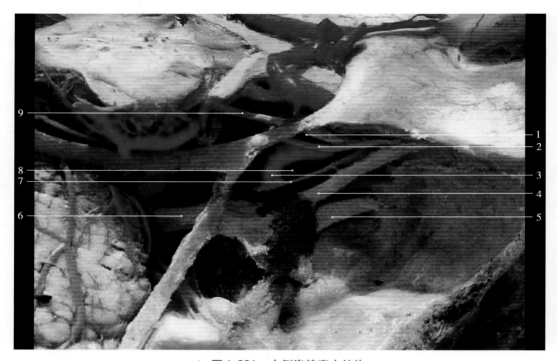

▲ 图 1-201　右侧海绵窦内结构
Fig. 1-201　Structures in the right cavernous sinus

1. 海绵窦外侧壁上三角 superior triangle in lateral wall of cavernous sinus
2. 滑车神经 trochlear nerve
3. 颈内动脉 internal carotid artery
4. 眼神经 ophthalmic nerve
5. 上颌神经 maxillary nerve
6. 三叉神经 trigeminal nerve
7. 展神经 abducent nerve
8. 海绵窦外侧壁下三角 inferior triangle in lateral wall of cavernous sinus（Parkinson triangle）
9. 动眼神经 oculomotor nerve

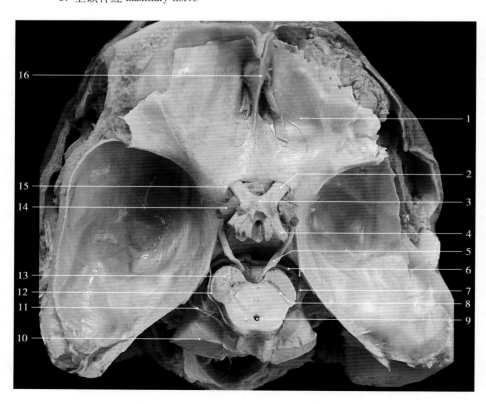

◄ 图 1-202　鞍隔上方结构
Fig. 1-202　Structures above the diaphragma

1. 眶板 orbital plate
2. 视神经 optic nerve
3. 视交叉 optic chiasma
4. 视束 optic tract
5. 动眼神经 oculomotor nerve
6. 大脑后动脉 posterior cerebral artery
7. 三叉神经 trigeminal nerve
8. 黑质 substantia nigra
9. 中脑导水管 mesencephalic aqueduct
10. 小脑上脚 superior cerebellar peduncle
11. 小脑上动脉 superior cerebellar artery
12. 滑车神经 trochlear nerve
13. 大脑脚 cerebral peduncle
14. 颈内动脉 internal carotid artery
15. 前床突 anterior clinoid process
16. 鸡冠 crista galli

海绵窦的应用解剖学要点

海绵窦位于蝶鞍两侧,呈前后狭长的不规则形,前方达眶上裂的内侧部,后方至颞骨岩尖部,上内侧抵前床突与后床突的连线,下外侧距圆孔与卵圆孔内缘连线 3~4mm。海绵窦长约 20mm,宽约 10mm,在经前、后床突中点作的冠状切面上呈近似直角三角形。颈内动脉在颞骨岩尖部走出颈动脉管,在蝶鞍的后下角,相当于后床突的外侧,突然转向前进入海绵窦,呈水平向前行 20mm,达前床突内侧再转向上穿出海绵窦的顶。因此,颈内动脉在海绵窦内形成 S 形双弯曲,称颈内动脉海绵窦部(又称虹吸部)。呈典型 S 形弯曲为 30%,呈直线行进的占 17%,呈中间型弯曲者为 53%。小儿常见为直线行程,随着年龄增长,其弯曲逐渐明显。动眼神经、滑车神经、三叉神经的眼神经和上颌神经均穿硬脑膜至海绵窦。在海绵窦外侧壁的硬脑膜内自上而下排列有动眼神经、滑车神经、眼神经和上颌神经。上颌神经紧贴于海绵窦的后下角,展神经在海绵窦居于眼神经内侧和颈内动脉的下方或下外侧,滑车神经从眼神经的外侧越至其上方。在海绵窦的后部,其外侧壁的上方为滑车神经,下方为眼神经,展神经居于颈内动脉的外侧。Parkinos 海绵窦三角:上界为动眼神经和滑车神经,下界为展神经和眼神经,后界为鞍背和斜坡的斜线。上界平均长约 13mm,下界为 14mm,后界为 6mm(图 1-192~图 1-202)。

应用解剖要点:

1. 颈内动脉在破裂孔处,恰好在海绵窦的近侧,位于三叉神经的下方,两者之间仅隔以薄骨片和硬脑膜,如骨片缺如,颈内动脉和三叉神经仅借硬脑膜相隔。颈内动脉在窦内被纤维小梁固定于窦壁,当颅底骨折时,动脉及其分支可破裂,血液流入窦内,引起海绵窦动、静脉瘘。

2. 颈内动脉居海绵窦的最内侧,紧邻垂体,其动脉的内侧缘与垂体外侧缘之间的距离为 2.3~7.0mm,有时颈内动脉海绵窦部弯曲而嵌入垂体,使脑垂体变形(28%)。这将给垂体手术带来巨大困难,术者一定要有应用解剖知识。

3. 运动眼球的动眼神经、滑车神经和展神经都与海绵窦的局部关系密切,故海绵窦栓塞时可出现眼球的运动障碍。

4. 外科手术治疗颈内动脉海绵窦瘘时,切开海绵窦外侧壁的位置应在 Parkinos 三角区,切开并显露颈内动脉及其分支时也不会损伤脑神经。

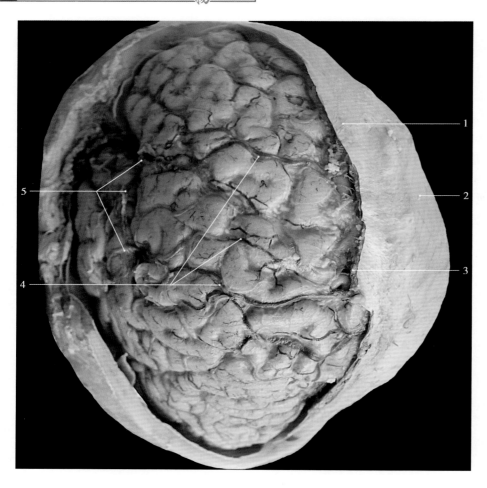

◀ 图 1-203　大脑浅静脉左侧面观

Fig. 1-203　Left aspect of the superficial cerebral veins

1. 上矢状窦 superior sagittal sinus
2. 硬脑膜 dura mater
3. 蛛网膜粒 arachnoid granulations
4. 大脑浅静脉上组 superior group of superficial cerebral vein
5. 大脑浅静脉下组 inferior group of superficial cerebral vein

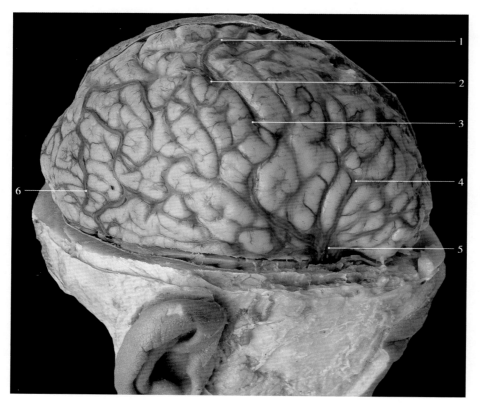

◀ 图 1-204　大脑浅静脉右侧面观

Fig. 1-204　Right aspect of the superficial cerebral veins

1. 大脑上静脉 superior cerebral vein
2. 顶叶静脉 parietal vein
3. 上吻合静脉 superior anastomotic vein
4. 额叶静脉 frontal vein
5. 大脑下静脉 inferior cerebral vein
6. 枕叶静脉 occipital vein

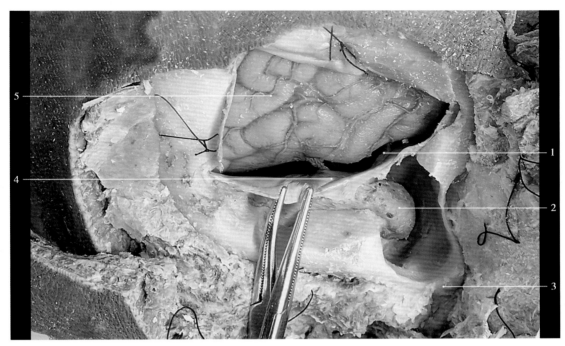

▲ 图 1-205 颞叶下静脉与横窦左侧面观

Fig. 1-205 Left aspect of the inferior temporal lobar vein and transverse sinus

1. 颞叶下静脉 inferior temporal vein
2. 乙状窦 sigmoid sinus
3. 乳窦 mastoid sinus
4. 横窦 transverse sinus
5. 颞叶 temporal lobe

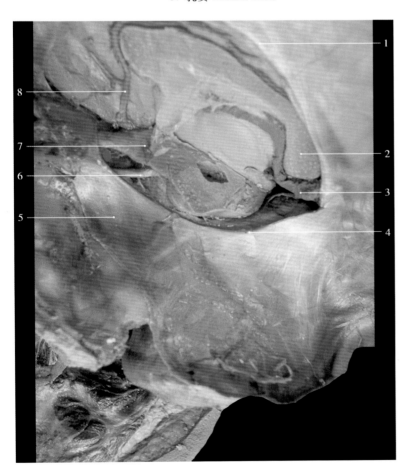

◀ 图 1-206 大脑深静脉(一)

Fig. 1-206 Deep cerebral vein (1)

1. 大脑镰 cerebral falx
2. 胼胝体压部 splenium of corpus callosum
3. 大脑深静脉 deep cerebral vein
4. 小脑幕切迹 tentorial notch
5. 小脑幕 tentorium of cerebellum
6. 动眼神经 oculomotor nerve
7. 视交叉 optic chiasma
8. 大脑前动脉 anterior cerebral artery

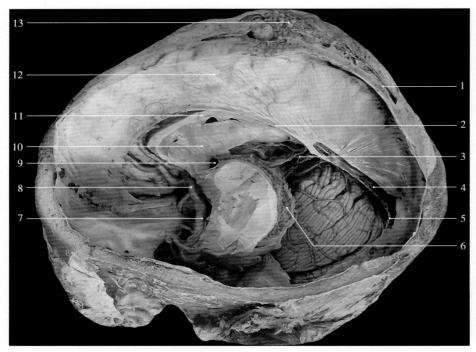

◀ 图 1-207　大脑深静脉
（二）
Fig. 1-207　Deep cerebral
vein（2）

1. 上矢状窦 superior sagit-
tal sinus
2. 下矢状窦 inferior sagittal
sinus
3. 大脑深静脉 deep cere-
bral vein
4. 直窦 straight sinus
5. 横窦 transverse sinus
6. 侧脑室脉络丛 choroid
plexus of lateral ventricle
7. 大脑中动脉 middle cere-
bral artery
8. 大脑前动脉 anterior cere-
bral artery
9. 室间孔 interventricular
foramen
10. 透明隔 septa pellucidum
11. 胼胝体 corpus callosum
12. 大脑镰 cerebral falx
13. 蛛网膜粒 arachnoid
granulations

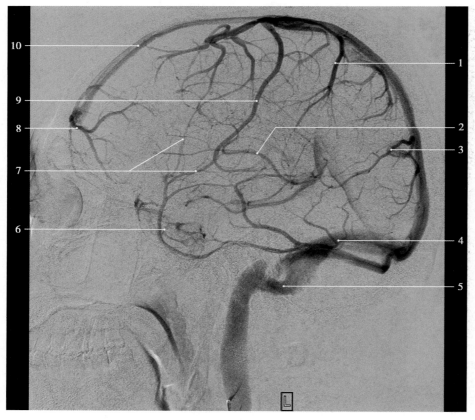

◀ 图 1-208　颈内动脉侧位
静脉期
Fig. 1-208　Lateral position
of the internal carotid artery
in the venous phase

1. 顶叶静脉 parietal vein
2. 大脑中、浅静脉 middle and
superficial cerebral veins
3. 枕叶静脉 occipital vein
4. 直窦 straight sinus
5. 乙状窦 sigmoid sinus
6. 颞下静脉 inferior tempo-
ral vein
7. 上吻合静脉 superior ana-
stomotic vein
8. 额前静脉 prefrontal vein
9. 中央沟静脉 vein of cen-
tral sulcus
10. 上矢状窦 superior sagit-
tal sinus

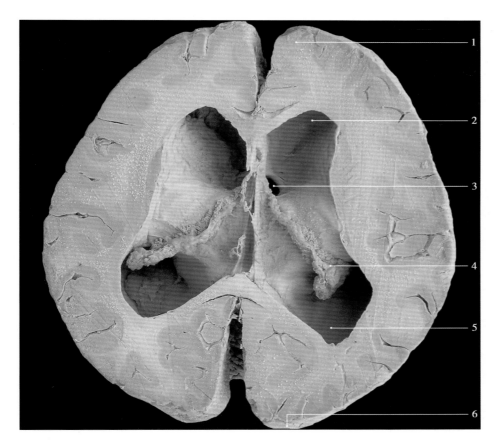

◀ 图 1-209　侧脑室脉络丛上面观

Fig. 1-209　Superior aspect of the choroid plexus in the lateral ventricle

1. 额叶 frontal lobe
2. 前角 anterior horn
3. 室间孔 interventricular foramen
4. 脉络丛 choroid plexus
5. 后角 posterior horn
6. 枕叶 occipital lobe

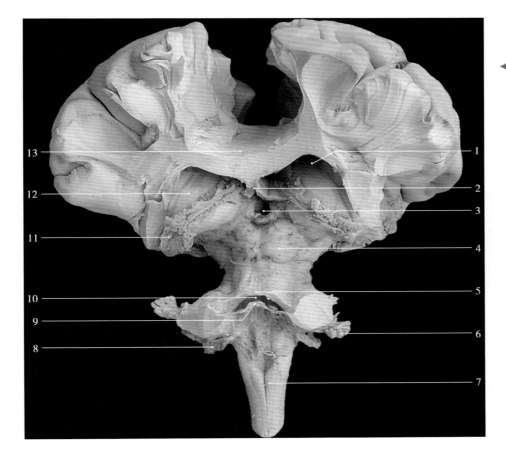

◀ 图 1-210　脑室系统后面观

Fig. 1-210　Posterior aspect of the ventricular system

1. 侧脑室 lateral ventricle
2. 透明隔 septum pellucidum
3. 第三脑室 third ventricle
4. 下丘 inferior colliculus
5. 上髓帆 superior medullary velum
6. 绒球 flocculus
7. 薄束结节 gracile tubercle
8. 第四脑室脉络丛 choroid plexus of fourth ventricle
9. 下髓帆 inferior medullary velum
10. 第四脑室 fourth ventricle
11. 侧脑室脉络丛 choroid plexus of lateral ventricle
12. 背侧丘脑 dorsal thalamus
13. 胼胝体 corpus callosum

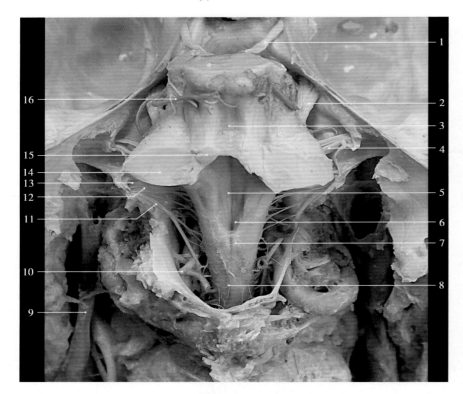

1. 动眼神经 oculomotor nerve
2. 三叉神经 trigeminal nerve
3. 上髓帆 superior medullary velum
4. 面神经、前庭蜗神经 facial nerve and vestibulocochlear nerve
5. 第四脑室 fourth ventricle
6. 舌下神经三角 hypoglossal triangle
7. 薄束结节 gracile tubercle
8. 延髓 medulla oblongata
9. 颈内静脉 internal jugular vein
10. 小脑下后动脉 posterior inferior cerebellar artery
11. 副神经 accessory nerve
12. 迷走神经 vagus nerve
13. 舌咽神经 glossopharyngeal nerve
14. 小脑中脚 middle cerebellar peduncle
15. 小脑上脚 superior cerebellar peduncle
16. 小脑上动脉 superior cerebellar artery

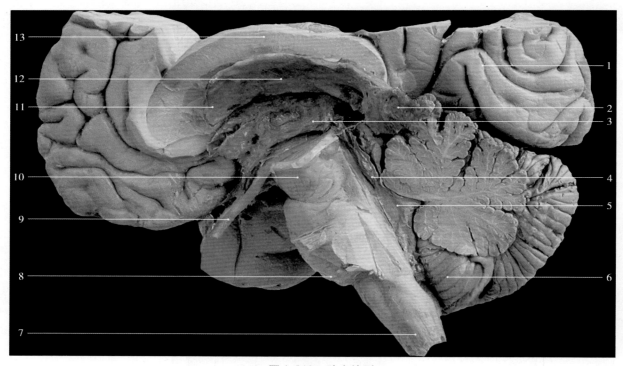

▲ 图 1-212 脑室铸型
Fig. 1-212 Cast of the ventricles

1. 枕叶 occipital lobe
2. 后角 posterior horn
3. 第三脑室 third ventricle
4. 中脑导水管 mesencephalic aqueduct
5. 第四脑室 fourth ventricle
6. 小脑扁桃体 tonsil of cerebellum
7. 延髓 medulla oblongata
8. 脑桥 pons
9. 视神经 optic nerve
10. 中脑 midbrain
11. 前角 anterior horn
12. 侧脑室 lateral ventricle
13. 胼胝体 corpus callosum

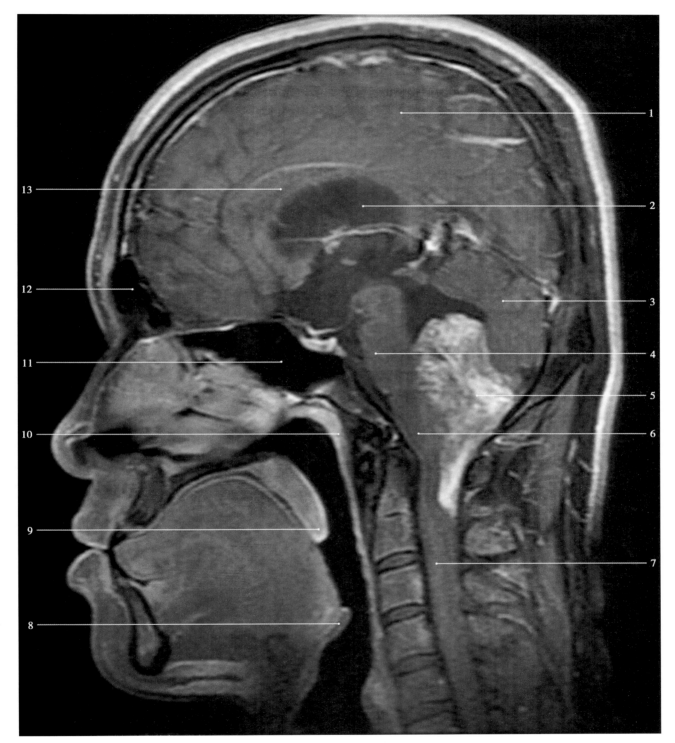

▲ 图 1-213 室管膜瘤
Fig. 1-213 Ependymoma

1. 顶叶 parietal lobe
2. 侧脑室 lateral ventricle
3. 小脑 cerebellum
4. 脑桥 pons
5. 室管膜瘤 ependymoma
6. 延髓 medulla oblongata
7. 颈髓 cervical spinal cord
8. 会厌软骨 epiglottic cartilage
9. 腭垂 uvula
10. 咽后壁 posterior wall of pharynx
11. 上颌窦 maxillary sinus
12. 额窦 frontal sinus
13. 胼胝体 corpus callosum

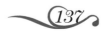

脑脊液及其循环的应用解剖学要点

脑脊液是充满于脑室、脊髓中央管和蛛网膜下隙内的无色透明的液体。脑脊液的功能是对中枢神经系统起缓冲、保护、营养、运输代谢产物和维持正常的颅内压的作用。成人脑脊液约150ml，处于不断地产生、循环和回流的平衡状态。脑脊液产生于脑室系统内的脉络丛。

脑脊液的循环：左、右侧脑室→室间孔→第三脑室→中脑水管→第四脑室→正中孔（1）、外侧孔（2）→蛛网膜下隙（以使脑、脊髓、脑神经根和脊神经根均浸泡在脑脊液之中）→蛛网膜粒→上矢状窦→窦汇→横窦→乙状窦→颈内静脉→头臂静脉→上腔静脉→右心房（图1-203～1-212）。

应用解剖要点：

1. 脑脊液经室间孔、中脑水管至第四脑室间的循环称脑脊液的脑内循环，其中任何一通道阻塞（如室间孔、中脑水管、正中孔或外侧孔）所引起的脑脊液循环障碍称脑内积水，而脑脊液经第四脑室的正中孔、外侧孔入蛛网膜下隙至上矢状窦内的蛛网膜粒，经蛛网膜粒渗入静脉。如蛛网膜粒发生阻塞引起脑脊液存于蛛网膜下隙内称颅内积水。

2. 脊髓蛛网膜衬于硬脊膜内面，并随脊神经前、后根延伸至脊神经，此处蛛网膜向硬膜下隙或硬膜外隙呈绒毛状突出称蛛网膜绒毛。蛛网膜绒毛可与硬膜外隙内的静脉丛相通，因此脊神经根的蛛网膜绒毛也属脑脊液的回流装置。

在椎间孔处行脊神经阻滞术时应避免刺入神经根，以防止药物注入蛛网膜下隙，这是在椎间孔处行脊神经阻滞术时引发脑脊液流出和引发脊髓麻醉的解剖学基础。

第七节　脑干和小脑

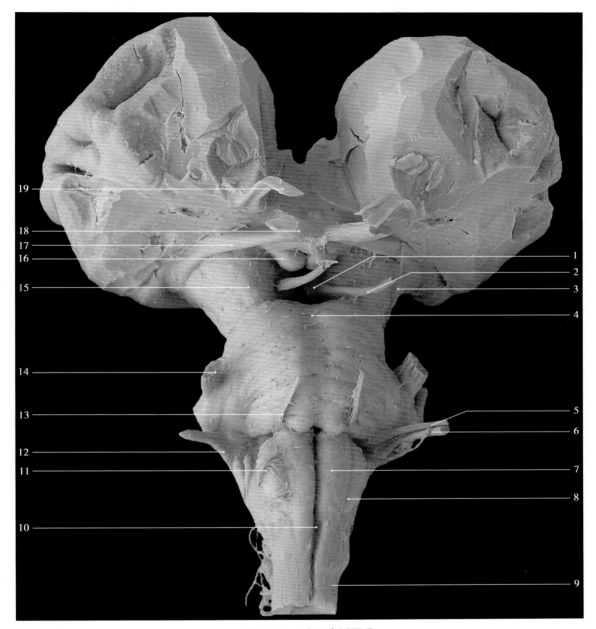

▲ 图 1-214　脑干腹侧面观

Fig. 1-214　Ventral aspect of the brain stem

1. 脚间窝 interpeduncular fossa
2. 动眼神经 oculomotor nerve
3. 滑车神经 trochlear nerve
4. 基底沟 basilar sulcus
5. 面神经 facial nerve
6. 前庭蜗神经 vestibulocochlear nerve
7. 锥体 pyramid
8. 橄榄 olive
9. 延髓 medulla oblongata
10. 前正中沟 anterior median groove
11. 舌下神经 hypoglossal nerve
12. 迷走神经 vagus nerve
13. 展神经 abducent nerve
14. 三叉神经 trigeminal nerve
15. 大脑脚 cerebral peduncle
16. 乳头体 mamillary body
17. 视束 optic tract
18. 视神经 optic nerve
19. 嗅束 olfactory tract

 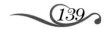

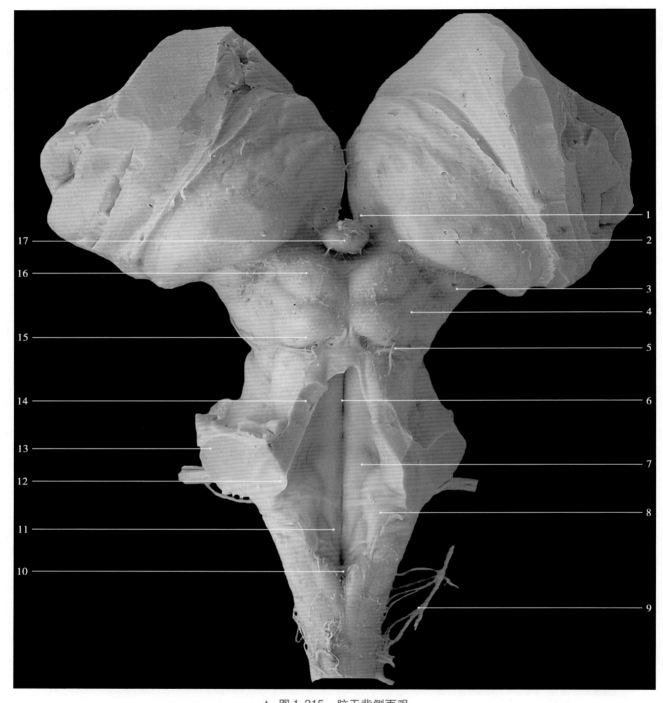

▲ 图1-215　脑干背侧面观
Fig. 1-215　Dorsal aspect of the brain stem

1. 缰三角 habenular trigone
2. 内侧膝状体 medial geniculate body
3. 外侧膝状体 lateral geniculate body
4. 下丘臂 brachium of inferior colliculus
5. 滑车神经 trochlear nerve
6. 菱形窝 rhomboid fossa
7. 内侧隆起 medial eminence
8. 髓纹 striae medullares
9. 副神经 accessory nerve
10. 闩 obex
11. 舌下神经三角 hypoglossal triangle
12. 绳状体 corpus restiforme
13. 桥臂 bridge arm
14. 结合臂 brachium conjunctivum
15. 下丘 inferior colliculus
16. 上丘 superior colliculus
17. 松果体 pineal body

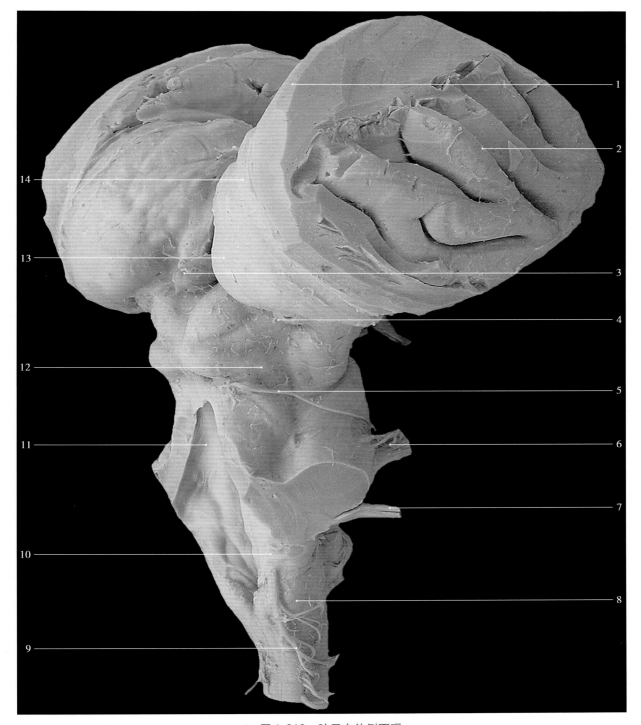

▲ 图 1-216 脑干右外侧面观

Fig. 1-216 Right lateral aspect of the brain stem

1. 内囊 internal capsule
2. 脑岛 insula
3. 松果体 pineal body
4. 外侧膝状体 lateral geniculate body
5. 滑车神经 trochlear nerve
6. 三叉神经 trigeminal nerve
7. 面神经 facial nerve
8. 橄榄 olive
9. 副神经 accessory nerve
10. 髓纹 striae medullares
11. 菱形窝 rhomboid fossa
12. 下丘臂 brachium of inferior colliculus
13. 丘脑枕 pulvinar
14. 尾状核 caudate nucleus

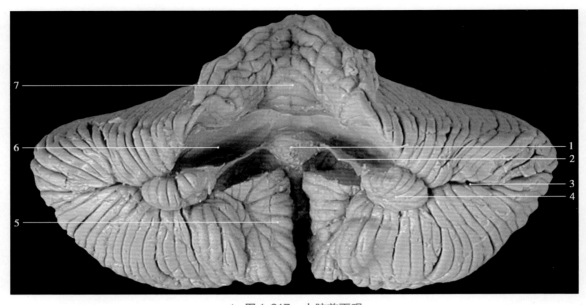

▲ 图 1-217　小脑前面观
Fig. 1-217　Anterior aspect of the cerebellum

1. 小结 nodule
2. 绒球脚 peduncle of flocculus
3. 后外侧裂 posterolateral fissure
4. 绒球 flocculus
5. 小脑扁桃体 tonsil of cerebellum
6. 第四脑室 fourth ventricle
7. 中央小叶 central lobule

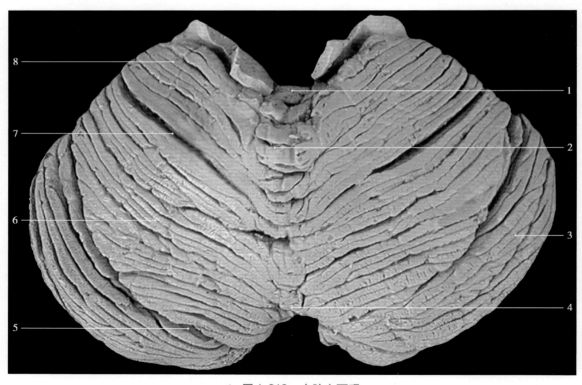

▲ 图 1-218　小脑上面观
Fig. 1-218　Superior aspect of the cerebellum

1. 中央小叶 central lobule
2. 小脑蚓 vermis
3. 下半月小叶 inferior semilunar lobule
4. 蚓叶 folium of vermis
5. 水平裂 horizontal fissure
6. 方形小叶后部 posterior quadrangular lobule
7. 原裂 primary fissure
8. 方形小叶前部 anterior quadrangular lobule

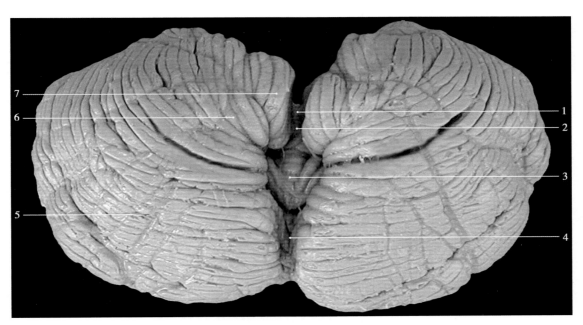

▲ 图 1-219　小脑下面观
Fig. 1-219　Inferior aspect of the cerebellum

1. 小结 nodule
2. 蚓垂 uvula of vermis
3. 蚓锥体 pyramid of vermis
4. 蚓结节 tuber of vermis
5. 下半月小叶 inferior semilunar lobule
6. 二腹小叶 biventral lobule
7. 小脑扁桃体 tonsil of cerebellum

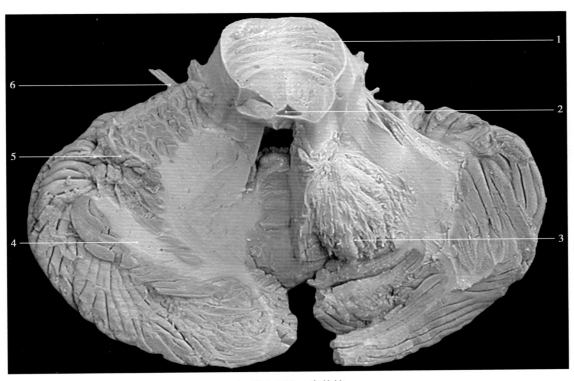

▲ 图 1-220　齿状核
Fig. 1-220　Dentate nucleus

1. 脑桥 pons
2. 中脑导水管 mesencephalic aqueduct
3. 齿状核 dentate nucleus
4. 小脑髓质 medulla of cerebellum
5. 小脑皮质 cortex of cerebellum
6. 前庭蜗神经 vestibulocochlear nerve

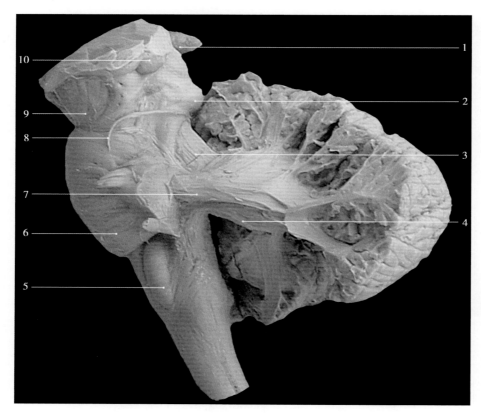

◀ 图1-221　小脑脚
Fig. 1-221　Cerebellar peduncle

1. 松果体 pineal body
2. 下丘 inferior colliculus
3. 小脑上脚 superior cerebellar peduncle
4. 小脑下脚 inferior cerebellar peduncle
5. 橄榄 olive
6. 脑桥 pons
7. 小脑中脚 middle cerebellar peduncle
8. 滑车神经 trochlear nerve
9. 大脑脚 cerebral peduncle
10. 外侧膝状体 lateral geniculate body

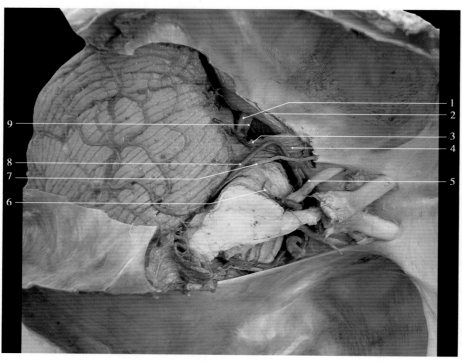

◀ 图1-222　左侧桥脑小脑角上面观
Fig. 1-222　Superior aspect of the left pontocerebellar trigone

1. 前庭蜗神经 vestibulocochlear nerve
2. 岩上窦 superior petrosal sinus
3. 桥脑小脑角 pontocerebellar trigone
4. 三叉神经 trigeminal nerve
5. 动眼神经 oculomotor nerve
6. 桥臂 bridge arm
7. 滑车神经 trochlear nerve
8. 小脑上动脉 superior cerebellar artery
9. 面神经 facial nerve

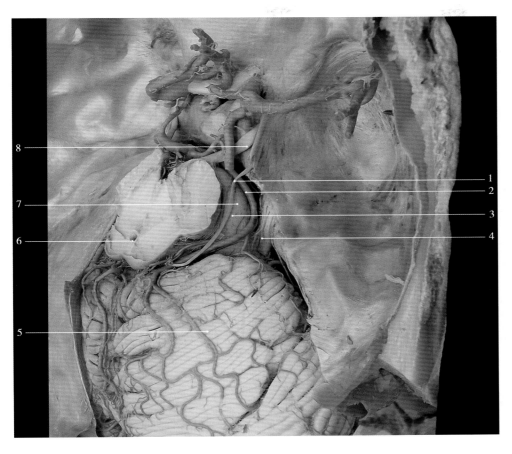

◀ 图 1-223　右侧桥脑小
脑角上面观
Fig. 1-223　Superior aspect of the right pontocerebellar trigone

1. 滑车神经 trochlear nerve
2. 小脑上动脉 superior cerebellar artery
3. 脑桥 pons
4. 三叉神经 trigeminal nerve
5. 小脑 cerebellum
6. 中脑导水管 mesencephalic aqueduct
7. 桥脑小脑角 pontocerebellar trigone
8. 动眼神经 oculomotor nerve

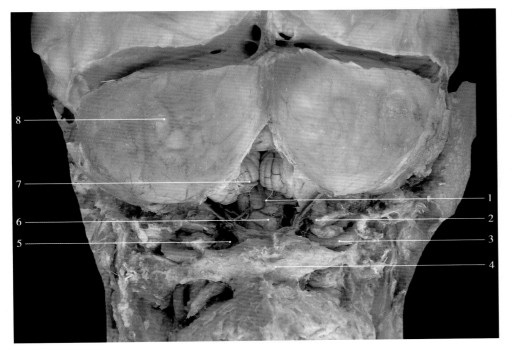

◀ 图 1-224　小脑扁桃体
与延髓后面观
Fig. 1-224　Posterior aspect of the tonsil of cerebellum and the medulla oblongata

1. 小脑下后动脉 posterior inferior cerebellar artery
2. 枕骨髁 occipital condyle
3. 椎动脉寰椎部 atlantic part of vertebral artery
4. 寰椎后结节 posterior tubercle of atlas
5. 枕骨大孔 foramen magnum of occipital bone
6. 延髓 medulla oblongata
7. 小脑扁桃体 tonsil of cerebellum
8. 硬脑膜 cerebral dura mater

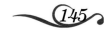

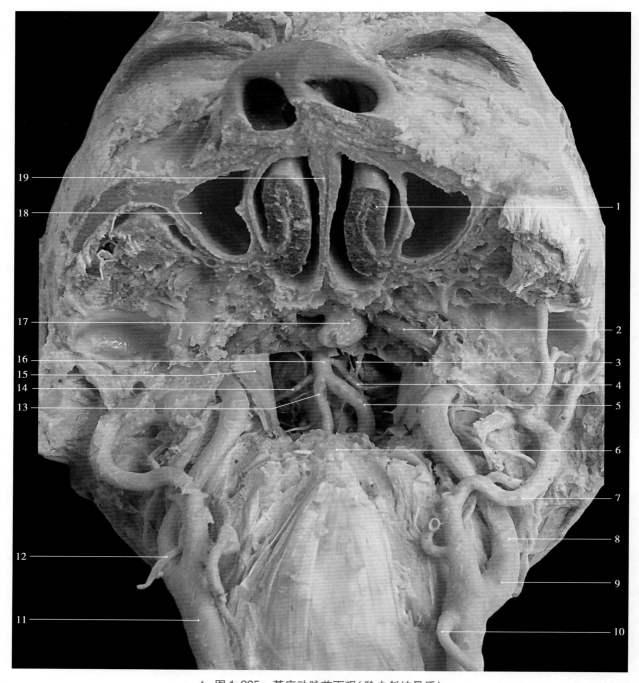

▲ 图 1-225　基底动脉前面观(除去斜坡骨质)

Fig. 1-225　Anterior aspect of the basilar artery(the clivus was removed)

1. 下鼻甲 inferior nasal concha
2. 颈内动脉岩部 petrosal part of internal carotid artery
3. 展神经 abducent nerve
4. 左侧小脑下前动脉 left anterior inferior cerebellar artery
5. 左侧椎动脉 left vertebral artery
6. 齿突 dens
7. 颈外动脉 external carotid artery
8. 颈内动脉 internal carotid artery
9. 颈动脉窦 carotid sinus
10. 甲状腺上动脉 superior thyroid artery
11. 颈总动脉 common carotid artery
12. 舌下神经 hypoglossal nerve
13. 右侧椎动脉 right vertebral artery
14. 右侧小脑下前动脉 right anterior inferior cerebellar artery
15. 硬膜(翻向外) dura mater (turned laterally)
16. 基底动脉 basilar artery
17. 垂体 hypophysis
18. 上颌窦 maxillary sinus
19. 鼻中隔 nasal septum

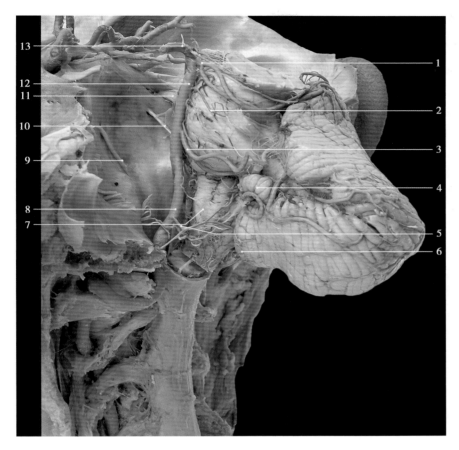

◀ 图 1-226　小脑动脉侧面观
Fig. 1-226　Lateral aspect of the cerebellar artery

1. 小脑上动脉 superior cerebellar artery
2. 桥支 branch of pons
3. 小脑下前动脉 anterior inferior cerebellar artery
4. 绒球 flocculus
5. 小脑下后动脉 posterior inferior cerebellar artery
6. 小脑扁桃体 tonsil of cerebellum
7. 延髓 medulla oblongata
8. 椎动脉 vertebral artery
9. 前庭蜗神经 vestibulocochlear nerve
10. 展神经 abducent nerves
11. 三叉神经 trigeminal nerves
12. 基底动脉 basilar artery
13. 大脑后动脉 posterior cerebral artery

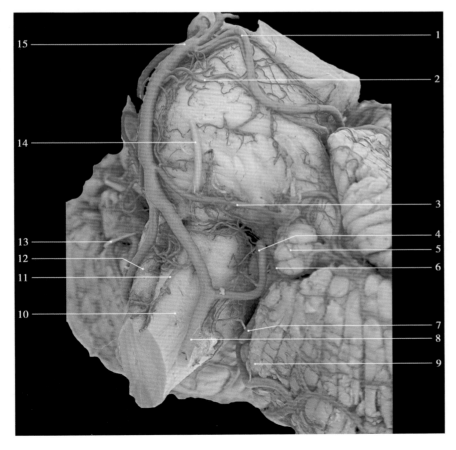

◀ 图 1-227　小脑和脑桥的动脉前外侧面观
Fig. 1-227　Anterolateral aspect of artery of the cerebellum and pons

1. 小脑上动脉 superior cerebellar artery
2. 桥支 branch of pons
3. 小脑下前动脉 anterior inferior cerebellar artery
4. 上袢 superior loop
5. 绒球 flocculus
6. 小脑下后动脉 posterior inferior cerebellar artery
7. 尾袢 tail loop
8. 椎动脉 vertebral artery
9. 小脑扁桃体 tonsil of cerebellum
10. 延髓 medulla oblongata
11. 脊髓前动脉 anterior spinal artery
12. 锥体 pyramid
13. 舌下神经 hypoglossal nerve
14. 展神经 abducent nerve
15. 基底动脉 basilar artery

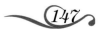

延髓腹外侧区血供的应用解剖学要点

解剖学和生理学上均认为延髓的腹外侧区(橄榄后沟的后外侧)的网状结构内有与呼吸和心血管调节相关的中枢,即相当于延髓内孤束核、疑核和巨细胞旁核的区域。脑桥小脑三角、岩斜区的手术时如不注意保护延髓腹外侧区血供,可能会引起严重的后果。

延髓腹外侧区营养动脉来自于小脑下前动脉、椎动脉、基底动脉、小脑下后动脉。分布于延髓腹外侧区的营养动脉,其起始处与前正中沟的距离在 8～10mm 之间。小脑下前动脉、椎动脉、基底动脉和小脑下后动脉发出至延髓腹外侧区脑组织的营养动脉的入脑处均在前庭蜗神经的内下方,其两者之间的距离在 6～10mm 之间。在位听神经瘤时,在听神经的内下方应保护发至延髓腹外侧区的营养动脉(图1-227)。

应用解剖要点:

在脑干腹侧、颅后窝,尤其是脑桥小脑三角区、岩斜区的病变(肿瘤等)实施手术切除时,除应避免过重牵拉延髓外,还应防止损伤供应延髓腹外侧区(生命中枢)的血管。小脑下前动脉、小脑下后动脉发出的营养动脉均在远离动脉起始处约2.0mm之后发出,在施行小脑下后动脉瘤手术时,应小心游离动脉瘤,对延髓供血的小动脉由延髓外侧段和背侧段分出,不要误当蛛网膜粘连而误伤它们。

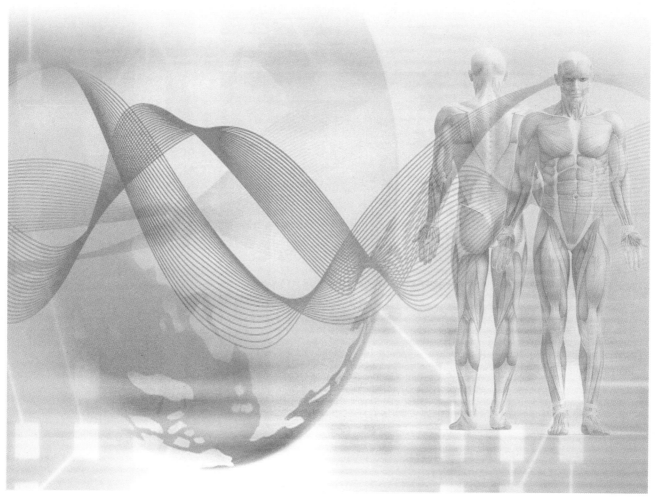

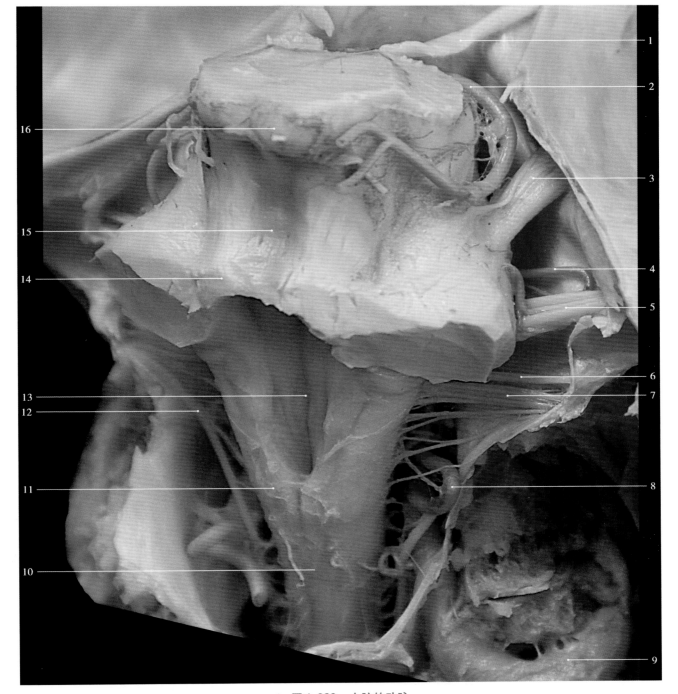

▲ 图 1-228　小脑的动脉
Fig. 1-228　Arteies of the cerebellum

1. 动眼神经 oculomotor nerve
2. 小脑上动脉 superior cerebellar artery
3. 三叉神经 trigeminal nerve
4. 小脑下前动脉 anterior inferior cerebellar artery
5. 面神经 facial nerve
6. 舌咽神经 glossopharyngeal nerve
7. 迷走神经 vagus nerve
8. 小脑下后动脉 posterior inferior cerebellar artery

9. 椎动脉 vertebral artery
10. 延髓 medulla oblongata
11. 薄束结节 gracile tubercle
12. 副神经 accessory nerve
13. 菱形窝 rhomboid fossa
14. 小脑上脚 superior cerebellar peduncle
15. 上髓帆 superior medullary velum
16. 下丘 inferior colliculus

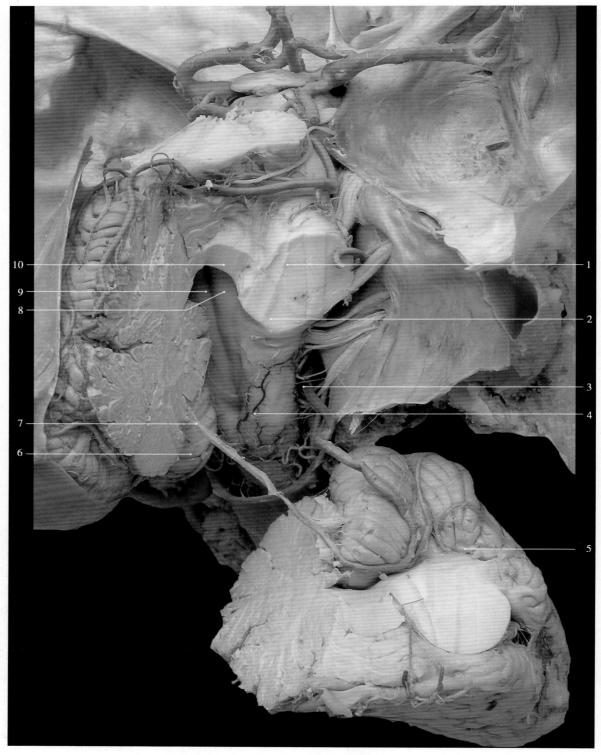

▲ 图 1-229 小脑下后动脉
Fig. 1-229 Posterior inferior cerebellar artery

1. 小脑中脚 middle cerebellar peduncle
2. 小脑下脚 inferior cerebellar peduncle
3. 小脑下后动脉 posterior inferior cerebellar artery
4. 延髓 medulla oblongata
5. 小脑半球（切开拉向下）cerebellar hemisphere
   （cut and pulled inferiorly）

6. 小脑扁桃体 tonsil of cerebellum
7. 扁桃体支 tonsillar branch
8. 面丘 facial colliculus
9. 第四脑室 fourth ventricle
10. 结合臂 brachium conjunctivum

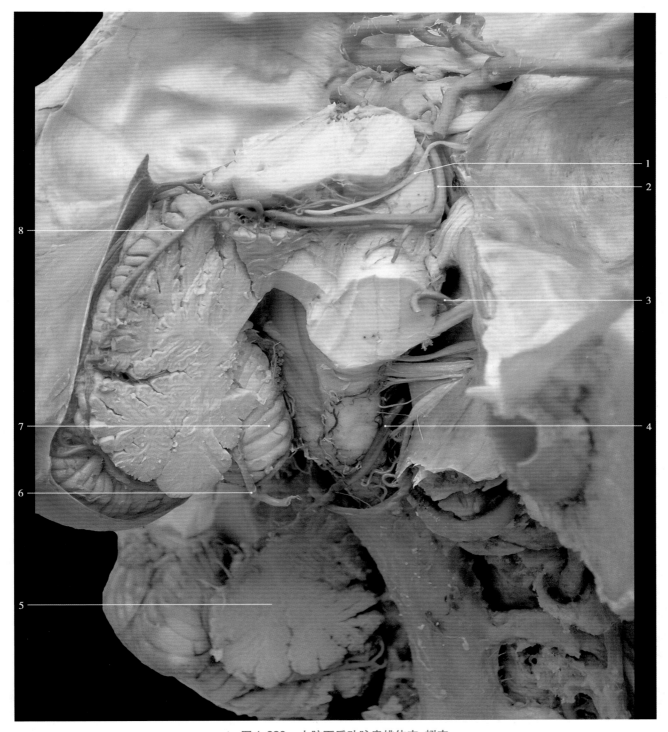

▲ 图 1-230　小脑下后动脉扁桃体支、蚓支

Fig. 1-230　Tonsillar and vermian branches of the posterior inferior cerebellar artery

1. 滑车神经 trochlear nerve
2. 小脑上动脉 superior cerebellar artery
3. 迷路动脉 labyrinthine artery
4. 小脑下后动脉 posterior inferior cerebellar artery
5. 小脑半球（切开翻向下）cerebellar hemisphere（cut and turned down）
6. 扁桃体支 tonsillar branch
7. 小脑扁桃体 tonsil of cerebellum
8. 蚓支 vermian branch

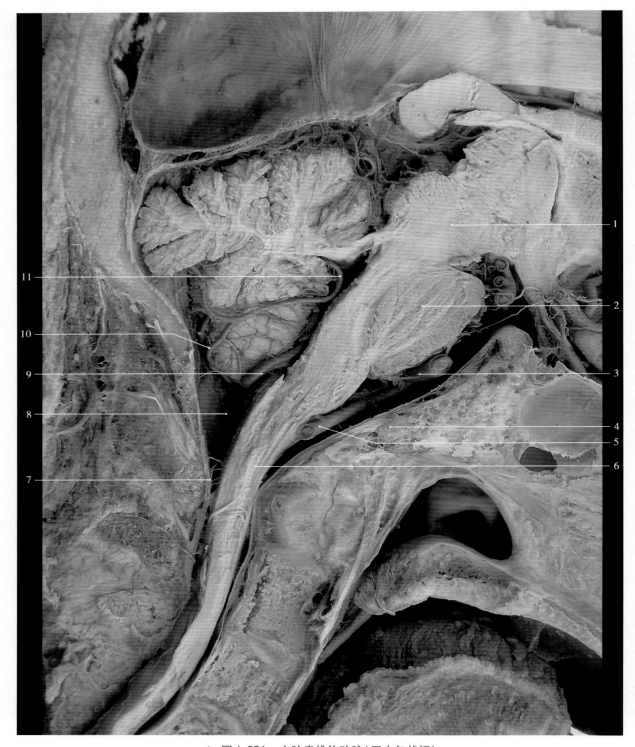

▲ 图 1-231　小脑扁桃体动脉（正中矢状切）

Fig. 1-231　Cerebellar tonsillar artery（median sagittal section）

1. 中脑 mesencephalon
2. 脑桥 pons
3. 基底动脉 basilar artery
4. 斜坡 clivus
5. 椎动脉 vertebral artery
6. 延髓 medulla oblongata
7. 枕骨大孔 foramen magnum of occipital bone
8. 小脑延髓池 cerebellomedullary cistern
9. 小脑下后动脉 posterior inferior cerebellar artery
10. 小脑扁桃体支 cerebellar tonsillar branch
11. 小脑下前动脉 anterior inferior cerebellar artery

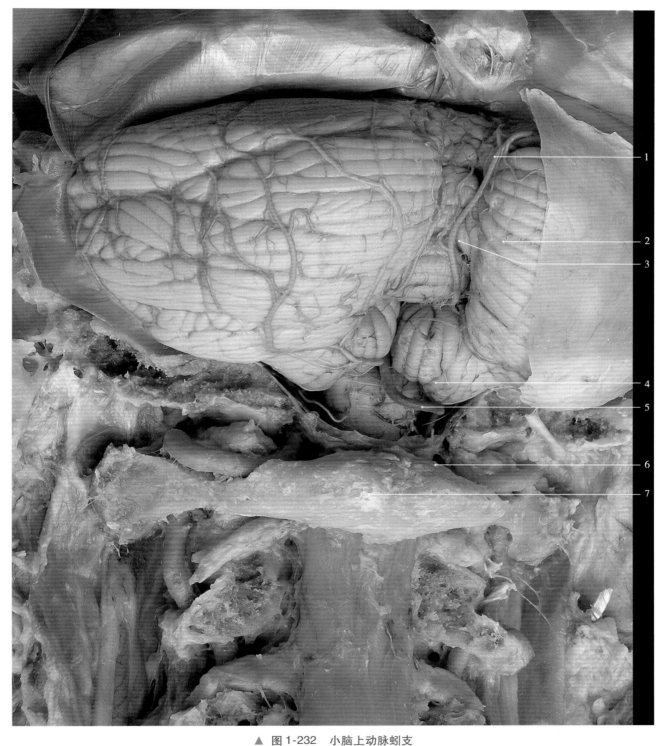

▲ 图 1-232　小脑上动脉蚓支

Fig. 1-232　Vermian branch of the superior cerebellar artery

1. 小脑上动脉蚓支 vermian branch of superior cerebellar artery

2. 小脑半球 cerebellar hemisphere

3. 小脑蚓 vermis

4. 小脑扁桃体 tonsil of cerebellum

5. 小脑下后动脉 posterior inferior cerebellar artery

6. 枕骨大孔 foramen magnum of occipital bone

7. 寰椎后结节 posterior tubercle of atlas

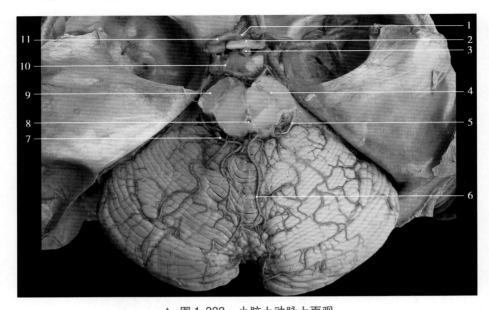

▲ 图 1-233　小脑上动脉上面观

Fig. 1-233　Superior aspect of the superior cerebellar artery

1. 前交通动脉 anterior communicating artery
2. 视交叉 optic chiasma
3. 垂体柄 hypophysial stalk
4. 黑质 substantia nigra
5. 滑车神经 trochlear nerve
6. 蚓支 vermian branch
7. 小脑上动脉 superior cerebellar artery
8. 中脑导水管 mesencephalic aqueduct
9. 大脑脚 cerebral peduncle
10. 后交通动脉 posterior communicating artery
11. 大脑前动脉 anterior cerebral artery

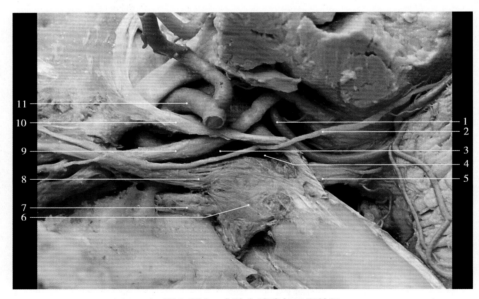

▲ 图 1-234　小脑上动脉与三叉神经

Fig. 1-234　Superior cerebellar artery and trigeminal nerve

1. 小脑上动脉 superior cerebellar artery
2. 滑车神经 trochlear nerve
3. 海绵窦外侧壁上三角 superior triangle in lateral wall of cavernous sinus
4. 海绵窦外侧壁下三角 inferior triangle in lateral wall of cavernous sinus
5. 三叉神经 trigeminal nerve
6. 三叉神经节 trigeminal ganglion
7. 上颌神经 maxillary nerve
8. 眼神经 ophthalmic nerve
9. 动眼神经 oculomotor nerve
10. 前床突 anterior clinoid process
11. 颈内动脉 internal carotid artery

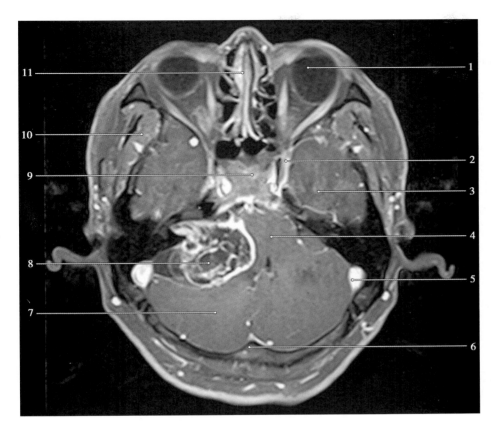

◀ 图 1-235 听神经瘤（一）
Fig. 1-235 Acoustic neuroma（1）

1. 眼球 eyeball
2. 视神经 optic nerve
3. 颞叶 temporal lobe
4. 脑桥 pons
5. 乙状窦 sigmoid sinus
6. 窦汇 confluence of sinus
7. 小脑半球 cerebellar hemisphere
8. 听神经瘤 acoustic neuroma
9. 蝶鞍 sella turcica
10. 颞肌 temporalis
11. 鼻中隔 nasal septum

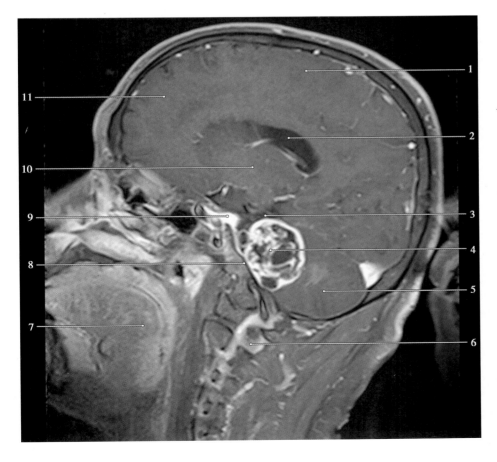

◀ 图 1-236 听神经瘤（二）
Fig. 1-236 Acoustic neuroma（2）

1. 顶叶 parietal lobe
2. 侧脑室 lateral ventricle
3. 脑桥小脑三角 pontocerebellar trigone
4. 听神经瘤 acoustic neuroma
5. 小脑半球 cerebellar hemisphere
6. 枢椎棘突 spinous process of axis
7. 舌 tongue
8. 斜坡 clivus
9. 蝶骨 sphenoid bone
10. 豆状核 lentiform nucleus
11. 额叶 frontal lobe

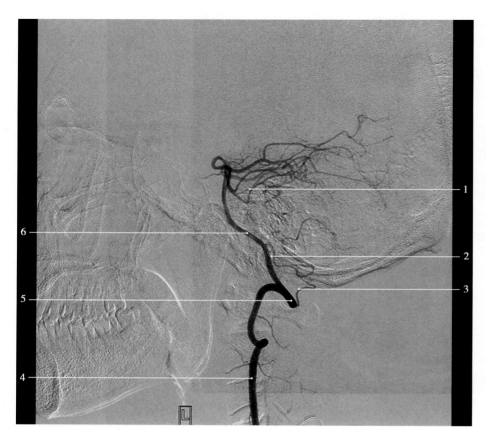

图 1-237 椎动脉侧位动脉期

Fig. 1-237 Lateral position of the vertebral artery in the arterial phase

1. 小脑上动脉 superior cerebellar artery
2. 小脑下前动脉 anterior inferior cerebellar artery
3. 小脑下后动脉 posterior inferior cerebellar artery
4. 椎动脉横突部 transverse part of vertebral artery
5. 椎动脉寰椎部 atlantic part of vertebral artery
6. 基底动脉 basilar artery

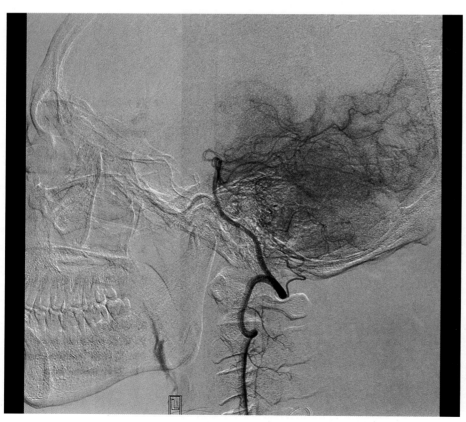

◀ 图 1-238 椎动脉侧位实质期

Fig. 1-238 Lateral position of the vertebral artery in the parenchymal phase

小脑上动脉的应用解剖学要点

小脑上动脉约在相当于脑桥上缘(平对基底动脉近终点)处发出,行向外侧。小脑上动脉与大脑后动脉相距仅为5mm左右。动眼神经从小脑上动脉和基底动脉间穿出行向前外。小脑上动脉行至中脑外侧绕大脑脚转向后内,转至中脑背侧,行于结合臂上方,小脑幕游离缘下方,经小脑前上缘至四叠体后部发出蚓支和半球支(图1-234)。

应用解剖要点:

小脑上动脉外径左侧为1.41mm,右侧为1.33mm,上行动脉经颞骨岩部位于三叉神经上方。正常两者相距仅为1.0mm,有30%三叉神经痛的患者经手术证实小脑上动脉在三叉神经根上有压迹,据此认为小脑上动脉行程中压于三叉神经上方是引起三叉神经痛的病因。经手术结扎或经介入治疗方法栓塞小脑上动脉和在三叉神经根与小脑上动脉之间隔以海绵垫均可使三叉神经痛的症状得到缓解。

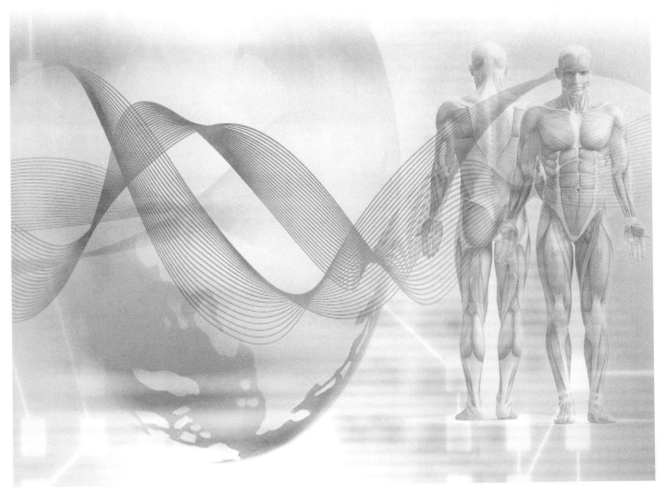

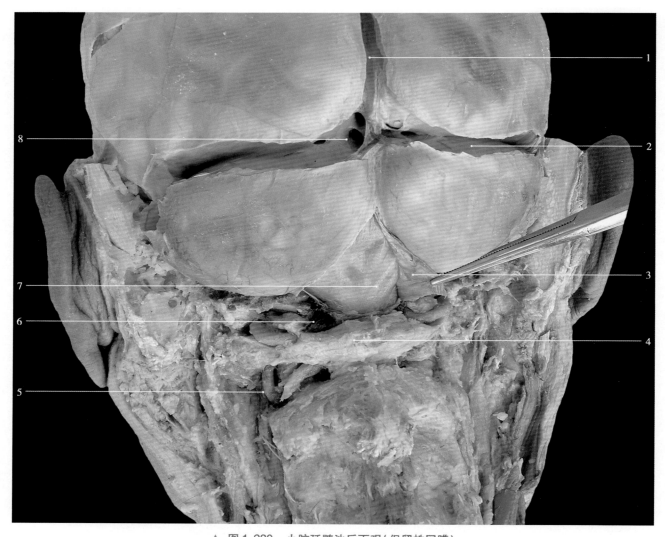

▲ 图 1-239　小脑延髓池后面观（保留蛛网膜）

Fig. 1-239　Posterior aspect of the cerebellomedullary cistern（the arachnoid was retained）

1. 上矢状窦 superior sagittal sinus
2. 横窦 transverse sinus
3. 硬脑膜（翻向外）cerebral dura mater（turned laterally）
4. 寰椎横突 transverse process of atlas
5. 椎动脉 vertebral artery
6. 枕骨大孔 foramen magnum of occipital bone
7. 小脑延髓池 cerebellomedullary cistern
8. 直窦开口 debouch of straight sinus

颅后窝外侧入路术的应用解剖学要点

对下斜坡区,枕骨大孔区和颈段腹侧和腹外侧区的肿瘤以及颈静脉孔区的肿瘤,临床上常采用颅后窝远外侧手术入路。该入路具有路径短,很少需要牵拉脑干,并可早期保护椎动脉等优点。由于该入路涉及后组脑神经、颈内动脉、椎动脉等重要结构,因此熟悉该区域的解剖结构对顺利完成手术是非常重要的(图1-224、图1-239)。

应用解剖要点:

1. 手术入路经过的层次为　皮肤→浅筋膜→深筋膜→斜方肌→夹肌(头夹肌、颈夹肌)→颈部静脉丛→棘肌(头半棘肌、颈半棘肌)→颈部深层静脉丛→枕下三角(头下斜肌、头上斜肌、头后大小直肌)→椎动脉虹吸部→寰椎横突→茎突→颈静脉孔(舌下神经、副神经、迷走神经、舌咽神经)→枕骨髁→颅后窝外侧部。

2. 应重视乳突至茎突、寰椎横突外侧和茎突至第1颈椎横突外侧的间距,三者之间的间距分别为30.67mm、24.15mm和15.20mm。乳突尖至舌咽神经、迷走神经、副神经和舌下神经的距离分别为26.13mm、24.27mm、21.17mm和24.64mm。手术入路中所要显示和保护的重要结构均在乳突尖、茎突尖和第1颈椎横突围成的三角内。颈内静脉、颈内动脉和后组脑神经均在手术视野中的茎突的前内侧。术中一定要辨认茎突、乳突和C1横突等结构。

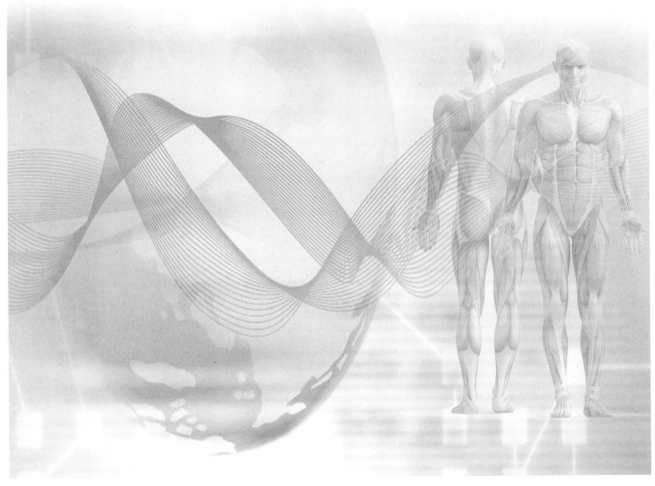

第八节 颅底结构

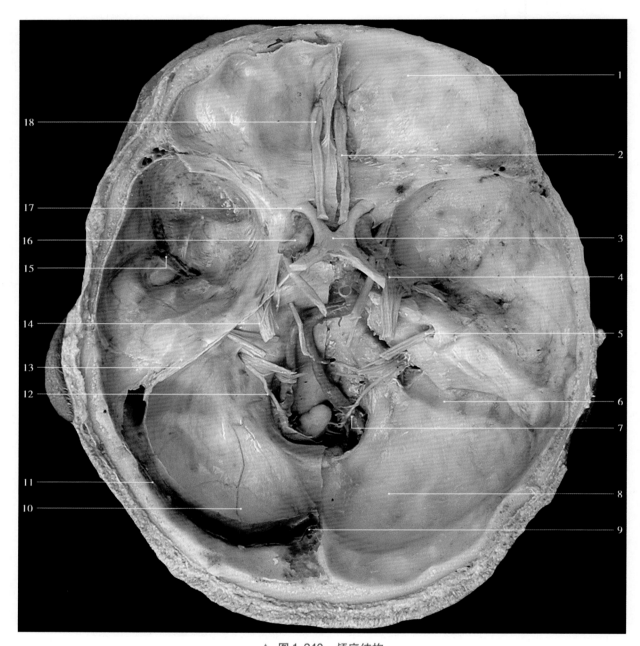

▲ 图 1-240　颅底结构
Fig. 1-240　Structures of the skull base

1. 颅前窝 anterior cranial fossa
2. 嗅束 olfactory tract
3. 视交叉 optic chiasma
4. 三叉神经节 trigeminal ganglion
5. 面神经 facial nerve
6. 乙状窦沟 sigmoid sulcus
7. 椎动脉 vertebral artery
8. 颅后窝 posterior cranial fossa
9. 窦汇 confluence of sinuses
10. 颅底硬脑膜 cerebral dura mater of skull base
11. 横窦 transverse sinus
12. 副神经 accessory nerve
13. 岩上窦 superior petrosal sinus
14. 三叉神经 trigeminal nerve
15. 脑膜中动脉 middle meningeal artery
16. 颈内动脉 internal carotid artery
17. 视神经 optic nerve
18. 嗅球 olfactory bulb

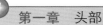

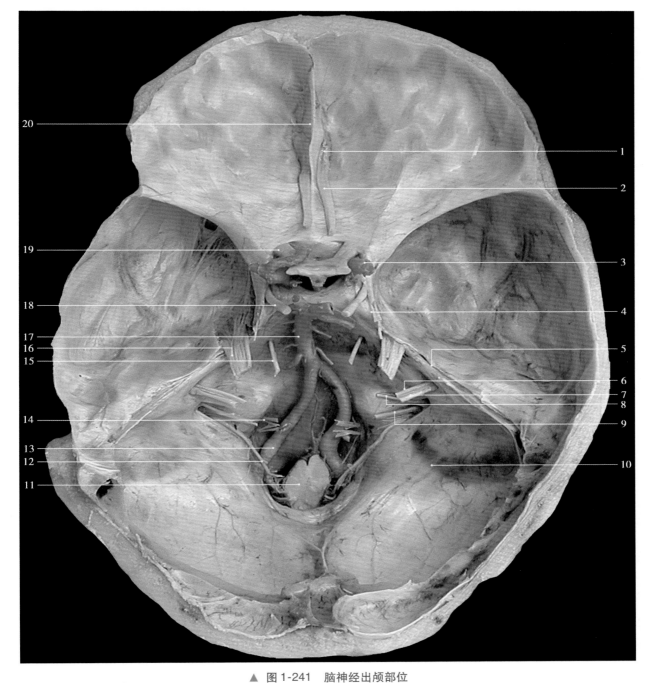

▲ 图 1-241　脑神经出颅部位

Fig. 1-241　Sites of the cranial nerves departing from the cranium

1. 嗅球 olfactory bulb
2. 嗅束 olfactory tract
3. 颈内动脉 internal carotid artery
4. 滑车神经 trochlear nerve
5. 岩上窦 superior petrosal sinus
6. 面神经 facial nerve
7. 前庭蜗神经 vestibulocochlear nerve
8. 舌咽神经 glossopharyngeal nerve
9. 迷走神经 vagus nerve
10. 乙状窦 sigmoid sinus
11. 延髓 medulla oblongata
12. 副神经 accessory nerve
13. 椎动脉 vertebral artery
14. 舌下神经 hypoglossal nerve
15. 展神经 abducent nerve
16. 三叉神经 trigeminal nerve
17. 基底动脉 basilar artery
18. 动眼神经 oculomotor nerve
19. 视神经 optic nerve
20. 鸡冠 crista galli

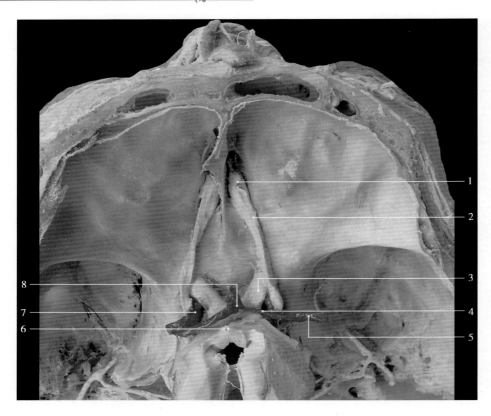

◀ 图1-242　颅前窝深层结构
Fig. 1-242　Deep structures of the anterior cranial fossa

1. 嗅球 olfactory bulb
2. 嗅束 olfactory tract
3. 视神经 optic nerve
4. 大脑前动脉 anterior cerebral artery
5. 大脑中动脉 middle cerebral artery
6. 视交叉 optic chiasma
7. 颈内动脉 internal carotid artery
8. 前交通动脉 anterior communicating artery

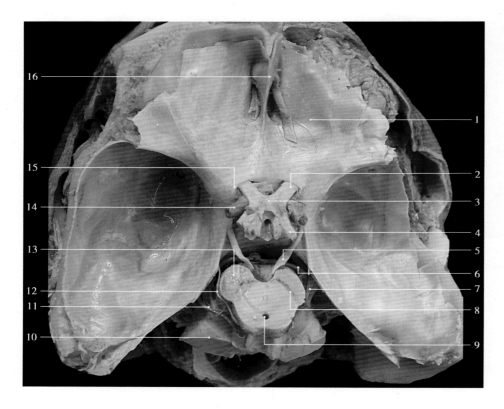

◀ 图1-243　颅中窝结构上面观
Fig. 1-243　Superior aspect of the structures in the middle cranial fossa

1. 眶板 orbital plate
2. 视神经 optic nerve
3. 视交叉 optic chiasma
4. 视束 optic tract
5. 动眼神经 oculomotor nerve
6. 大脑后动脉 posterior cerebral artery
7. 三叉神经 trigeminal nerve
8. 黑质 substantia nigra
9. 中脑导水管 mesencephalic aqueduct
10. 小脑上脚 superior cerebellar peduncle
11. 小脑上动脉 superior cerebellar artery
12. 滑车神经 trochlear nerve
13. 大脑脚 cerebral peduncle
14. 颈内动脉 internal carotid artery
15. 前床突 anterior clinoid process
16. 鸡冠 crista galli

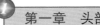

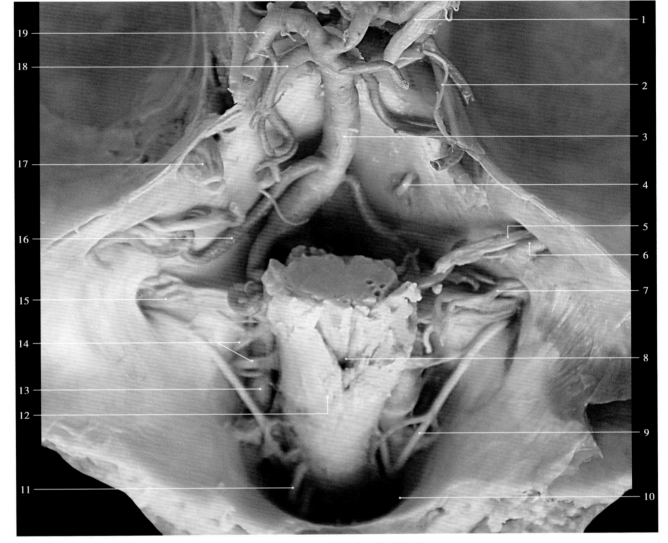

▲ 图 1-244　颅后窝结构后面观

Fig. 1-244　Posterior aspect of the structures in the posterior cranial fossa

1. 动眼神经 oculomotor nerve
2. 滑车神经 trochlear nerve
3. 基底动脉 basilar artery
4. 展神经 abducent nerve
5. 面神经 facial nerve
6. 前庭蜗神经 vestibulocochlear nerve
7. 舌咽神经 glossopharyngeal nerve
8. 菱形窝 rhomboid fossa
9. 副神经 accessory nerve
10. 枕骨大孔 foramen magnum of occipital bone
11. 第 1 脊神经 the 1st spinal nerve
12. 薄束结节 gracile tubercle
13. 椎动脉 vertebral artery
14. 舌下神经 hypoglossal nerve
15. 迷走神经 vagus nerve
16. 小脑下前动脉 anterior inferior cerebellar artery
17. 三叉神经 trigeminal nerve
18. 小脑上动脉 superior cerebellar artery
19. 大脑后动脉 posterior cerebral artery

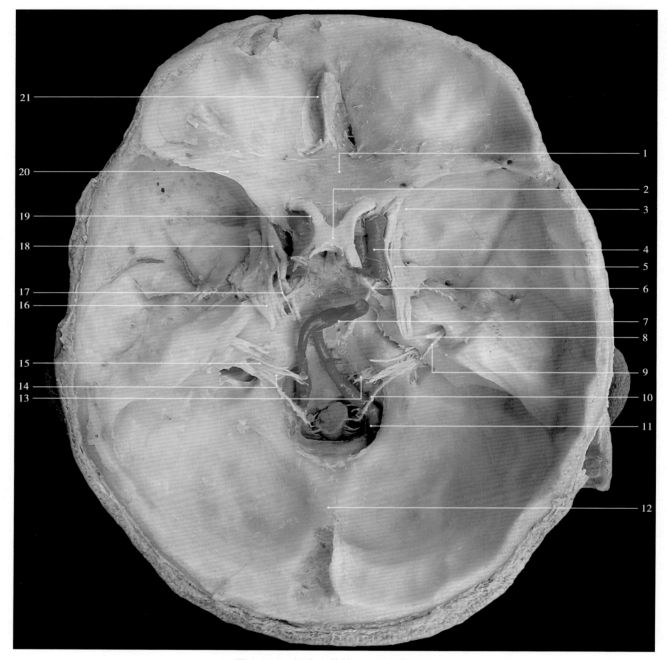

▲ 图 1-245　颅底血管神经（硬脑膜已去除）

Fig. 1-245　Vessels and nerves of the skull base (the dura mater was removed)

1. 眶板 orbital plate
2. 视交叉 optic chiasma
3. 筛板 cribriform plate
4. 颈内动脉海绵窦部 cavernous part of internal carotid artery
5. 上颌神经 maxillary nerve
6. 展神经 abducent nerve
7. 基底动脉 basilar artery
8. 面神经 facial nerve
9. 前庭蜗神经 vestibulocochlear nerve
10. 副神经 accessory nerve
11. 椎动脉 vertebral artery

12. 枕内隆嵴 internal occipital protuberance
13. 舌下神经 hypoglossal nerve
14. 迷走神经 vagus nerve
15. 舌咽神经 glossopharyngeal nerve
16. 三叉神经 trigeminal nerve
17. 滑车神经 trochlear nerve
18. 动眼神经 oculomotor nerve
19. 视神经 optic nerve
20. 蝶骨小翼 small wing of sphenoid bone
21. 鸡冠 crista galli

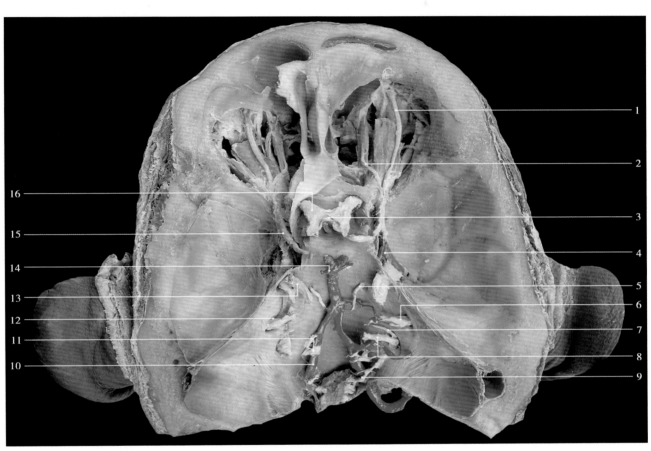

▲ 图 1-246 颅底血管神经(眶板已打开)

Fig. 1-246 Vessels and nerves of the skull base (the orbital plate was opened)

1. 额神经 frontal nerve
2. 滑车神经 trochlear nerve
3. 视交叉 optic chiasma
4. 三叉神经节 trigeminal ganglion
5. 展神经 abducent nerve
6. 前庭蜗神经 vestibulocochlear nerve
7. 舌咽神经 glossopharyngeal nerve
8. 迷走神经 vagus nerve
9. 副神经 accessory nerve
10. 椎动脉 vertebral artery
11. 舌下神经 hypoglossal nerve
12. 面神经 facial nerve
13. 三叉神经 trigeminal nerve
14. 基底动脉 basilar artery
15. 动眼神经 oculomotor nerve
16. 视神经 optic nerve

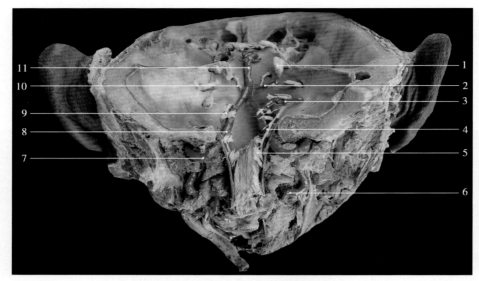

▲ 图 1-247　椎动脉和基底动脉
Fig. 1-247　Vertebral artery and basilar artery

1. 三叉神经 trigeminal nerve
2. 迷路动脉 labyrinthine artery
3. 小脑下前动脉 anterior inferior cerebellar artery
4. 副神经 accessory nerve
5. 第1脊神经后根 posterior root of the 1st spinal nerve
6. 椎动脉横突部 transverse part of vertebral artery

7. 椎动脉寰椎部 atlantic part of vertebral artery
8. 椎动脉颅内部 intracranial part of vertebral artery
9. 舌下神经 hypoglossal nerve
10. 展神经 abducent nerve
11. 基底动脉 basilar artery

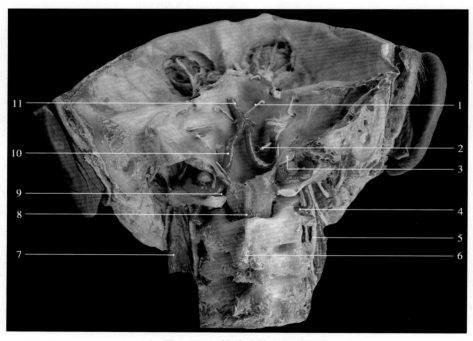

▲ 图 1-248　椎动脉颅内部后面观
Fig. 1-248　Posterior aspect of the intracranial part of vertebral artery

1. 展神经 abducent nerve
2. 舌下神经 hypoglossal nerve
3. 枕骨髁 occipital condyle
4. 椎动脉 vertebral artery
5. 迷走神经 vagus nerve
6. 枢椎棘突 spinous process of axis

7. 颈内静脉 internal jugular vein
8. 硬脊膜 spinal dura mater
9. 枕骨大孔 foramen magnum of occipital bone
10. 椎动脉颅内部 intracranial part of vertebral artery
11. 基底动脉 basilar artery

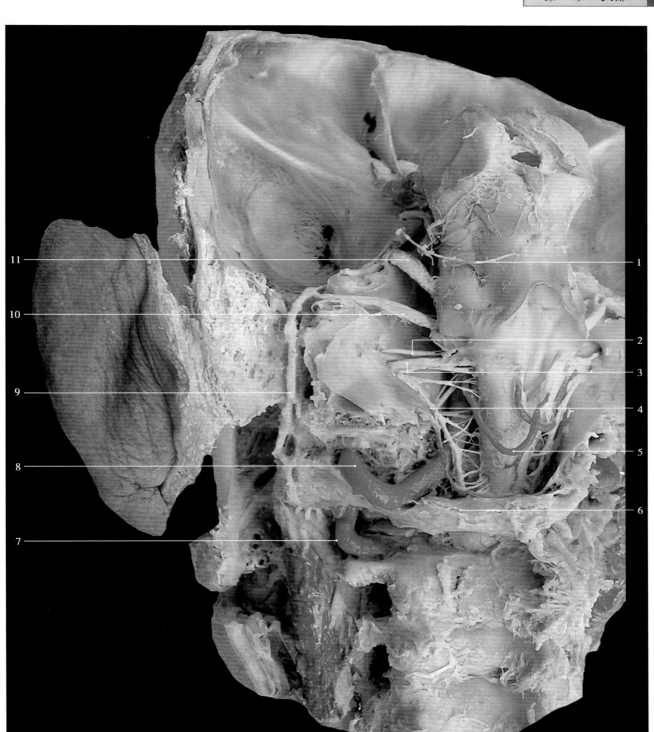

▲ 图 1-249 椎动脉寰椎部
Fig. 1-249 Atlantic part of the vertebral artery

1. 滑车神经 trochlear nerve
2. 舌咽神经 glossopharyngeal nerve
3. 迷走神经 vagus nerve
4. 副神经 accessory nerve
5. 小脑下后动脉 posterior inferior cerebellar artery
6. 寰椎后结节 posterior tubercle of atlas
7. 椎动脉 vertebral artery
8. 椎动脉寰椎部 atlantic part of vertebral artery
9. 面神经 facial nerve
10. 前庭蜗神经 vestibulocochlear nerve
11. 三叉神经 trigeminal nerve

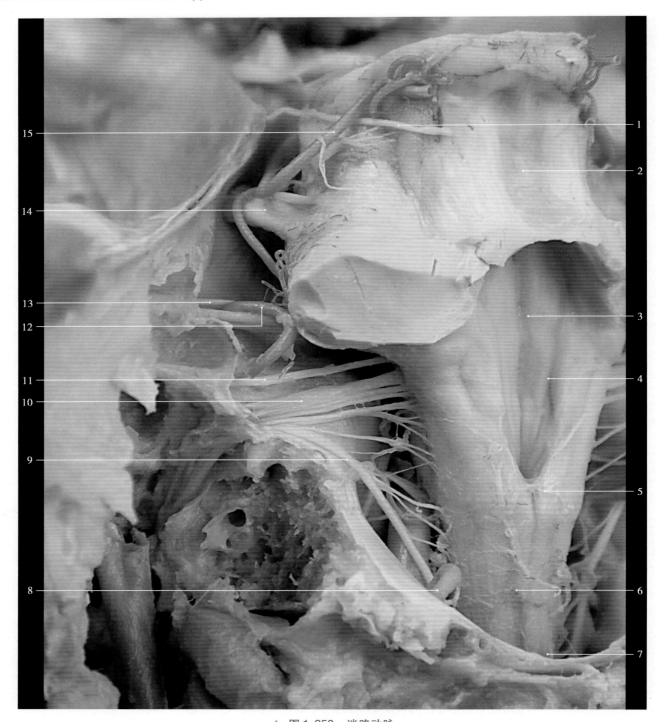

▲ 图 1-250　迷路动脉
Fig. 1-250　Labyrinthine artery

1. 滑车神经 trochlear nerve
2. 上髓帆 superior medullary velum
3. 菱形窝 rhomboid fossa
4. 界沟 terminal sulcus
5. 薄束结节 gracile tubercle
6. 延髓 medulla oblongata
7. 枕骨大孔 foramen magnum of occipital bone
8. 小脑下后动脉 posterior inferior cerebellar artery

9. 副神经 accessory nerve
10. 迷走神经 vagus nerve
11. 舌咽神经 glossopharyngeal nerve
12. 迷路动脉 labyrinthine artery
13. 面神经 facial nerve
14. 三叉神经 trigeminal nerve
15. 小脑上动脉 superior cerebellar artery

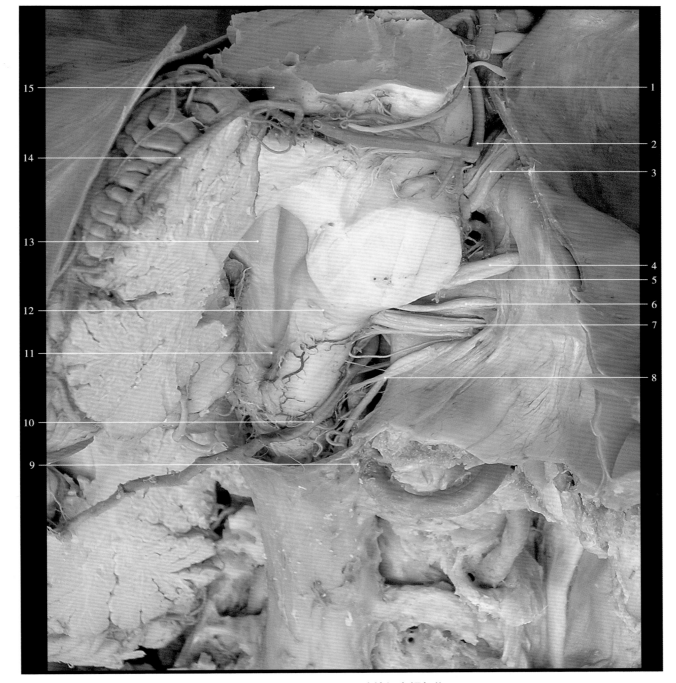

▲ 图 1-251 V、Ⅶ-Ⅺ脑神经出颅部位

Fig. 1-251 Sites of the cranial nerve Ⅴ, Ⅶ-Ⅺ departing from the cranium

1. 滑车神经 trochlear nerve
2. 小脑上动脉 superior cerebellar artery
3. 三叉神经 trigeminal nerve
4. 面神经 facial nerve
5. 前庭蜗神经 vestibulocochlear nerve
6. 舌咽神经 glossopharyngeal nerve
7. 迷走神经 vagus nerve
8. 副神经 accessory nerve
9. 枕骨大孔 foramen magnum of occipital bone
10. 小脑下后动脉 posterior inferior cerebellar artery
11. 闩 obex
12. 前庭区 vestibular area
13. 第四脑室 fourth ventricle
14. 蚓支 vermian branch
15. 下丘 inferior colliculus

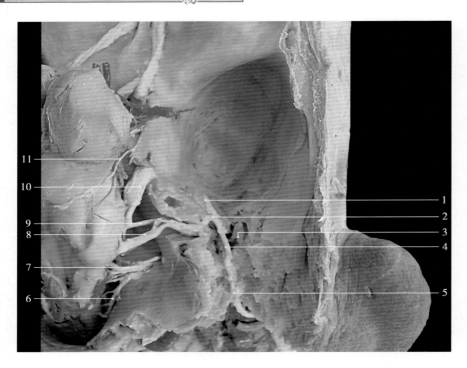

◀ 图 1-252　面神经鼓窦后段
Fig. 1-252　Posterior segment of the facial nerve in the tympanic sinus

1. 岩大神经 greater petrosal nerve
2. 面神经膝 genu of facial nerve
3. 砧骨 incus
4. 面神经鼓窦后段 posterior segment of facial nerve in tympanic sinus
5. 面神经管内段 internal segment of facial canal
6. 副神经 accessory nerve
7. 迷走神经 vagus nerve
8. 前庭蜗神经 vestibulocochlear nerve
9. 面神经 facial nerve
10. 三叉神经 trigeminal nerve
11. 滑车神经 trochlear nerve

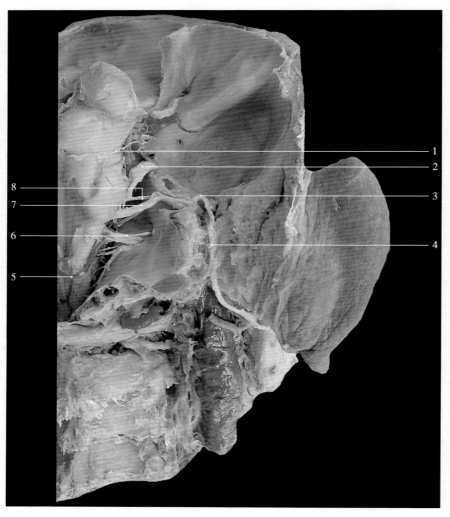

◀ 图 1-253　面神经膝
Fig. 1-253　Genu of the facial nerve

1. 滑车神经 trochlear nerve
2. 三叉神经 trigeminal nerve
3. 面神经膝 genu of facial nerve
4. 面神经管内段 internal segment of facial canal
5. 小脑下后动脉 posterior inferior cerebellar artery
6. 迷走神经 vagus nerve
7. 前庭蜗神经 vestibulocochlear nerve
8. 面神经 facial nerve

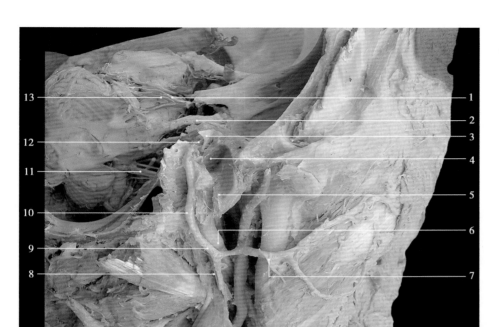

图 1-254 面神经鼓窦后段右侧面观
Fig. 1-254 Right aspect of the posterior segment of the facial nerve in the tympanic sinus

1. 滑车神经 trochlear nerve
2. 三叉神经 trigeminal nerve
3. 锤骨 malleus
4. 鼓膜 tympanic membrane
5. 外耳道 external acoustic meatus
6. 茎突 styloid process
7. 腮腺内丛 intraparotid plexus
8. 颈支 cervical branch
9. 面神经 facial nerve
10. 面神经鼓窦后段 posterior segment of facial nerve in tympanic sinus
11. 迷走神经 vagus nerve
12. 鼓室 tympanic cavity
13. 小脑上动脉 superior cerebellar artery

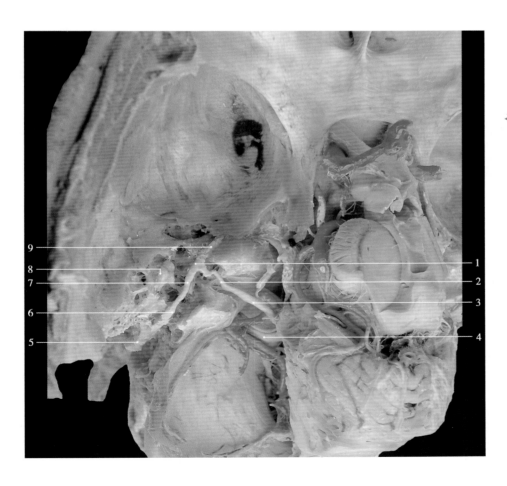

图 1-255 左侧面神经颅内段和管内段上面观
Fig. 1-255 Superior aspect of the intracranial and intraductal segment of the left facial nerve

1. 面神经膝 genu of facial nerve
2. 面神经内耳道段 internal auditory canal segment of facial nerve
3. 面神经颅内段 intracranial segment of facial nerve
4. 迷走神经 vagus nerve
5. 面神经降段 descending segment of facial nerve
6. 面神经水平段 horizontal segment of facial nerve
7. 面神经鼓室段 tympanic segment of facial nerve
8. 砧骨 incus
9. 岩大神经 greater petrosal nerve

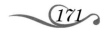

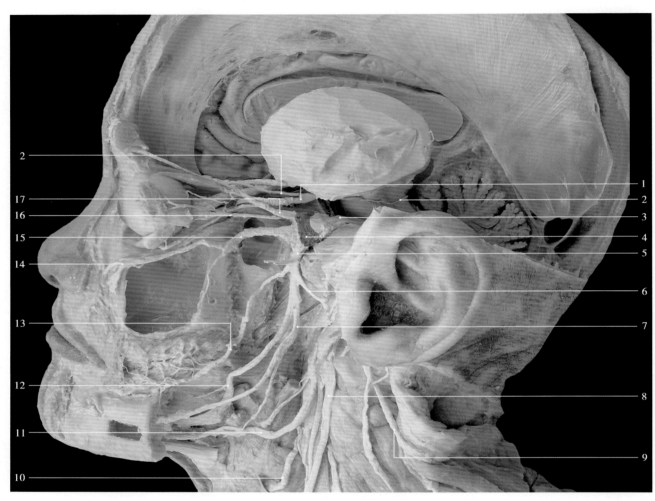

▲ 图 1-256 脑神经
Fig. 1-256 Cranial nerves

1. 动眼神经 oculomotor nerve
2. 滑车神经 trochlear nerve
3. 三叉神经 trigeminal nerve
4. 三叉神经节 trigeminal ganglion
5. 下颌神经 mandibular nerve
6. 耳颞神经 auriculotemporal nerve
7. 下牙槽神经 inferior alveolar nerve
8. 迷走神经 vagus nerve
9. 副神经 accessory nerve

10. 喉上神经内支 internal branch of superior laryngeal nerve
11. 舌下神经 hypoglossal nerve
12. 舌神经 lingual nerve
13. 颊神经 buccal nerve
14. 眶下神经 infraorbital nerve
15. 上颌神经 maxillary nerve
16. 展神经 abducent nerve
17. 眼神经 ophthalmic nerve

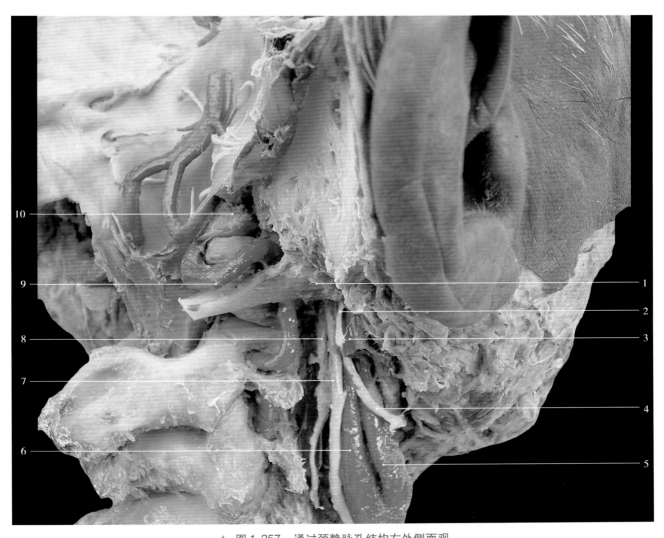

▲ 图 1-257　通过颈静脉孔结构右外侧面观

Fig. 1-257　Right aspect of the structures through the jugular foramen

1. 寰椎横突 transverse process of atlas
2. 副神经 accessory nerve
3. 颈内静脉 internal jugular vein
4. 舌下神经 hypoglossal nerve
5. 颈外动脉 external carotid artery
6. 颈内动脉 internal carotid artery
7. 迷走神经 vagus nerve
8. 颈上神经节 superior cervical ganglion
9. 椎动脉寰椎部 atlantic part of vertebral artery
10. 枕骨髁 occipital condyle

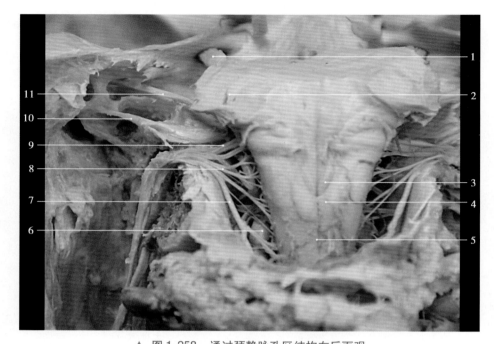

▲ 图 1-258　通过颈静脉孔区结构左后面观

Fig. 1-258　Left posterior aspect of the structures through the jugular foramen

1. 三叉神经 trigeminal nerve
2. 小脑中脚 middle cerebellar peduncle
3. 舌下神经三角 hypoglossal triangle
4. 薄束结节 gracile tubercle
5. 延髓 medulla oblongata
6. 椎动脉 vertebral artery
7. 副神经 accessory nerve
8. 迷走神经 vagus nerve
9. 舌咽神经 glossopharyngeal nerve
10. 中脑导水管 mesencephalic aqueduct
11. 面神经 facial nerve

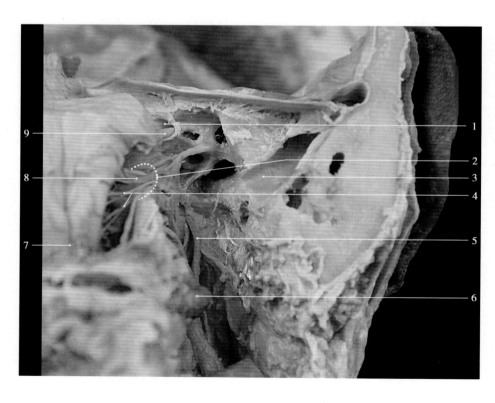

◀ 图 1-259　通过颈静脉孔区结构右后面观

Fig. 1-259　Right posterior aspect of the structures through the jugular foramen

1. 内耳门 internal acoustic pore
2. 颈静脉孔（虚线内区域）jugular foramen（area in dashed line）
3. 乙状窦沟 sigmoid sulcus
4. 迷走神经 vagus nerve
5. 副神经 accessory nerve
6. 椎动脉寰椎部 atlantic part of vertebral artery
7. 延髓 medulla oblongata
8. 舌咽神经 glossopharyngeal nerve
9. 前庭蜗神经 vestibulocochlear nerve

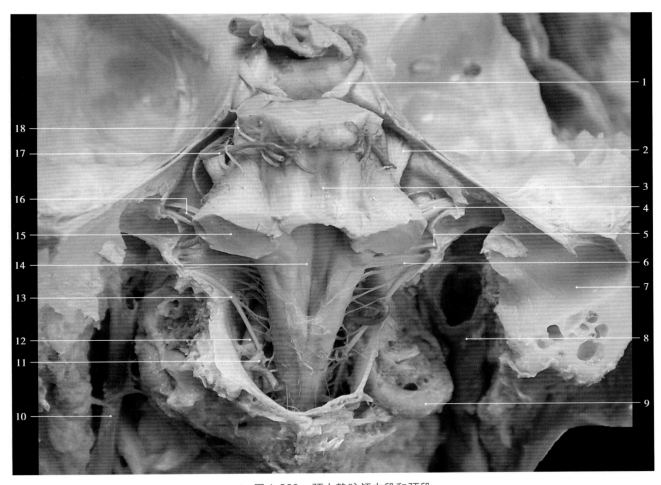

▲ 图 1-260　颈内静脉颅内段和颈段

Fig. 1-260　Intracranial and cervical part of the internal jugular vein

1. 动眼神经 oculomotor nerve
2. 三叉神经 trigeminal nerve
3. 上髓帆 superior medullary velum
4. 前庭蜗神经 vestibulocochlear nerve
5. 舌咽神经 glossopharyngeal nerve
6. 迷走神经 vagus nerve
7. 乙状窦 sigmoid sinus
8. 颈内静脉颅内段 intracranial part of internal jugular vein
9. 椎动脉寰椎部 atlantic part of vertebral artery
10. 颈内静脉颈段 cervical part of internal jugular vein
11. 小脑下后动脉 posterior inferior cerebellar artery
12. 椎动脉 vertebral artery
13. 副神经 accessory nerve
14. 内侧隆起 medial eminence
15. 小脑中脚 middle cerebellar peduncle
16. 迷路动脉 labyrinthine artery
17. 小脑上动脉 superior cerebellar artery
18. 滑车神经 trochlear nerve

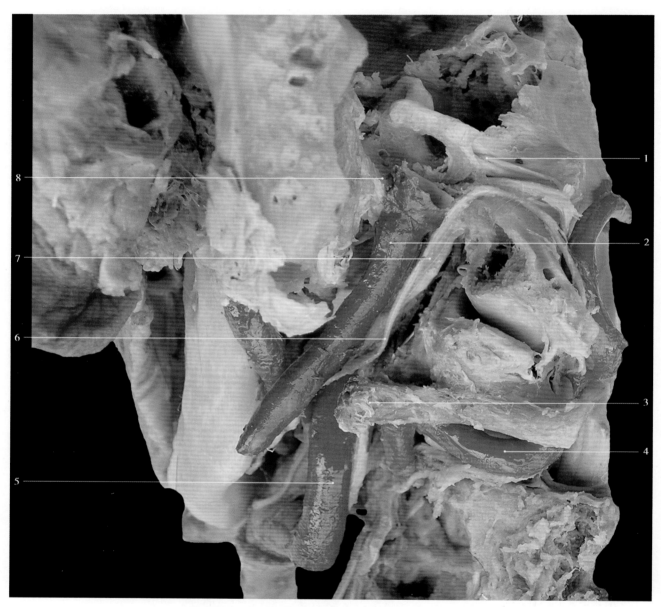

▲ 图 1-261　经过颈静脉孔前内侧的神经（椎动脉行程变异）
Fig. 1-261　Anteromedial nerves through the jugular foramen（with variant course of the vertebral artery）

1. 舌咽神经 glossopharyngeal nerve
2. 颈内静脉 internal jugular vein
3. 寰椎横突 transverse process of atlas
4. 椎动脉 vertebral artery
5. 颈内动脉 internal carotid artery
6. 副神经 accessory nerve
7. 迷走神经 vagus nerve
8. 颈静脉孔 jugular foramen

颈静脉孔区的应用解剖学要点

颅底外面可见颞骨岩部的后外侧有颈动脉管外口。颈动脉管外口的后外侧有颈静脉窝,窝的内侧有颈静脉孔。颈静脉孔前部通过的结构有岩下窦、咽升动脉的脑膜支;中部通过的结构有舌咽神经、迷走神经和副神经;后部有颈内静脉、枕动脉的脑膜支、迷走神经的脑膜支及淋巴管通过。颈静脉孔内外径右侧比左侧大者为60%,左侧比右侧大者为39%;前后径右侧比左侧大者为69%,左侧比右侧大者为31%。颈静脉孔骨间桥出现率为46%,其中14%为连续型骨间桥,其余32%为非连续型骨间桥。

颈静脉孔右侧的内外径为(14.47±2.52)mm,前后径为(8.80±1.63)mm,深度为(13.79±3.67)mm,颈静脉窝有顶者为56%,无顶者为44%;左侧的内外径为(13.90±2.44)mm,前后径为(7.90±2.01)mm,深度为(12.28±2.41)mm,颈静脉窝有顶者为48%,无顶者为52%。颈静脉窝无顶者其颈静脉球的顶部直接与颅底的硬膜相邻。

颈静脉孔与周边结构的解剖关系:孔的后外方为颞骨的乳突,乳突尖与颈静脉孔的后外缘的间距左侧为(23.47±2.65)mm,右侧为(22.84±2.88)mm;孔的外侧为茎突,茎突根部与孔的外缘间距左侧为(5.48±1.33)mm,右侧为(5.00±2.88)mm;茎突根部的后外方为茎乳孔,茎乳孔与颈静脉孔外缘的间距左侧为(7.44±1.36)mm,右侧为(6.78±1.61)mm。颈静脉孔内侧为枕骨大孔前外方,有一呈肾形突起的枕骨髁,髁后端外侧常有导静脉孔。髁的前后长度左侧为(22.67±2.41)mm,右侧为(22.80±2.35)mm;中点处宽度左侧为(12.07±1.49)mm,右侧为(12.17±1.53)mm;髁中点外侧缘与舌下神经管外口的直线间距左侧为(6.78±1.51)mm,右侧为(6.72±1.49)mm;髁中点内侧缘距舌下神经管内口下缘的间距左侧为(10.40±1.75)mm,右侧为(10.32±2.00)mm。颈静脉孔外口前缘与颈动脉管外口后缘的间距左侧为(3.64±1.19)mm,右侧为(3.62±1.43)mm。(图1-257~图1-261)。

应用解剖要点:

颈静脉孔区的肿瘤可出现在孔的外侧或内侧,也可沿颈静脉壁的外侧或内侧自颅后窝经孔延伸至颅底的外面。神经外科根据肿瘤与颈静脉的位置关系,其手术入路常可分为外侧或远外侧入路和内侧入路。

1. 远外侧入路 皮肤切口:自枕外隆凸水平向耳后横行切开,再沿耳郭纵行切至乳突尖,将皮片翻向内下方。再依次经过皮下组织、斜方肌、胸锁乳突肌(注意保护胸锁乳突肌后缘的枕小神经)、夹肌、半棘肌、头上斜肌。注意事项:切除寰椎横突时防止伤及椎动脉,磨除颈静脉孔外侧部的颅底骨质时注意不能太深以免进入中耳腔底和伤及面神经。如肿瘤沿颈内静脉球体外侧延伸至颈静脉孔的外侧,可将孔外侧与乳突间骨质磨除,在磨除外侧的骨质时要防止伤及面神经和鼓索。

2. 内侧入路 皮肤切口:至颅底同远外侧入路。如切除肿瘤需要,可磨除颈静脉内侧枕骨髁的后部。枕骨髁后部至舌下神经管外口的间距左侧为(11.09±2.75)mm,右侧为(14.39±1.85)mm;舌下神经管外口前缘至枕骨髁外缘的间距左侧为(14.46±1.24)mm,右侧为(11.41±1.91)mm。在磨除枕骨髁时要防止伤及横过髁中部深面的舌下神经。

3. 颈静脉孔前缘或前上缘的肿瘤,可采用经口至咽磨开枕骨基底部的咽结节达颅后窝,向外下方可磨除舌下神经管内口上方的颈静脉结节,结节的后外侧即为颈静脉窝的前上部。颈静脉结节的顶部距舌下神经管内口上方的距离左侧为(8.99±1.79)mm,右侧为(8.50±1.56)mm;此距离即为颈静脉结节可磨除的厚度,5mm以内可防止伤及横过结节深部的舌下神经。

第九节　颞骨相关结构

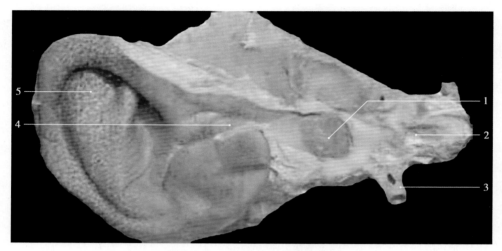

▲ 图 1-262　外耳、外耳道和鼓膜（右）
Fig. 1-262　External ear, external acoustic meatus and tympanic membrane (right)

1. 鼓膜 tympanic membrane
2. 岩尖 petrous apex
3. 颈内动脉 internal carotid artery
4. 外耳道 external acoustic meatus
5. 耳郭 auricle

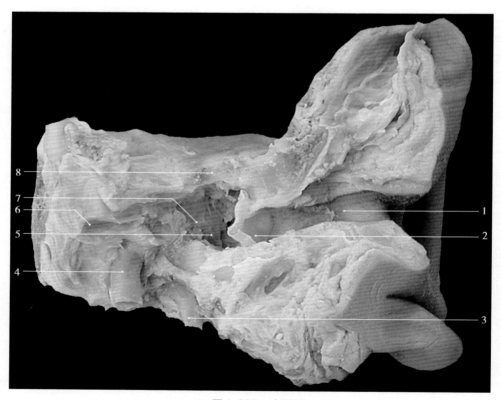

▲ 图 1-263　中耳腔
Fig. 1-263　Middle ear cavity

1. 外耳道 external acoustic meatus
2. 鼓膜 tympanic membrane
3. 颈内静脉 internal jugular vein
4. 颈内动脉 internal carotid artery
5. 中耳腔 middle ear cavity
6. 咽鼓管 auditory tube
7. 岬 promontory
8. 鼓室盖壁 tegmental wall of tympanic cavity

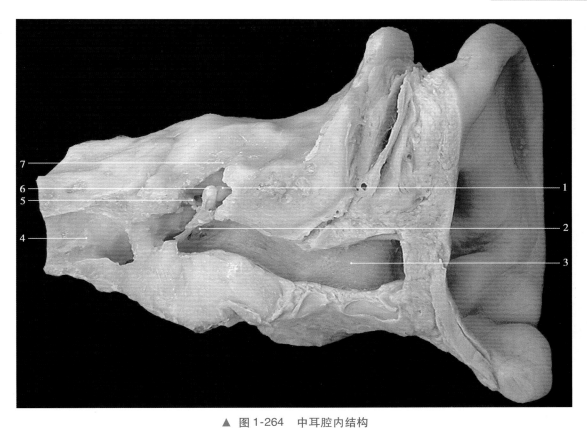

▲ 图 1-264 中耳腔内结构

Fig. 1-264 Internal structures of the middle ear cavity

1. 砧骨 incus
2. 鼓膜 tympanic membrane
3. 外耳道 external acoustic meatus
4. 颈动脉管 carotid canal
5. 镫骨 stapes
6. 锤骨 malleus
7. 盖壁 tegmental wall

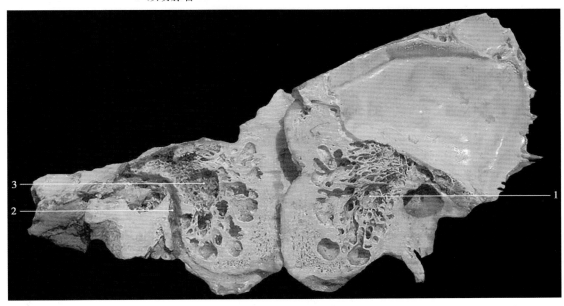

▲ 图 1-265 颞骨内部结构(沿岩部作冠状切开)

Fig. 1-265 Internal structures of the temporal bone (coronal sectioning along the petrosal part)

1. 乳突小房 mastoid cells
2. 面神经管 facial canal
3. 乳突窦 mastoid antrum

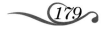

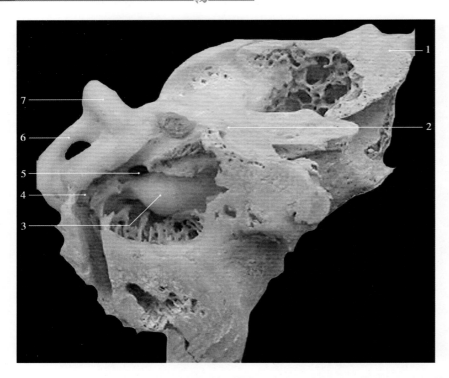

◀ 图 1-266　鼓室内侧壁结构
Fig. 1-266　Structures of the medial wall of the tympanic cavity

1. 岩尖 petrous apex
2. 岩部 petrosal part
3. 鼓室岬 promontory
4. 面神经管 facial canal
5. 前庭窗 fenestra vestibuli
6. 外骨半规管 lateral semicircular canal
7. 前骨半规管 anterior semicircular canal

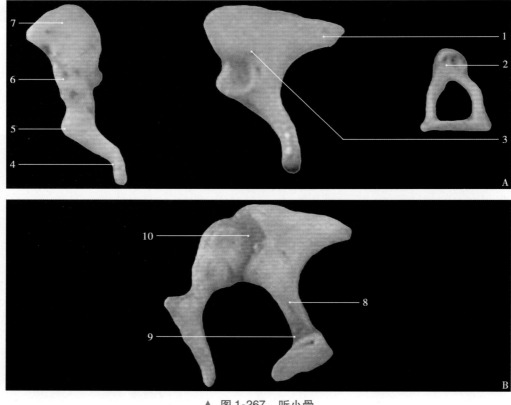

▲ 图 1-267　听小骨
Fig. 1-267　Auditory ossicles

1. 短脚 short crus
2. 镫骨头 head of stapes
3. 砧骨体 body of incus
4. 锤骨柄 manubrium of malleus
5. 前突 anterior process
6. 锤骨颈 neck of malleus
7. 锤骨头 head of malleus
8. 长脚 long crus
9. 砧镫关节 incudostapedial joint
10. 砧锤关节 incudomalleolar joint

鼓室的应用解剖学要点

鼓室是中耳的组成部分,居于颞骨岩部,是位于鼓膜与内耳之间的不规则的含气空腔,容积约 1 ~ 2ml,前方借咽鼓管与咽相通,后方借鼓室窦与乳突小房通连。鼓室可分为上、下、前、后、内、外六壁(图 1-264 ~ 图 1-267)。

1. 上壁 即鼓室的顶,由颞骨岩部的鼓室盖构成,将鼓室与颅中窝隔开。

2. 下壁 即鼓室的底,也称颈静脉壁,将鼓室和颈静脉(上)球分隔开。

3. 前壁 颈动脉壁,由颈动脉管的后外壁形成,前壁上部有鼓膜张肌半管和咽鼓管的开口。咽鼓管鼓室口与鼓室后壁的鼓室窦口相对,并在一个水平。

4. 外侧壁 由骨部和膜部构成。骨部即鼓室的外侧壁,位于骨性外耳道上壁水平之上,由颞骨鳞部外板构成。膜部即鼓膜。

5. 后壁 又称乳突壁。后壁与上壁交界处有鼓窦开口,鼓室经鼓窦口与乳突小房相通。

6. 内壁 又称迷路壁,由内耳骨迷路的外侧壁构成,内壁上有如下结构:①鼓岬;②前庭窗(卵圆窗);③蜗窗(圆窗);④面神经管凸。

应用解剖要点:

1. 鼓室上壁厚度约 3 ~ 4mm,有的菲薄如纸。在小儿(2 岁以前)位于此壁上的岩鳞裂由于骨化不全可未闭,则鼓室黏膜与硬脑膜相贴;在成人也偶有未闭者,鼓室的静脉通过此裂注入岩上窦。幼儿的咽鼓管较成人的短而平,腔径相对较大,流质食物(如乳汁)易从咽鼓管流入中耳,咽部的感染也易沿此管进入鼓室,诱发化脓性感染称中耳炎。发生化脓性中耳炎时,鼓室内的脓液可穿透鼓膜经外耳道流出;向后经乳突窦蔓延至乳突小房造成乳突炎;脓液向上可穿破鼓室盖(上壁)侵入颅内,造成耳源性脑脓肿。

2. 下壁的厚度与颈静脉球的大小有关,通常约 10mm,下壁一般为一薄板,有的此壁尚未骨化,仅借黏膜与纤维组织分隔,因而颈静脉球的蓝色透过鼓膜下隐约可见。有异常的高位颈静脉球经鼓室下壁裂隙突入鼓室,从而影响听骨链的正常活动,故在中耳手术时应注意这种先天性异常,以免损伤颈静脉球造成大量出血。

3. 前壁下部以极薄的骨板与颈内动脉相隔,骨板厚度不到 0.5mm,裂隙的出现率为 1%,鼓室内颈内动脉畸形患者多有听力下降、搏动性耳鸣和眩晕。

4. 乳突壁上的鼓窦入口底部有砧骨窝,容纳砧骨短突,此窝恰在面神经水平段与垂直段交界处的外侧,为中耳手术的重要标志之一。

5. 迷路壁上的面神经管的后上方有外半规管隆凸,它的骨质比较平滑而坚硬,其与面神经水平段之间的距离为 0.5 ~ 1.5mm。故也是寻找面神经的重要标志。

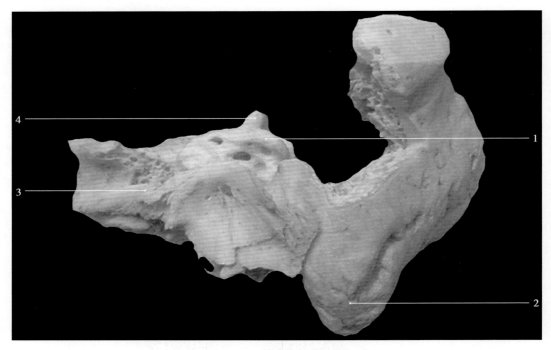

▲ 图 1-268　骨迷路位置外侧面观

Fig. 1-268　Lateral aspect of the position of the bony labyrinth

1. 外骨半规管 lateral semicircular canal　　3. 岩部 petrous part
2. 乳突 mastoid process　　　　　　　　　4. 前骨半规管 anterior semicircular canal

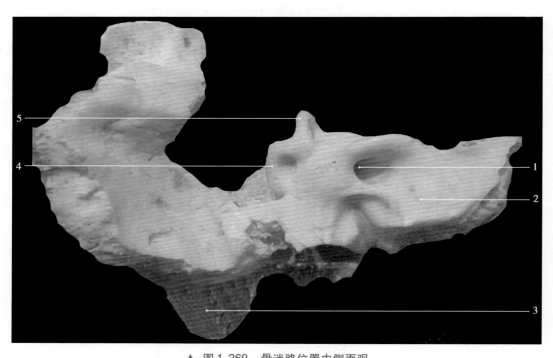

▲ 图 1-269　骨迷路位置内侧面观

Fig. 1-269　Medial aspect of the position of the bony labyrinth

1. 内耳门 internal acoustic pore　　　4. 后骨半规管 posterior semicircular canal
2. 岩部 petrous part　　　　　　　　5. 前骨半规管 anterior semicircular canal
3. 乳突 mastoid process

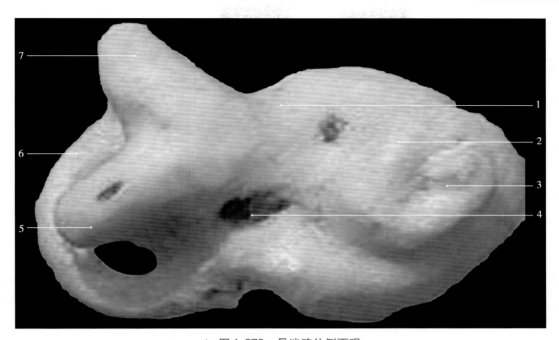

▲ 图 1-270 骨迷路外侧面观

Fig. 1-270 Lateral aspect of the bony labyrinth

1. 前庭 vestibule
2. 耳蜗 cochlea
3. 蜗顶 cupula of cochlea
4. 前庭窗 fenestra vestibuli
5. 后骨半规管 posterior semicircular canal
6. 外骨半规管 lateral semicircular canal
7. 前骨半规管 anterior semicircular canal

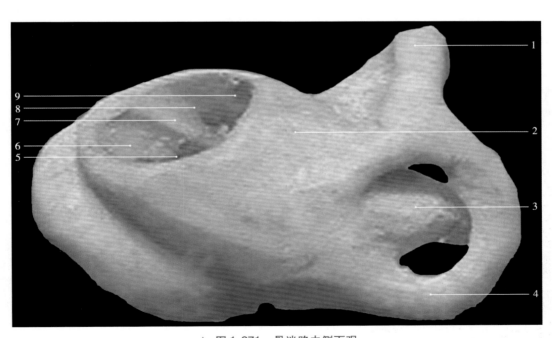

▲ 图 1-271 骨迷路内侧面观

Fig. 1-271 Medial aspect of the bony labyrinth

1. 前骨半规管 anterior semicircular canal
2. 前庭 vestibule
3. 外骨半规管 lateral semicircular canal
4. 后骨半规管 posterior semicircular canal
5. 前庭下区 inferior vestibular area
6. 蜗区 cochlear area
7. 横嵴 transverse crest
8. 面神经区 area of facial nerve
9. 前庭上区 superior vestibular area of fundus of internal acoustic meatus

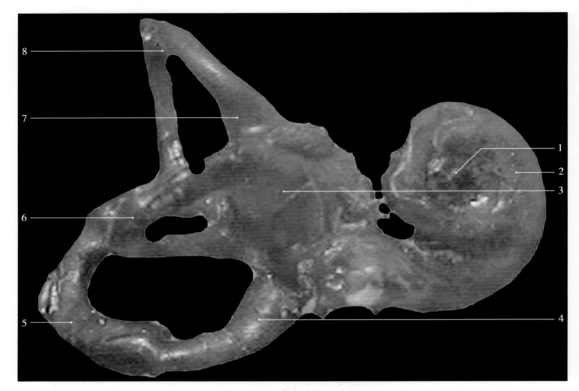

▲ 图 1-272 膜迷路铸型内侧面观

Fig. 1-272 Medial aspect of the cast of the membranous labyrinth

1. 蜗顶 cupula of cochlea
2. 蜗管 cochlear duct
3. 椭圆囊 utricle
4. 后膜壶腹 posterior membranous ampulla

5. 后膜半规管 posterior semicircular duct
6. 外膜半规管 lateral semicircular duct
7. 前膜壶腹 anterior membranous ampulla
8. 前膜半规管 anterior semicircular duct

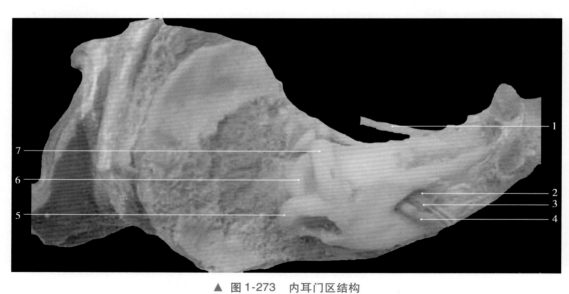

▲ 图 1-273 内耳门区结构

Fig. 1-273 Structures around the internal acoustic pore

1. 三叉神经 trigeminal nerve
2. 内耳门 internal acoustic pore
3. 面神经 facial nerve
4. 前庭蜗神经 vestibulocochlear nerve

5. 后骨半规管 posterior semicircular canal
6. 外骨半规管 lateral semicircular canal
7. 前骨半规管 anterior semicircular canal

内耳的应用解剖学要点

内耳位于颞骨岩部,由一系列复杂的管腔组成,故又称迷路,迷路可分为骨迷路和膜迷路。骨迷路是骨性管道,膜迷路为膜性管道。膜迷路是套在骨性管道内的膜性管道和囊。骨迷路与膜迷路之间的间隙内含有外淋巴,膜迷路内含有内淋巴,内、外淋巴之间互不相通。听觉和位置觉感受器位于膜迷路内(图1-268～1-273)。

(一) 骨迷路

1. 骨半规管　前骨半规管、后骨半规管和外骨半规管,每个骨半规管均有两脚,其中一个膨大称壶腹,前后骨半规管的两个脚合成一个脚,因此骨半规管共有五个脚连于前庭。

2. 前庭　前庭的外侧壁上有前庭窗和蜗窗。

3. 耳蜗　呈底朝内、顶朝外的蜗牛形。由蜗管绕蜗轴转约2.5圈而成。

(二) 膜迷路

包括膜半规管、椭圆囊、球囊和蜗管。每个骨壶腹内有一个膨大的膜壶腹,内有位置觉感受器。椭圆囊和球囊位于前庭内。两囊腔内有突出的椭圆囊斑和球囊斑,是头部静止位置觉感受器所在之处。蜗管的基底膜上有听觉感受器。

应用解剖要点:

前庭和半规管是人体头部空间位置感受器,参与调节人体静止及运动状态的平衡。当头的位置改变或做变速运动时,椭圆囊和球囊内的淋巴流动,同时膜半规管内的淋巴也会相应地流动,从而引起椭圆囊、球囊和壶腹嵴上毛细胞的摆动,进而转化为神经冲动,由前庭神经传入中枢,从而感知头部的位置,调节身体平衡。

各种原因引起的内淋巴循环障碍均可导致内耳功能失调,产生强烈的眩晕、耳鸣或呕吐和内耳性眩晕(梅尼埃病)。当前庭位置觉感受器受到过长、过强的刺激,或刺激并不强,但前庭功能过于敏感时,会引起恶心、呕吐、眩晕、出汗和皮肤苍白等症状,如晕船、晕车。

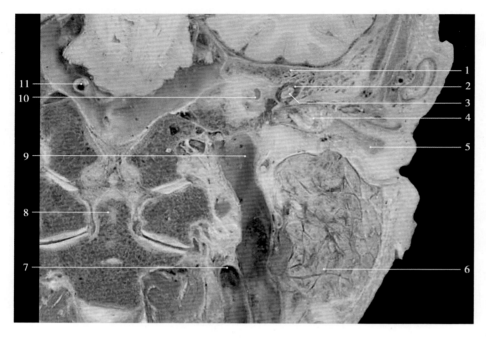

◀ 图 1-274　颞骨冠状切（示中耳腔）
Fig. 1-274　Coronary section of the temporal bone (showing the middle ear cavity)

1. 鼓室盖 tegmen tympani
2. 中耳腔 middle ear cavity
3. 砧骨 incus
4. 鼓膜 tympanic membrane
5. 外耳道 external acoustic meatus
6. 腮腺 parotid gland
7. 颈内动脉 internal carotid artery
8. 齿突 dens
9. 颈内静脉 internal jugular vein
10. 骨迷路 bony labyrinth
11. 椎动脉 vertebral artery

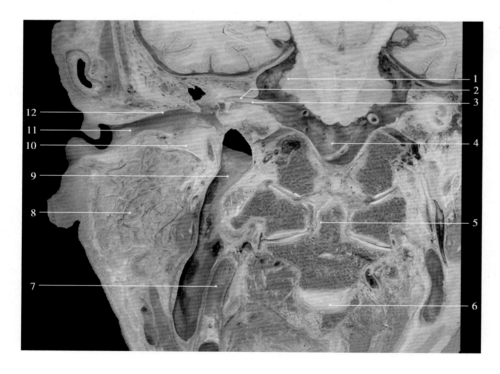

◀ 图 1-275　颞骨在体冠状切（示外耳道、内耳道）
Fig. 1-275　Coronary section of the temporal bone in situ (showing the external and internal acoustic meatus)

1. 小脑中脚 middle cerebellar peduncle
2. 内耳道 internal acoustic meatus
3. 前庭蜗神经 vestibulocochlear nerve
4. 延髓 medulla oblongata
5. 齿突 dens
6. 椎间盘 intervertebral disc
7. 颈内动脉 internal carotid artery
8. 腮腺 parotid gland
9. 颈内静脉 internal jugular vein
10. 外耳道骨部 bony auditory meatus
11. 外耳道 external acoustic meatus
12. 外耳道软骨部 cartilaginous auditory meatus

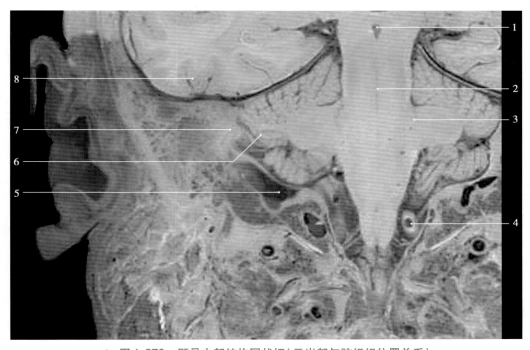

▲ 图 1-276 颞骨内部结构冠状切（示岩部与脑组织位置关系）

Fig. 1-276 Coronal plane of the internal structures of the temporal bone（showing positional relation of petrous part and brain tissue）

1. 中脑导水管 mesencephalic aqueduct
2. 脑桥 pons
3. 小脑中脚 middle cerebellar peduncle
4. 椎动脉 vertebral artery
5. 乙状窦 sigmoid sinus
6. 小脑半球 cerebellar hemisphere
7. 颞骨岩部 petrous part of temporal bone
8. 颞叶 temporal lobe

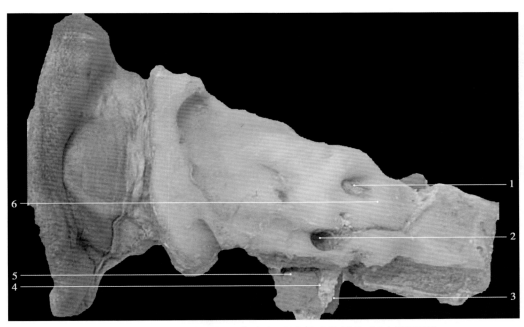

▲ 图 1-277 颞骨岩部与颈内动脉、颈内静脉位置关系（内侧面观）

Fig. 1-277 Positional relation of the petrous part of temporal bone, the internal carotid artery and the internal jugular vein（medial aspect）

1. 内耳门 internal acoustic pore
2. 颈静脉孔内口 inner debouch of jugular foramen
3. 颈内动脉颈部 cervical part of internal carotid artery
4. 迷走神经 vagus nerve
5. 颈内静脉 internal jugular vein
6. 颈内动脉岩部 petrosal part of internal carotid artery

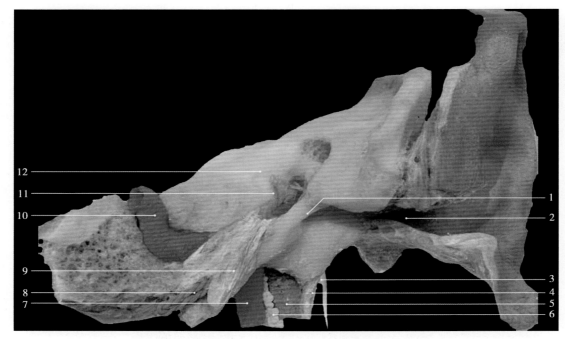

▲ 图 1-278　颞骨岩部与颈内动脉、颈内静脉位置关系（外侧面观）
Fig. 1-278　Positional relation of the petrous part of temporal bone，the internal carotid artery and the internal jugular vein（lateral aspect）

1. 鼓膜 tympanic membrane
2. 外耳道 external acoustic meatus
3. 面神经 facial nerve
4. 茎突 styloid process
5. 颈内静脉 internal jugular vein
6. 迷走神经 vagus nerve
7. 颈内动脉颈部 cervical part of internal carotid artery
8. 咽鼓管探条 bougies in auditory tube
9. 咽鼓管 pharyngotympanic tube
10. 颈内动脉岩部 petrosal part of internal carotid artery
11. 中耳腔 middle ear cavity
12. 颞骨岩部 petrous part of temporal bone

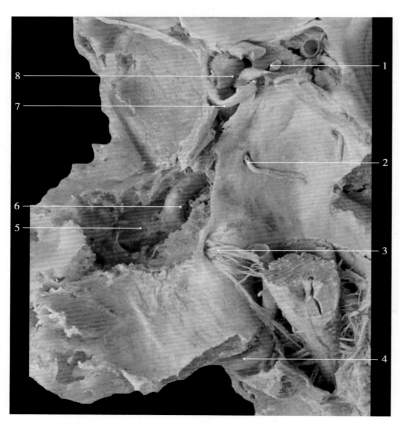

◀ 图 1-279　颞骨岩部与颈内动脉关系（示颈内动脉岩部）
Fig. 1-279　Positional relation of the petrous part of temporal bone and internal carotid artery（showing the petrosal part of internal carotid artery）

1. 垂体柄 hypophysial stalk
2. 展神经 abducent nerve
3. 迷走神经 vagus nerve
4. 椎动脉 vertebral artery
5. 乳突窦 mastoid antrum
6. 颈内动脉岩部 petrosal part of internal carotid artery
7. 动眼神经 oculomotor nerve
8. 颈内动脉海绵窦部 cavernous part of internal carotid artery

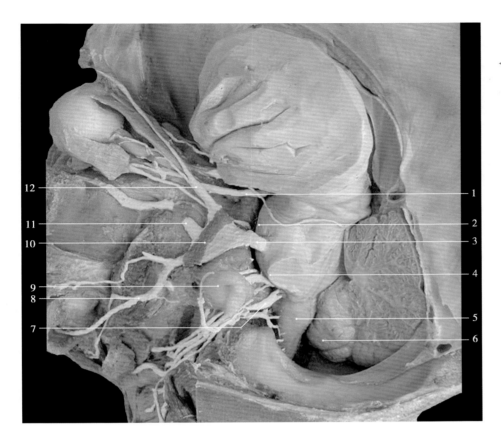

◀ 图 1-280 颞骨与脑干、脑神经的毗邻关系
Fig. 1-280 Adjacent relation of the temporal bone, brain stem and cranial nerves

1. 动眼神经 oculomotor nerve
2. 脑桥 pons
3. 三叉神经 trigeminal nerve
4. 小脑中脚 middle cerebellar peduncle
5. 延髓 medulla oblongata
6. 小脑扁桃体 tonsil of cerebellum
7. 迷走神经 vagus nerve
8. 下颌神经 submandibular nerve
9. 颞骨岩部 petrous part of temporal bone
10. 三叉神经节 trigeminal ganglion
11. 上颌神经 maxillary nerve
12. 眼神经 ophthalmic nerve

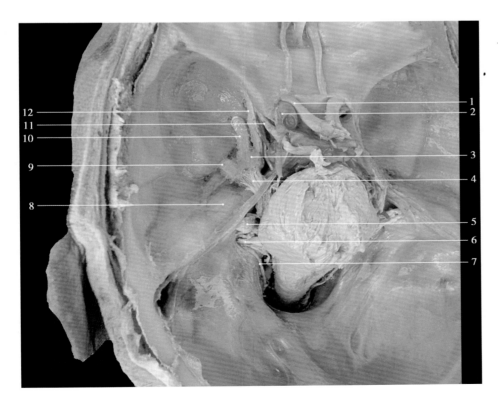

◀ 图 1-281 颞骨与脑神经的关系(左)
Fig. 1-281 Relation between the temporal bone and cranial nerves(left)

1. 视神经 optic nerve
2. 颈内动脉大脑部 cerebral part of internal carotid artery
3. 三叉神经节 trigeminal ganglion
4. 三叉神经 trigeminal nerve
5. 前庭蜗神经 vestibulocochlear nerve
6. 迷走神经 vagus nerve
7. 副神经 accessory nerve
8. 颞骨岩部 petrous part of temporal bone
9. 下颌神经 mandibular nerve
10. 上颌神经 maxillary nerve
11. 动眼神经 oculomotor nerve
12. 眼神经 ophthalmic nerve

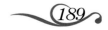

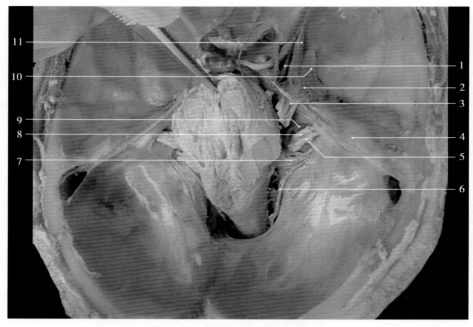

▲ 图 1-282 颞骨与脑神经的关系（右）
Fig. 1-282 Relation between the temporal bone and cranial nerves（right）

1. 展神经 abducent nerve
2. 三叉神经节 trigeminal ganglion
3. 三叉神经 trigeminal nerve
4. 颞骨岩部 petrous part of temporal bone
5. 前庭蜗神经 vestibulocochlear nerve
6. 副神经 accessory nerve
7. 迷走神经 vagus nerve
8. 面神经 facial nerve
9. 迷路动脉 labyrinthine artery
10. 上颌神经 maxillary nerve
11. 眼神经 ophthalmic nerve

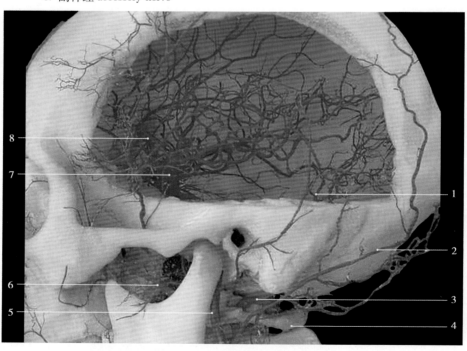

▲ 图 1-283 颅内、外动脉铸型（颅骨左壁已打开）
Fig. 1-283 Cast of the intracranial and extracranial artery（left wall of the skull was removed）

1. 大脑后动脉 posterior cerebral artery
2. 枕动脉 occipital artery
3. 椎动脉 vertebral artery
4. 寰椎 atlas
5. 颈外动脉 external carotid artery
6. 上颌动脉 maxillary artery
7. 大脑中动脉 middle cerebral artery
8. 大脑前动脉 anterior cerebral artery

第二章 颈 部

第一节 概 述

颈部位于头与胸部之间,连接头、躯干和上肢。颈部的支架是脊柱的颈段,前方有呼吸、消化道的颈段,两侧有纵行的大血管和神经,颈根部有胸膜顶和肺尖,并有通过斜角肌间隙的血管和神经。颈部诸结构之间填充有疏松结缔组织,并形成若干与临床诊治有密切关系的筋膜和筋膜间隙。

一、颈部的境界和分区

(一)境界

上界为下颌骨下缘、下颌角、乳突尖、上项线和枕外隆凸的连线;下界为胸骨的颈静脉切迹、胸锁关节、锁骨、肩峰至第 7 颈椎棘突的连线。

(二)分区

颈部以斜方肌前缘为界分为前、后两部。斜方肌前缘以前的部分称为颈前外侧部或称固有颈部。斜方肌前缘以后的部分称颈后部或项部。

颈前外侧部以二腹肌和肩胛舌骨肌上腹分成数个三角:

1. 颏下三角　位于两侧二腹肌前腹之间。

2. 下颌下三角　位于下颌骨下缘与二腹肌两腹之间。

3. 颈动脉三角　位于胸锁乳突肌前缘、二腹肌后腹与肩胛舌骨肌上腹之间。

4. 肌三角　位于肩胛舌骨肌上腹下缘、胸锁乳突肌下段前缘与前正中线之间。

5. 胸锁乳突肌区　胸锁乳突肌在颈部所在的区域。

6. 颈后三角以肩胛舌骨肌下腹分为:

(1) 枕三角:位于斜方肌前缘、胸锁乳突肌后缘与肩胛舌骨肌下腹上缘之间。

(2) 锁骨上大窝:位于肩胛舌骨肌下腹下缘、锁骨上缘和胸锁乳突肌下段后缘之间。

二、颈部的表面解剖

1. 舌骨　舌骨体后方平对第 3 颈椎,舌骨大角是手术寻找舌动脉和舌下神经的解剖标志。

2. 甲状软骨　位于舌骨体的下方,男性甲状软骨前部明显突出称喉结。甲状软骨上缘平对第 4 颈椎,此平面为颈总动脉的分叉处及颈外动脉发出甲状腺上动脉的部位。

3. 环状软骨　相当于第 6 颈椎水平,在此平面,椎动脉进入第 6 颈椎横突孔。

4. 颈动脉结节　即第 6 颈椎横突前结节,位于环状软骨的两侧。

5. 胸锁乳突肌　位于颈侧部,是颈部外科的重要标志。

6. 锁骨上窝　位于胸骨颈静脉切迹上方的凹陷,是触诊气管的部位。

7. 锁骨上大窝　是锁骨中 1/3 上方的凹陷,在窝底可摸到第 1 肋骨。臂丛自内上向外下经过此窝的上部。锁骨上臂丛阻滞麻醉术通常在锁骨中点上方 1.5cm 处进针。紧靠锁骨上内方可摸及锁骨下动脉的搏动。

三、颈部结构的表面投影

1. 颈总动脉和颈外动脉　自下颌角与乳突尖连线的中点,右侧至胸锁关节、左侧至锁骨上小窝的连线。

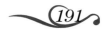

191

该线平甲状软骨上缘以下的一段为颈总动脉体表投影。在甲状软骨上缘以上的一段为颈外动脉体表投影。

2. 副神经　自乳突尖与下颌角连线的中点,经胸锁乳突肌后缘上、中 1/3 交点,至斜方肌前缘中、下 1/3 交点的连线。

3. 胸膜顶和肺尖　位于锁骨内侧 1/3 的上方,相当于胸锁乳突肌的胸骨头与锁骨头之间,其最高处一般距锁骨上缘 2～3cm。

4. 锁骨下动脉　相当于右侧自胸锁关节、左侧自锁骨上小窝向外上至锁骨上缘中点的弧线。最高点距锁骨上缘约 1.0cm。

5. 臂丛　自胸锁乳突肌后缘中、下 1/3 交点至锁骨中、外 1/3 交点稍内侧的连线。

四、舌骨下肌群及其神经支配

舌骨下肌群有 4 对,肩胛舌骨肌和胸骨舌骨肌为浅层,深层自下而上为胸骨甲状肌和甲状舌骨肌,它们均为扁薄的带状肌。胸骨舌骨肌、肩胛舌骨肌上腹和胸骨甲状肌三者因紧贴甲状腺前面,故又称之为甲状腺前肌。

舌骨下肌群的神经支配:来自于颈神经第 1～3 的前支构成的颈袢。颈袢上根(舌下神经降支)由第 1、2 颈神经前支的纤维构成。成人颈袢上根有 80.3% 经颈内动脉及颈总动脉的前外侧浅面;19.3% 行经颈内动脉与颈内静脉之间。上根约在甲状软骨中部至环状软骨下缘这一段的距离内,向内侧发出分支从深面进入肩胛舌骨肌上腹、胸骨舌骨肌及胸骨甲状肌的上部。

颈袢下根由第 2、3 颈神经的前支纤维构成,由外往内经颈内静脉浅面 59% 或深面 41%,与颈袢上根连结成袢,向下发出较粗大的肌支至胸骨舌骨肌和胸骨甲状肌的下部,另发一小肌支至肩胛舌骨肌下腹。

施行甲状腺手术之际,若遇腺体过大或上极过高导致显露不佳、操作困难时,常将甲状腺前肌完全切断以利甲状腺的显露。术中如损伤甲状腺前肌的支配神经,有关的肌在术后将发生萎缩,可致气管突出。为了防止在切断甲状腺前肌时伤及肌的支配神经,建议在 1、2 气管软骨环高度,由正中线往外夹住并切断甲状腺前肌。因为甲状腺前肌中部被切断后,其上半部和下半部仍有支配肌的神经进入。此外还应特别注意避免损伤在胸骨甲状肌外侧缘与颈内静脉之间的颈袢下行支。

第二节 颈椎及其连接

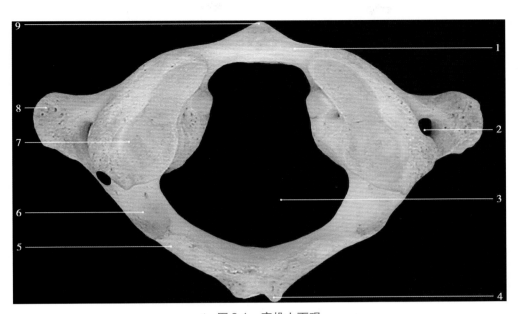

▲ 图 2-1 寰椎上面观

Fig. 2-1 Superior aspect of the atlas

1. 前弓 anterior arch
2. 横突孔 transverse foramen
3. 椎孔 vertebral foramen
4. 后结节 posterior tubercle
5. 后弓 posterior arch
6. 椎动脉沟 groove for vertebral artery
7. 上关节凹 superior articular fovea
8. 横突 transverse process
9. 前结节 anterior tubercle

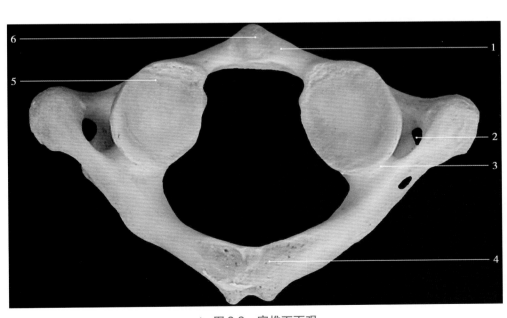

▲ 图 2-2 寰椎下面观

Fig. 2-2 Inferior aspect of the atlas

1. 前弓 anterior arch
2. 横突孔 transverse foramen
3. 侧块 lateral mass
4. 后弓 posterior arch
5. 下关节面 inferior articular surface
6. 前结节 anterior tubercle

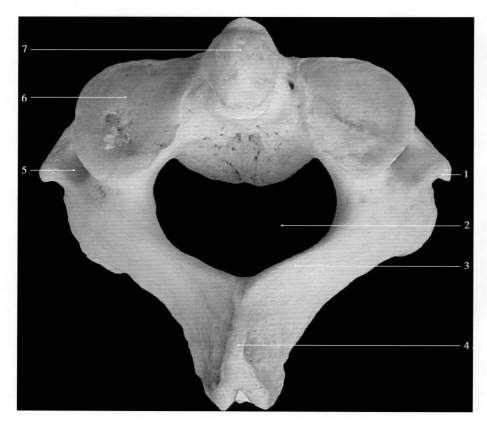

◀ 图2-3 枢椎上面观
Fig. 2-3 Superior aspect of the axis

1. 横突 transverse process
2. 椎孔 vertebral foramen
3. 椎弓 vertebral arch
4. 棘突 spinous process
5. 横突孔 transverse foramen
6. 上关节面 superior articular surface
7. 齿突 dens

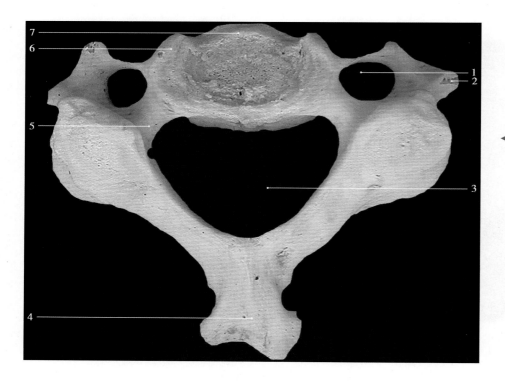

◀ 图2-4 第3颈椎上面观
Fig. 2-4 Superior aspect of the 3rd cervical vertebra

1. 横突孔 transverse foramen
2. 横突后结节 posterior tubercle of transverse process
3. 椎孔 vertebral foramen
4. 棘突 spinous process
5. 椎弓根 pedicle of vertebral arch
6. 椎体钩 uncus of vertebral body
7. 椎体 vertebral body

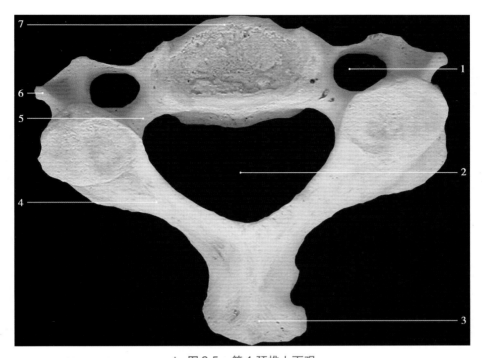

▲ 图 2-5　第 4 颈椎上面观

Fig. 2-5　Superior aspect of the 4th cervical vertebra

1. 横突孔 transverse foramen
2. 椎孔 vertebral foramen
3. 棘突 spinous process
4. 椎弓 vertebral arch
5. 椎弓根 pedicle of vertebral arch
6. 横突后结节 posterior tubercle of transverse process
7. 椎体 vertebral body

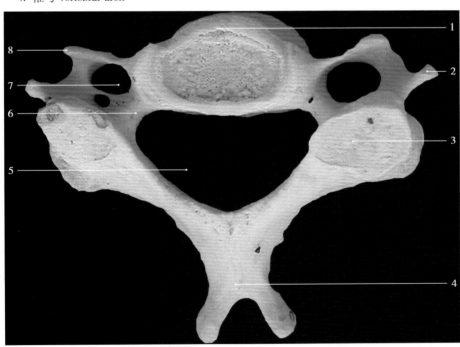

▲ 图 2-6　第 5 颈椎上面观

Fig. 2-6　Superior aspect of the 5th cervical vertebra

1. 椎体 vertebral body
2. 横突后结节 posterior tubercle of transverse
3. 上关节突 superior articular process
4. 棘突 spinous process
5. 椎孔 vertebral foramen
6. 椎弓根 pedicle of vertebral arch
7. 横突孔 transverse foramen
8. 横突前结节 anterior tubercle of transverse process

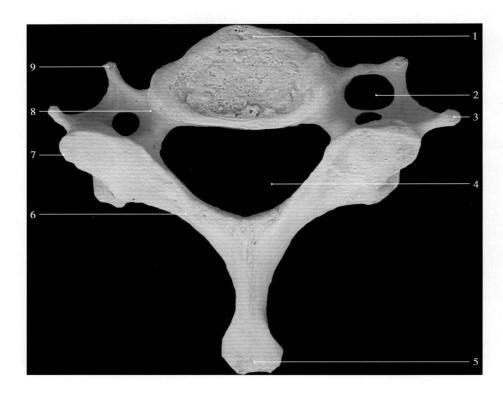

◀ 图2-7　第6颈椎上面观
Fig. 2-7　Superior aspect of the 6th cervical vertebra

1. 椎体 vertebral body
2. 横突孔 transverse foramen
3. 横突后结节 posterior tubercle of transverse process
4. 椎孔 vertebral foramen
5. 棘突 spinous process
6. 椎弓 vertebral arch
7. 上关节突 superior articular process
8. 脊神经沟 sulcus for spinal nerve
9. 横突前结节 anterior tubercle of transverse

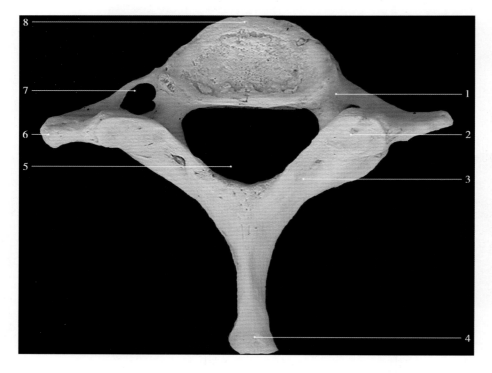

◀ 图2-8　第7颈椎(隆椎)
上面观
Fig. 2-8　Superior aspect of the 7th cervical vertebra (vertebra prominens)

1. 脊神经沟 sulcus for spinal nerve
2. 上关节突 superior articular process
3. 椎弓板 lamina of vertebra arch
4. 棘突 spinous process
5. 椎孔 vertebral foramen
6. 横突 transverse process
7. 横突孔 transverse foramen
8. 椎体 vertebral body

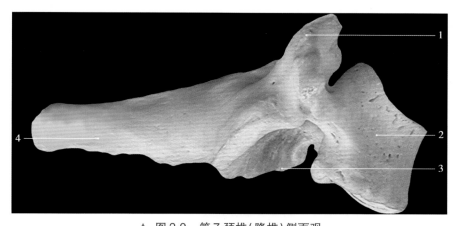

▲ 图2-9 第7颈椎(隆椎)侧面观
Fig. 2-9 Lateral aspect of the 7th cervical vertebra (vertebra prominens)

1. 上关节突 superior articular process
2. 椎体 vertebral body
3. 下关节突 inferior articular process
4. 棘突 spinous process

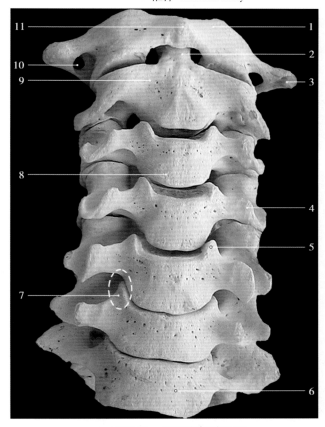

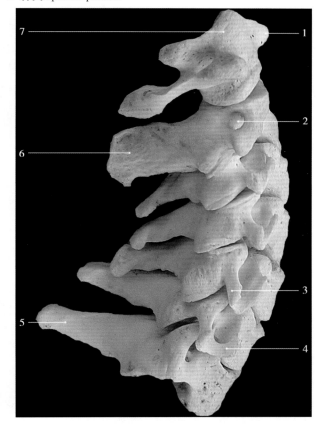

▲ 图2-10 颈段脊椎前面观
Fig. 2-10 Anterior aspect of the cervical vertebrae

1. 寰椎 atlas
2. 齿突 dens
3. 横突 transverse process
4. 横突前结节 anterior tubercle of transverse process
5. 椎体钩 uncus of vertebral body
6. 隆椎 vertebra prominens
7. 钩突关节 joint of uncinate process
8. 第3颈椎 the third cervical vertebra
9. 枢椎 axis
10. 横突孔 transverse foramen
11. 前结节 anterior tubercle

▲ 图2-11 颈段脊椎侧面观
Fig. 2-11 Lateral aspect of the cervical vertebrae

1. 前结节 anterior tubercle
2. 横突孔 transverse foramen
3. 横突后结节 posterior tubercle of transverse process
4. 横突前结节 anterior tubercle of transverse process
5. 第7颈椎棘突 spinous process of the 7th cervical vertebra
6. 枢椎棘突 spinous process of axis
7. 寰椎 atlas

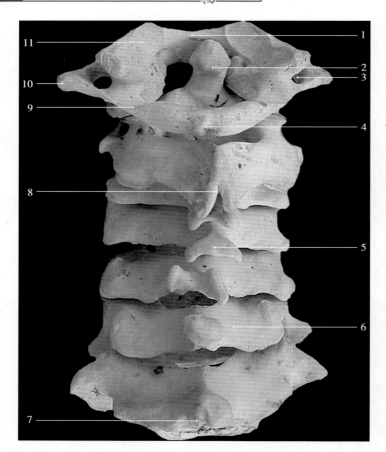

◀ 图2-12　颈段脊椎后面观
Fig. 2-12　Posterior aspect of the cervical vertebrae

1. 寰椎 atlas
2. 齿突 dens
3. 横突孔 transverse foramen
4. 后结节 posterior tubercle
5. 第 4 颈椎棘突 spinous process of the 4th cervical
vertebra
6. 椎弓板 lamina of vertebral arch
7. 第 7 颈椎棘突 spinous process of the seventh cervical vertebra
8. 枢椎棘突 spinous process of axis
9. 椎动脉沟 groove for vertebral artery
10. 横突 transverse process
11. 上关节凹 anterior articular fovea

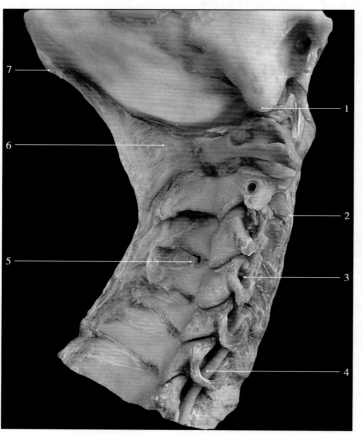

◀ 图2-13　项韧带
Fig. 2-13　Ligamentum nuchae

1. 乳突 mastoid process
2. 前纵韧带 anterior longitudinal ligament
3. 横突孔 transverse foramen
4. 椎动脉 vertebral artery
5. 棘间韧带 interspinous ligament
6. 项韧带 ligamentum nuchae
7. 枕外隆凸 external occipital protuberance

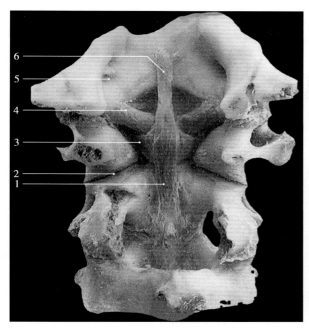

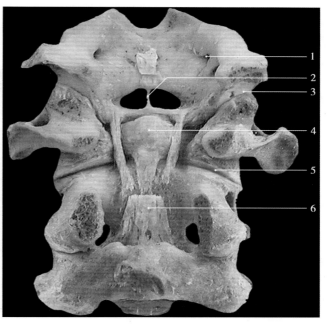

▲ 图 2-14 寰椎十字韧带（寰椎后弓已切除）
Fig. 2-14 Cruciform ligament of the atlas（the posterior arch of the atlas was excised）

1. 纵束 longitudinal bands
2. 寰枢外侧关节 lateral atlantoaxial joint
3. 寰椎横韧带 transverse ligament of atlas
4. 翼状韧带 alar ligaments
5. 舌下神经管 hypoglossal canal
6. 齿突尖韧带 apical ligament of dens

▲ 图 2-15 寰枕和寰枢关节（寰椎后弓已切除）
Fig. 2-15 Atlantooccipital and atlantoaxial joint（the posterior arch of the atlas was excised）

1. 舌下神经管 hypoglossal canal
2. 齿突尖韧带 apical ligament of dens
3. 寰枕关节 atlantooccipital joint
4. 寰椎十字韧带 cruciform ligament of atlas
5. 寰枢外侧关节 lateral atlantoaxial joint
6. 覆膜 tectorial membrane

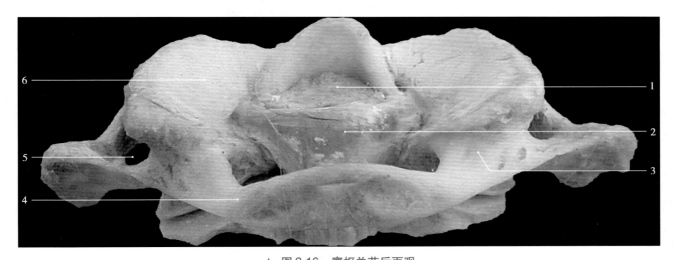

▲ 图 2-16 寰枢关节后面观
Fig. 2-16 Posterior aspect of the atlantoaxial joint

1. 齿突 dens
2. 寰椎横韧带 transverse ligament of atlas
3. 椎动脉沟 groove for vertebral artery
4. 寰椎后弓 posterior arch of atlas
5. 横突孔 transverse foramen
6. 上关节面 superior articular surface

第三节 颈前外侧区的肌、血管和神经

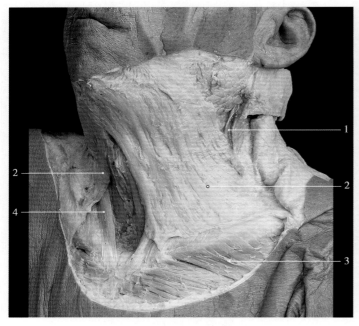

▲ 图 2-17 颈阔肌
Fig. 2-17 Platysma

1. 颈外静脉 external jugular vein
2. 颈阔肌 platysma
3. 胸大肌锁骨部 clavicular part of pectoralis major
4. 胸锁乳突肌 sternocleidomastoid

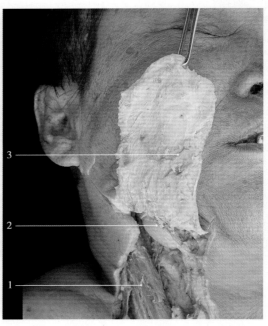

▲ 图 2-18 颈阔肌（皮）瓣
Fig. 2-18 Platysmal（skin）flap

1. 胸锁乳突肌 sternocleidomastoid
2. 下颌下腺 submandibular gland
3. 面动脉颈阔肌支 platysmal branch of facial artery

颈阔肌肌（皮）瓣的应用解剖学要点

颈阔肌血供丰富，由多条小动脉提供营养，主要的营养动脉来自于颈横动脉、甲状腺上动脉和面动脉发出的肌皮支。其中面动脉和颏下动脉大部分的分支从肌上部进入颈阔肌，以上部为蒂的颈阔肌肌皮瓣可用于修复口内、颊、腭、口底、舌以及唇面部的软组织缺损（图 2-18）。

应用解剖要点：

颈阔肌肌（皮）瓣如受区的面积较大和所需蒂较长时，为了保证组织瓣的血供，可将甲状腺上动脉（远端）与面动脉（远端）行端-端吻合，以增加肌皮瓣的长度。颈阔肌肌瓣可覆盖下颌骨裸露的骨面，当下颌骨移植骨时，包绕植骨块，加厚骨块与口底黏膜之间的厚度，有利于骨块生长。

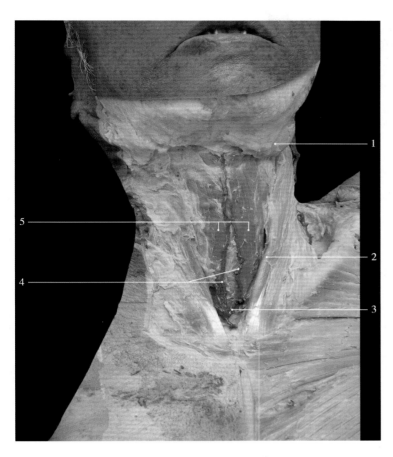

◀ 图 2-19 颈前静脉
Fig. 2-19 Anterior jugular vein

1. 下颌下腺 submandibular gland
2. 胸锁乳突肌 sternocleidomastoid
3. 颈静脉弓 jugular venous arch
4. 颈前静脉 anterior jugular vein
5. 胸骨舌骨肌 sternohyoid

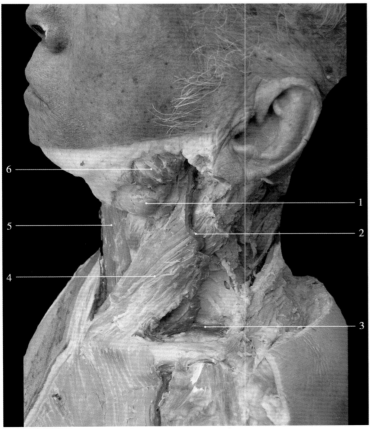

◀ 图 2-20 颈外静脉
Fig. 2-20 External jugular vein

1. 下颌下腺 submandibular gland
2. 颈外静脉 external jugular vein
3. 颈横静脉 transverse cervical vein
4. 胸锁乳突肌 sternocleidomastoid
5. 胸骨舌骨肌 sternohyoid
6. 咬肌 masseter

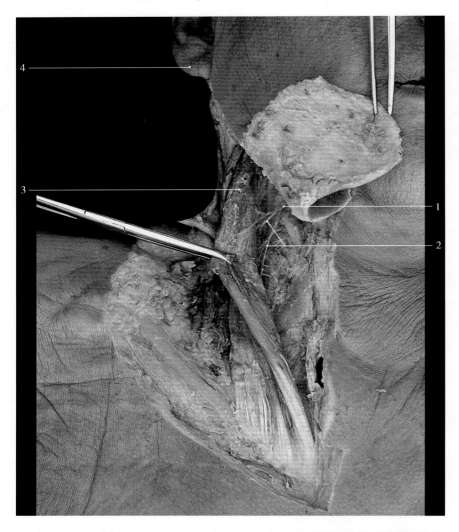

▶ 图 2-21　胸锁乳突肌（皮）瓣
Fig. 2-21　Sternocleidomastoid(skin)flap

1. 甲状腺上动脉 superior thyroid artery
2. 胸锁乳突肌支 sternocleidomastoid branches
3. 胸锁乳突肌 sternocleidomastoid
4. 耳垂 auricular lobule

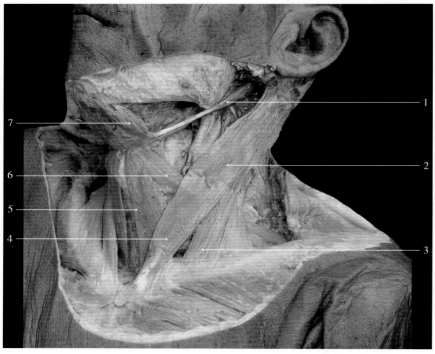

▶ 图 2-22　胸锁乳突肌
Fig. 2-22　Sternocleidomastoid

1. 二腹肌后腹 posterior belly of digastric
2. 胸锁乳突肌 sternocleidomastoid
3. 锁骨头 clavicle head
4. 胸骨头 sternum head
5. 胸骨舌骨肌 sternohyoid
6. 肩胛舌骨肌上腹 superior belly of omohyoid
7. 二腹肌前腹 anterior belly of digastric

胸锁乳突肌肌(皮)瓣的应用解剖学要点

胸锁乳突肌主要由枕动脉、颈外动脉和甲状腺上动脉的肌支供应。胸锁乳突肌肌(皮)瓣多选用上部为蒂的肌皮瓣,为向内上转移修复口底、舌、颊黏膜、扁桃体区、口咽侧壁和软腭等部口腔组织缺损的理想供区。肌瓣可用于下颌骨裸露骨面的覆盖和充填腮腺区术后凹陷畸形,复合肌瓣则可用于治疗咀嚼肌瘫痪症(图2-21、图2-22)。

应用解剖要点:

胸锁乳突肌位于颈侧面,以内、外两头起于胸骨上缘深面和锁骨内侧半,止于乳突部。肌的上部血供主要来自枕动脉的肌支,中部来自甲状腺上动脉发出的肌支,下部血供来自颈横动脉。以枕动脉为蒂的肌皮瓣可向上、内方旋转,以颈横动脉为蒂的胸锁乳突肌肌(皮)瓣可向下旋转。胸锁乳突肌受副神经和颈丛中颈3、4的分支支配,副神经在肌深面分为肌内支和肌外支,切取肌瓣时应注意保护。

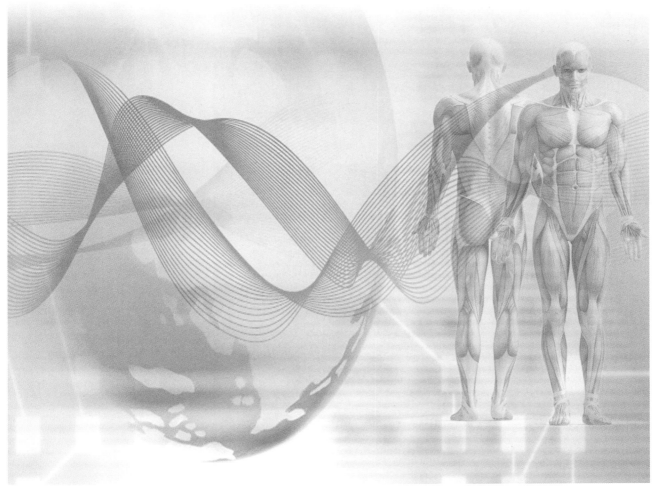

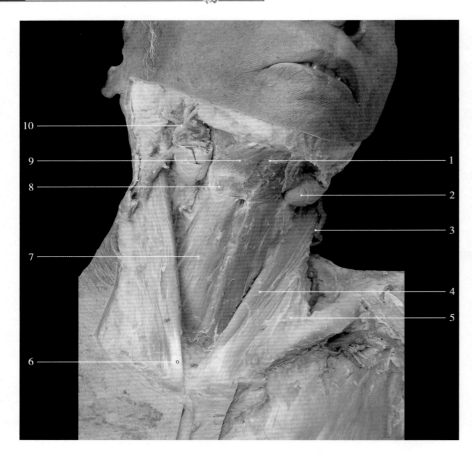

◀ 图 2-23　颈浅肌群
Fig. 2-23　Superficial muscles of the neck

1. 下颌舌骨肌 mylohyoid
2. 下颌下腺 submandibular gland
3. 颈外静脉 external jugular vein
4. 胸锁乳突肌 sternocleidomastoid
5. 锁骨头 clavicle head
6. 胸骨头 sternum head
7. 胸骨舌骨肌 sternohyoid
8. 舌骨 hyoid bone
9. 二腹肌前腹 anterior belly of digastric
10. 面动脉 facial artery

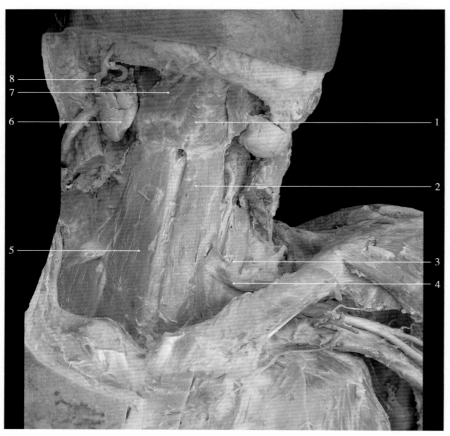

◀ 图 2-24　颈前肌
Fig. 2-24　Anterior muscles of the neck

1. 下颌舌骨肌 mylohyoid
2. 胸骨舌骨肌 sternohyoid
3. 颈内静脉 internal jugular vein
4. 肩胛舌骨肌下腹 inferior belly of omohyoid
5. 胸骨舌骨肌 sternohyoid
6. 下颌下腺 submandibular gland
7. 二腹肌前腹 anterior belly of digastric
8. 面动脉 facial artery

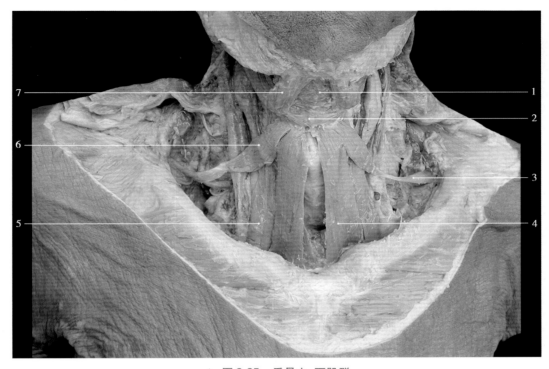

▲ 图 2-25 舌骨上、下肌群

Fig. 2-25 Suprahyoid and infrahyoid muscles

1. 下颌舌骨肌 mylohyoid
2. 舌骨 hyoid bone
3. 肩胛舌骨肌下腹 inferior belly of omohyoid
4. 胸骨舌骨肌 sternohyoid
5. 胸骨甲状肌 sternothyroid
6. 肩胛舌骨肌上腹 superior belly of omohyoid
7. 二腹肌前腹 anterior belly of digastric

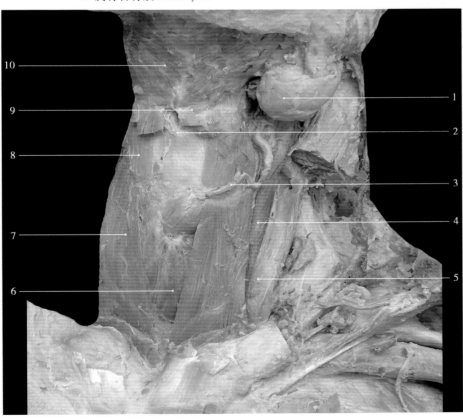

◀ 图 2-26 胸骨甲状肌、甲状舌骨肌

Fig. 2-26 Sternothyroid and thyrohyoid

1. 下颌下腺 submandibular gland
2. 喉结 laryngeal prominence
3. 喉上动脉 superior laryngeal artery
4. 颈内动脉 internal carotid artery
5. 颈内静脉 internal jugular vein
6. 甲状腺 thyroid gland
7. 胸骨甲状肌 sternothyroid
8. 甲状舌骨肌 thyrohyoid
9. 舌骨 hyoid bone
10. 下颌舌骨肌 mylohyoid

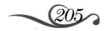

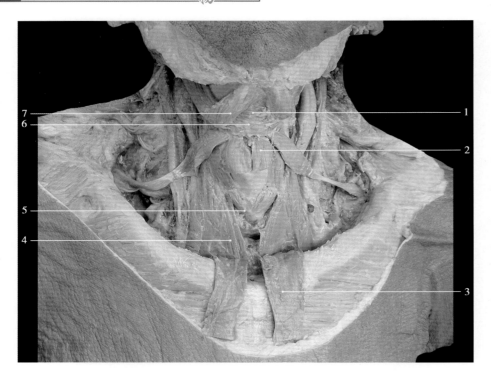

◀ 图 2-27　舌骨下肌群深层
Fig. 2-27　Deep layer of the infrahyoid muscles

1. 下颌舌骨肌 mylohyoid
2. 甲状舌骨肌 thyrohyoid
3. 胸骨舌骨肌 sternohyoid
4. 胸骨甲状肌 sternothyroid
5. 环甲肌 cricothyroid muscle
6. 舌骨 hyoid bone
7. 二腹肌前腹 anterior belly of digastric

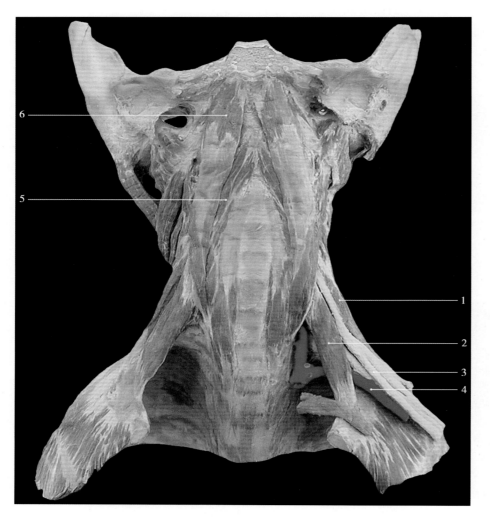

◀ 图 2-28　颈深肌群
Fig. 2-28　Deep muscle of the neck

1. 中斜角肌 scalenus medius
2. 前斜角肌 scalenus anterior
3. 臂丛 brachial plexus
4. 锁骨下动脉 subclavian artery
5. 颈长肌 longus colli
6. 头长肌 longus capitis

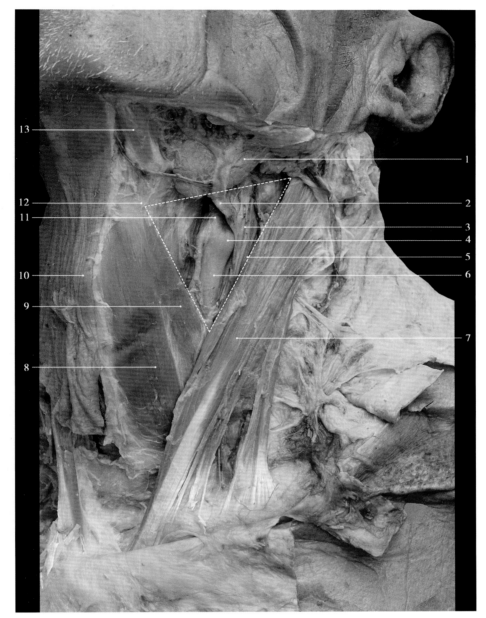

▲ 图2-29 颈动脉三角
Fig. 2-29 Carotid triangle

1. 下颌下腺 submandibular gland
2. 面总静脉 common facial vein
3. 颈内静脉 internal jugular vein
4. 颈动脉窦 carotid sinus
5. 颈动脉三角 carotid triangle
6. 颈总动脉 common carotid artery
7. 胸锁乳突肌 sternocleidomastoid
8. 胸骨舌骨肌 sternohyoid
9. 肩胛舌骨肌 omohyoid
10. 喉结 laryngeal prominence
11. 颈外动脉 external carotid artery
12. 舌骨 hyoid bone
13. 二腹肌前腹 anterior belly of digastric

舌骨下肌群肌皮瓣的应用解剖学要点

　　舌骨下肌群肌皮瓣主要是以甲状腺浅层肌及其表面的颈阔肌和皮肤构成的组织瓣,主要血管来自于甲状腺上动脉与伴行的静脉,其肤色、厚度与口腔颌面部很接近,是修复口腔、舌、颊部缺损的理想供区之一(图2-23～图2-27)。

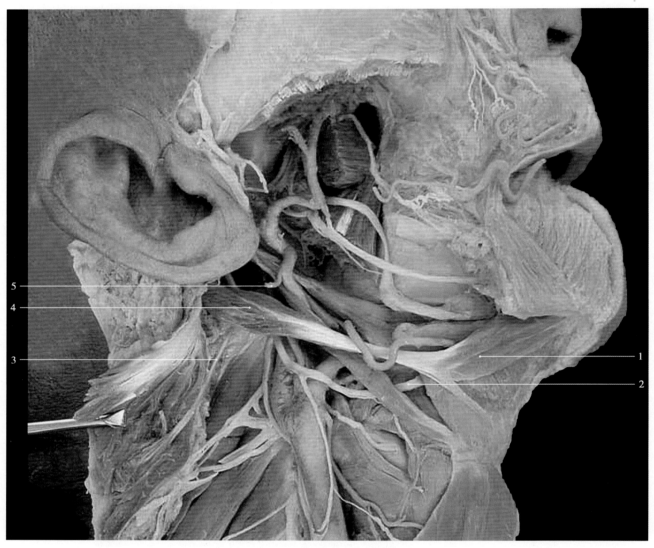

▲ 图 2-30 二腹肌瓣
Fig. 2-30 Digastric flap

1. 二腹肌前腹 anterior belly of digastric
2. 舌下神经 hypoglossal nerve
3. 副神经 accessory nerve
4. 二腹肌后腹 posterior belly of digastric
5. 二腹肌支 digastric branch

二腹肌肌瓣的应用解剖学要点

　　二腹肌属于舌骨上肌群,其作用为牵引颏部向后下,参与张口活动。临床上可利用其收缩功能,进行肌腹移植或移位治疗中央性舌麻痹与矫治口轮匝肌的瘫痪(图 2-30)。

　　应用解剖要点:

　　二腹肌有两个肌腹组成,较长的后腹起于颞骨乳突切迹,行向前下,较短的前腹起于下颌骨二腹肌窝,行向后下,二腹会合于中间腱。中间腱借颈深筋膜构成的吊带,即腱环,与舌骨大角和舌骨体侧面相连。因舌下神经功能丧失,使患者进食和语言功能丧失时,可将二腹肌移植在舌根深层肌肉内,利用二腹肌肌腹收缩的功能,帮助患者完成进食和提高语言功能。

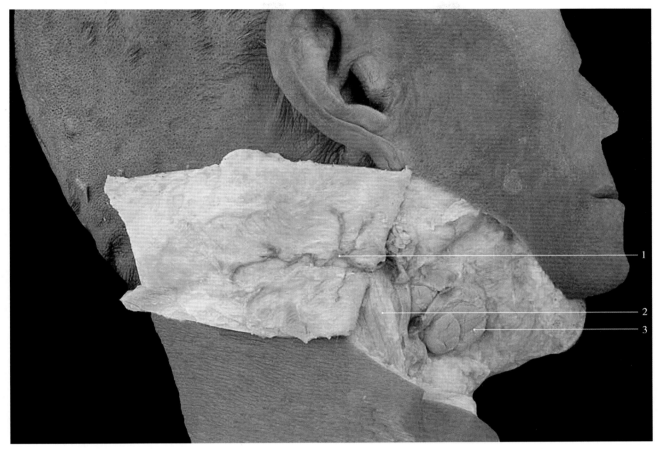

▲ 图 2-31 颏下皮瓣
Fig. 2-31　Submental skin flap

1. 颏下动脉 submental artery
2. 胸锁乳突肌 sternocleidomastoid
3. 下颌下腺 submandibular gland

颏下皮瓣的应用解剖学要点

颏下皮瓣是以颏下动脉为蒂,供区位于颏下部,位置隐蔽,皮瓣肤色与面部近似,如果颏下脂肪或皱纹过多,皮瓣切取后供区可作为 I 期缝合。根据临床应用的实际需要,该区可作成皮瓣、筋膜瓣和骨皮瓣。局部转移可修复口腔颌面部的软组织缺损(图 2-31)。

应用解剖要点:

颏下动脉是面动脉颈部最大的分支。当面动脉即将转至面部时发出,沿下颌舌骨肌表面前进至颏部。颏下动脉起始处的外径为 1.8mm,起始点距下颌骨下缘 1.1mm,距下颌角 2.6cm,血管沿下颌下腺浅部上缘与下颌骨下缘深面之间的结缔组织内向前行约 2.6cm,发支至下颌窝处的皮肤、皮下组织、下颌骨骨膜等处。皮瓣最大的切取面积可达 15cm×7cm。

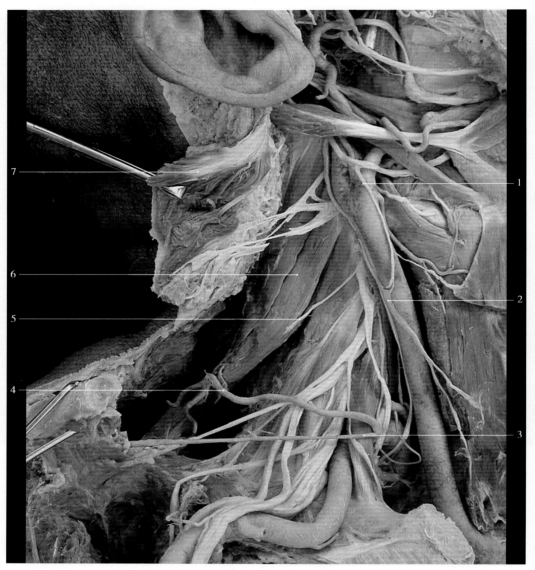

▲ 图 2-32　肩胛提肌瓣

Fig. 2-32　Levator scapulae flap

1. 颈袢上根 superior root of cervical ansa
2. 颈袢 cervical ansa
3. 肩胛上动脉 suprascapular artery
4. 颈横动脉 transverse cervical artery
5. 肩胛提肌神经 nerve of levator scapulae
6. 肩胛提肌 levator scapulae
7. 胸锁乳突肌 sternocleidomastoid

肩胛提肌肌瓣的应用解剖学要点

　　肩胛提肌位于颈部两侧,肌的上部位于胸锁乳突肌的深面,下部位于斜方肌的深面,为一对带状肌。肩胛提肌起自上位四个颈椎横突的后结节,肌纤维斜向下稍外方,止于肩胛骨的上角和肩胛骨内侧缘的上部。此肌收缩时,上提肩胛骨,同时使肩胛骨下角转向内;肩胛骨固定时,使颈向同侧屈曲并后仰。肩胛提肌肌瓣可用于颈部肿瘤根治术后覆盖和保护颈动脉及修复口咽部和面颊部的缺损(图 2-32)。

　　应用解剖要点:

　　肩胛提肌长 129.13mm,中部宽 19.01mm,厚 6.90mm。肌的上部血供主要由颈升动脉发支供应,肌的下部主要由颈横动脉和肩胛上动脉发支供应,肩胛提肌受脊神经 C_3、C_4 直接分支和肩胛背神经(C_5)支配。

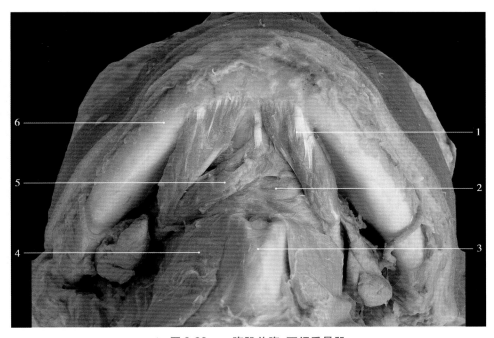

▲ 图 2-33 二腹肌前腹、下颌舌骨肌
Fig. 2-33 Anterior belly of the digastric and mylohyoid

1. 二腹肌前腹 anterior belly of digastric
2. 下颌舌骨肌 mylohyoid
3. 喉结 laryngeal prominence
4. 胸骨舌骨肌 sternohyoid
5. 变异下颌舌骨肌 variant mylohyoid
6. 下颌骨 mandible

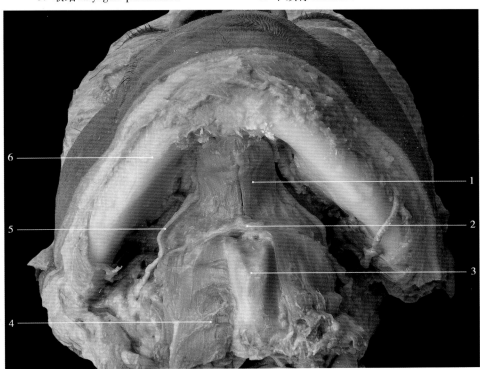

▲ 图 2-34 颏舌骨肌
Fig. 2-34 Geniohyoid

1. 颏舌骨肌 geniohyoid
2. 舌骨体 body of hyoid bone
3. 喉结 laryngeal prominence
4. 胸骨舌骨肌 sternohyoid
5. 舌下神经 hypoglossal nerve
6. 下颌骨 mandible

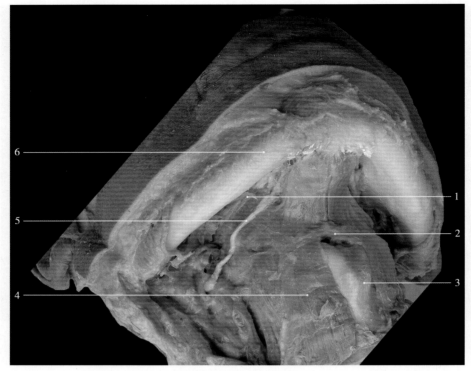

▲ 图 2-35　舌骨舌肌
Fig. 2-35　Hyoglossus

1. 舌骨舌肌 hyoglossus
2. 舌骨体 body of hyoid bone
3. 喉结 laryngeal prominence
4. 胸骨舌骨肌 sternohyoid
5. 舌下神经 hypoglossal nerve
6. 下颌骨 mandible

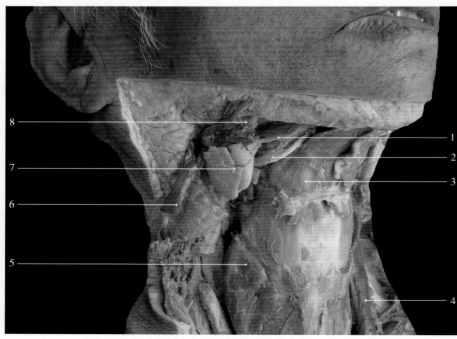

▲ 图 2-36　舌下神经和舌骨舌肌
Fig. 2-36　Hypoglossal nerve and hyoglossus

1. 舌动脉 lingual artery
2. 舌下神经 hypoglossal nerve
3. 舌骨舌肌 hyoglossus
4. 颈内静脉 internal jugular vein
5. 甲状腺上极 upper pole of thyroid gland
6. 颈外静脉 external jugular vein
7. 下颌下腺 submandibular gland
8. 面动脉 facial artery

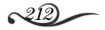

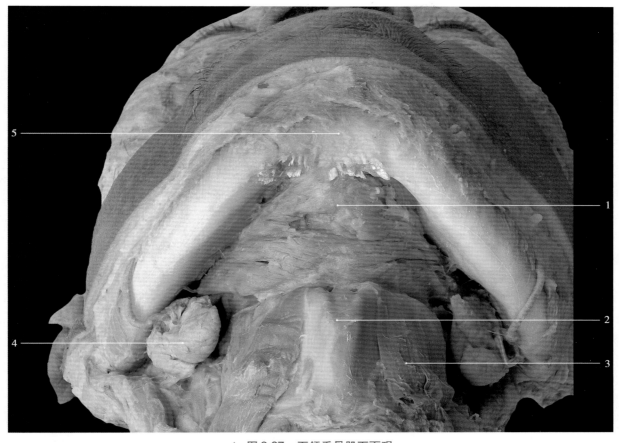

▲ 图 2-37 下颌舌骨肌下面观

Fig. 2-37 Inferior aspect of the mylohyoid

1. 下颌舌骨肌 mylohyoid   4. 下颌下腺 submandibular gland
2. 喉结 laryngeal prominence   5. 下颌骨 mandible
3. 胸骨舌骨肌 sternohyoid

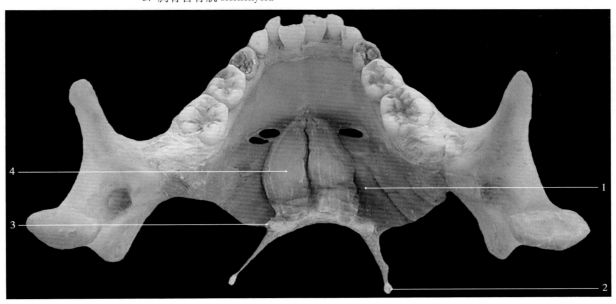

▲ 图 2-38 口底肌上面观

Fig. 2-38 Superior aspect of the muscles of the mouth floor

1. 下颌舌骨肌 mylohyoid   3. 舌骨小角 lesser cornu of hyoid bone
2. 舌骨大角 greater cornu of hyoid bone   4. 颏舌骨肌 geniohyoid

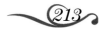

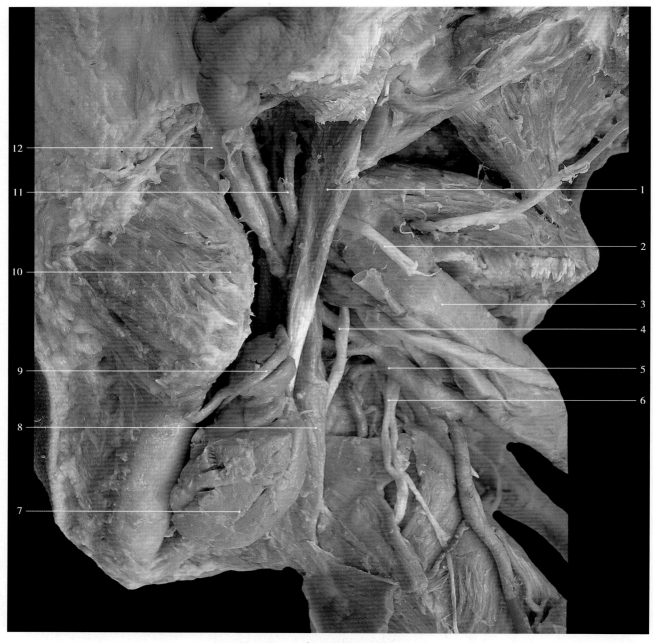

▲ 图 2-39　二腹肌后腹深面结构（左侧）

Fig. 2-39　Profundal structures of the posterior belly of digastric（left）

1. 二腹肌后腹 posterior belly of digastric
2. 副神经 accessory nerve
3. 颈内静脉 internal jugular vein
4. 舌下神经 hypoglossal nerve
5. 颈外动脉 external carotid artery
6. 喉上神经 superior laryngeal nerve
7. 下颌下腺 submandibular gland
8. 茎突舌骨肌 stylohyoid
9. 面动脉 facial artery
10. 下颌角 angle of mandible
11. 枕动脉 occipital artery
12. 下颌后静脉 retromandibular vein

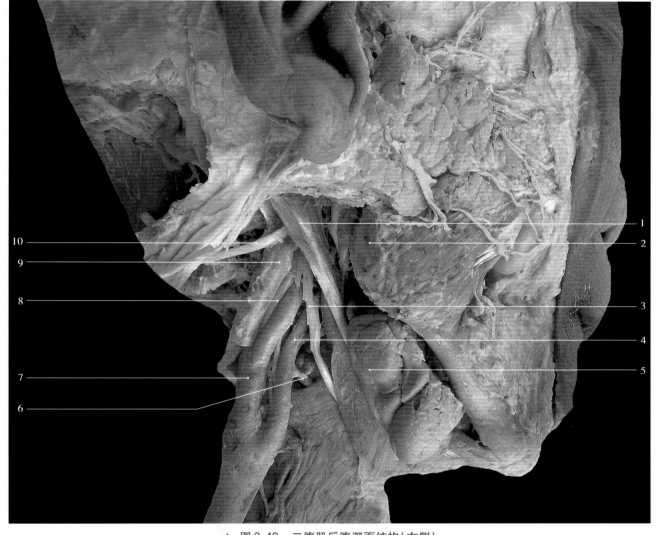

▲ 图2-40 二腹肌后腹深面结构(右侧)

Fig. 2-40 Profundal structures of the posterior belly of digastric(right)

1. 二腹肌后腹 posterior belly of digastric	6. 舌动脉 lingual artery
2. 下颌角 angle of mandible	7. 颈内动脉 internal carotid artery
3. 舌下神经 hypoglossal nerve	8. 迷走神经 vagus nerve
4. 颈外动脉 external carotid artery	9. 颈内静脉 internal jugular vein
5. 下颌下腺 submandibular gland	10. 副神经 accessory nerve

二腹肌后腹的应用解剖学要点

二腹肌为舌骨上肌群浅层肌,位于下颌骨的下方,起于乳突切迹,止于下颌骨二腹肌窝。有前、后两肌腹,两肌腹间有中间腱连于舌骨。二腹肌前腹由下牙槽神经的下颌舌骨肌神经支配,后腹由面神经的二腹肌肌支支配(图2-39～图2-42)。

应用解剖要点:

二腹肌后腹是下颌下三角与颈动脉三角的分界,也是颌面部手术与颈部手术的重要标志。所有位于颈动脉三角内与面部及颅内相通的结构均由此通过:表面有耳大神经、下颌后静脉及面神经颈支;深面有颈内动脉、颈内静脉、颈外动脉、迷走神经、副神经和舌下神经以及颈上神经节、颈交感干;二腹肌后腹的上缘有耳后动脉、面神经及舌咽神经;二腹肌后腹的下缘有枕动脉和舌下神经。

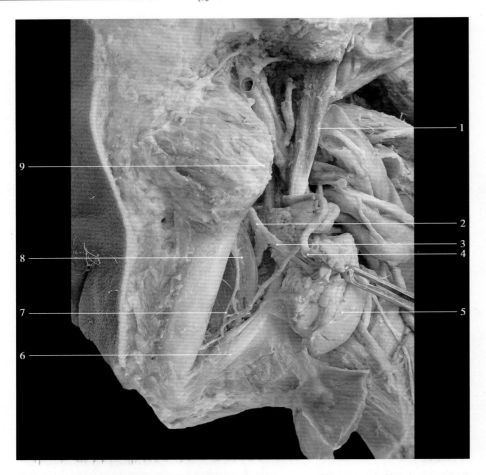

◀ 图 2-41　左侧下颌下神经节
Fig. 2-41　Left submandibular ganglion

1. 二腹肌后腹 posterior belly of digastric
2. 舌神经 lingual nerve
3. 下颌下神经节 submandibular ganglion
4. 面动脉 facial artery
5. 下颌下腺 submandibular gland
6. 二腹肌前腹 anterior belly of digastric
7. 二腹肌支 digastric branch
8. 下颌舌骨肌 mylohyoid
9. 下颌角 angle of mandible

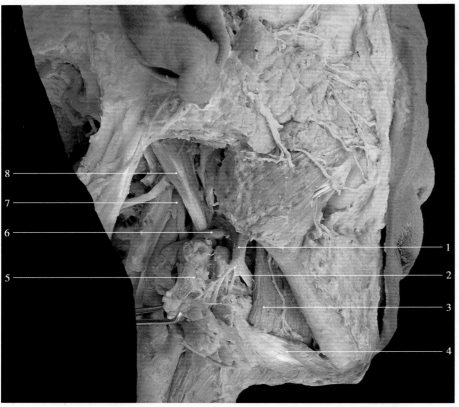

◀ 图 2-42　右侧下颌下神经节
Fig. 2-42　Right submandibular ganglion

1. 舌神经 lingual nerve
2. 下颌下神经节 submandibular ganglion
3. 下颌舌骨肌 mylohyoid
4. 二腹肌前腹 anterior belly of digastric
5. 下颌下腺 submandibular gland
6. 面动脉 facial artery
7. 舌下神经 hypoglossal nerve
8. 二腹肌后腹 posterior belly of digastric

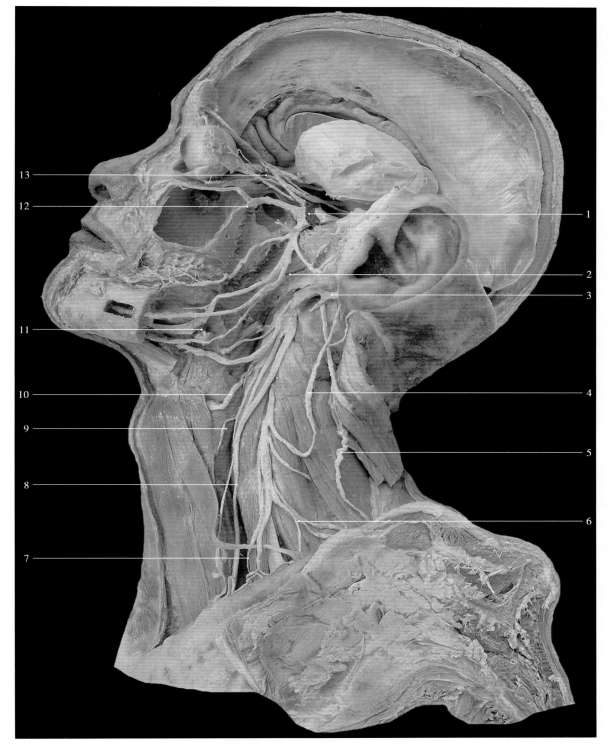

▲ 图2-43 头部副交感神经节

Fig. 2-43 Parasympathetic ganglia of the head

1. 三叉神经节 trigeminal ganglion
2. 鼓索 chorda tympanic
3. 面神经 facial nerve
4. 耳大神经 great auricular nerve
5. 副神经 accessory nerve
6. 锁骨上神经 supraclavicular nerve
7. 膈神经 phrenic nerve
8. 迷走神经 vagus nerve
9. 喉上神经外支 external branch of superior laryngeal nerve
10. 喉上神经内支 internal branch of superior laryngeal nerve
11. 下颌下神经节 submandibular ganglion
12. 翼腭神经 pterygopalatine nerve
13. 睫状神经节 ciliary ganglion

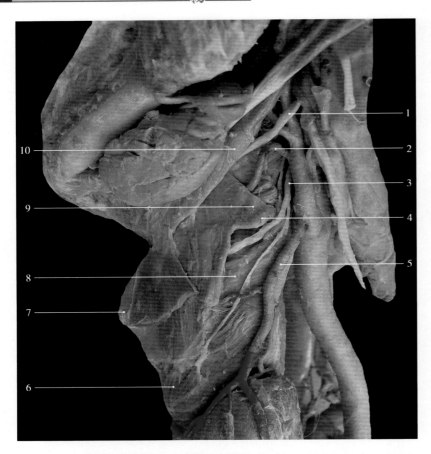

◀ 图 2-44　左侧舌骨大角周围结构
Fig. 2-44　Structures around the left
great cornu of hyoid bone

1. 舌下神经 hypoglossal nerve
2. 舌动脉 lingual artery
3. 喉上神经 superior laryngeal nerve
4. 舌骨大角 greater cornu of hyoid bone
5. 甲状腺上动脉 superior thyroid artery
6. 环甲肌 cricothyroid muscle
7. 喉结 laryngeal prominence
8. 咽上缩肌 superior constrictor of pharynx
9. 下颌舌骨肌 mylohyoid
10. 茎突舌骨肌 stylohyoid

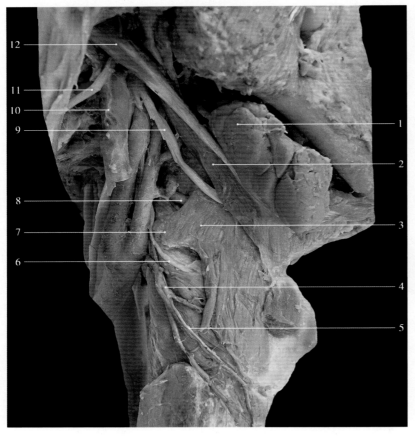

◀ 图 2-45　右侧舌骨大角周围结构
Fig. 2-45　Structures around the right
great cornu of hyoid bone

1. 下颌下腺 submandibular gland
2. 茎突舌骨肌 stylohyoid
3. 下颌舌骨肌 mylohyoid
4. 甲状腺上动脉 superior thyroid artery
5. 喉上神经外支 external branch of superior laryngeal nerve
6. 喉上神经内支 medial branch of l superior laryngeal nerve
7. 舌骨大角 greater cornu of hyoid bone
8. 舌动脉 lingual artery
9. 舌下神经 hypoglossal nerve
10. 颈内静脉 internal jugular vein
11. 副神经 accessory nerve
12. 二腹肌后腹 posterior belly of digastric

舌骨大角的应用解剖学要点

舌骨属于面颅骨中的一块,借肌肉与韧带悬挂在颈部前正中,分为体、大角和小角。舌骨体为舌骨中部的方形骨板,前面凸隆,后面光滑而凹陷,体的上缘较锐、下缘较钝。大角成对,自体的外侧端凸向后方,中部扁薄,根部肥厚,末端呈结节状。舌骨体和舌骨大角在颈部皮下均可摸及,是颈部的常用标志之一(图2-44、图2-45)。

应用解剖要点:

舌骨大角后上方有咽上缩肌附着,前上缘有舌骨舌肌附着,下缘有甲状舌骨肌附着。舌骨大角内上方约10mm处有舌动脉经舌骨舌肌的后上缘自浅层穿入深层;在舌动脉的内上方约7.0mm处有舌下神经经颈外动脉前外侧,沿茎突舌骨肌下缘,行于舌骨舌肌浅面。在舌骨大角下内方约15mm处,喉上神经内支沿咽中缩肌上缘,行于甲状舌骨肌深面,穿甲状舌骨膜分布于喉黏膜;喉上神经外支沿其内支的前外侧下行,穿咽中缩肌,在甲状软骨下缘距前正中线约27.5mm处,在环甲肌的外上方分细支入环甲肌。

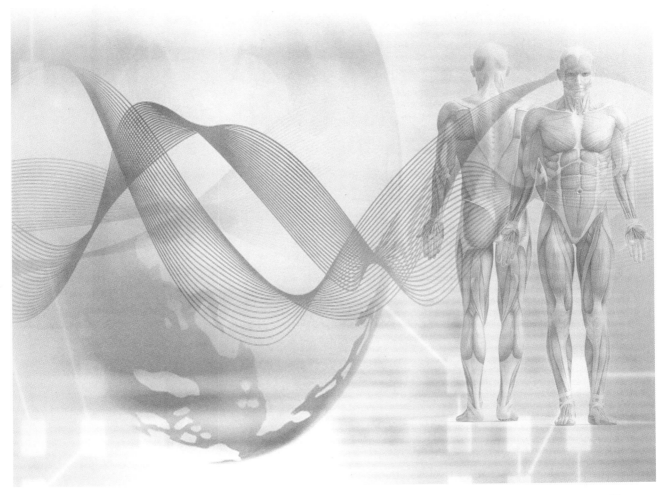

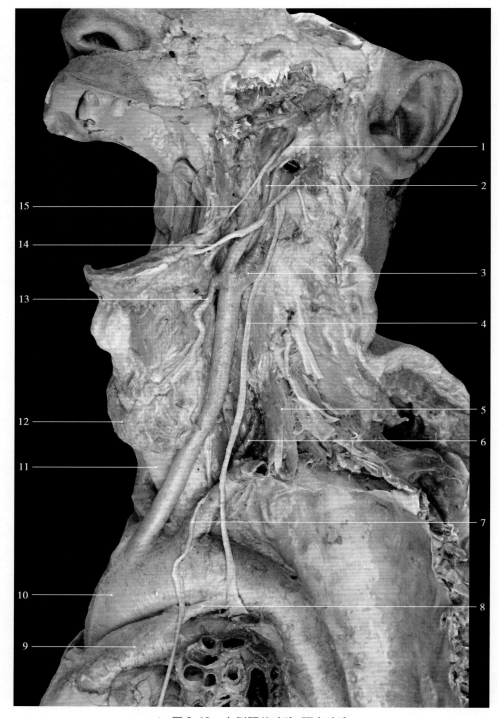

▲ 图 2-46 左侧颈总动脉、颈内动脉
Fig. 2-46 Left common carotid artery and internal carotid artery

1. 茎突 styloid process
2. 颈内动脉 internal carotid artery
3. 颈动脉窦 carotid sinus
4. 迷走神经 vagus nerve
5. 前斜角肌 scalenus anterior
6. 椎动脉 vertebral artery
7. 膈神经 phrenic nerve
8. 动脉韧带 arterial ligament
9. 肺动脉 pulmonary artery
10. 主动脉弓 aortic arch
11. 气管 trachea
12. 甲状腺 thyroid gland
13. 甲状腺上动脉 superior thyroid artery
14. 舌下神经 hypoglossal nerve
15. 舌咽神经 glossopharyngeal nerve

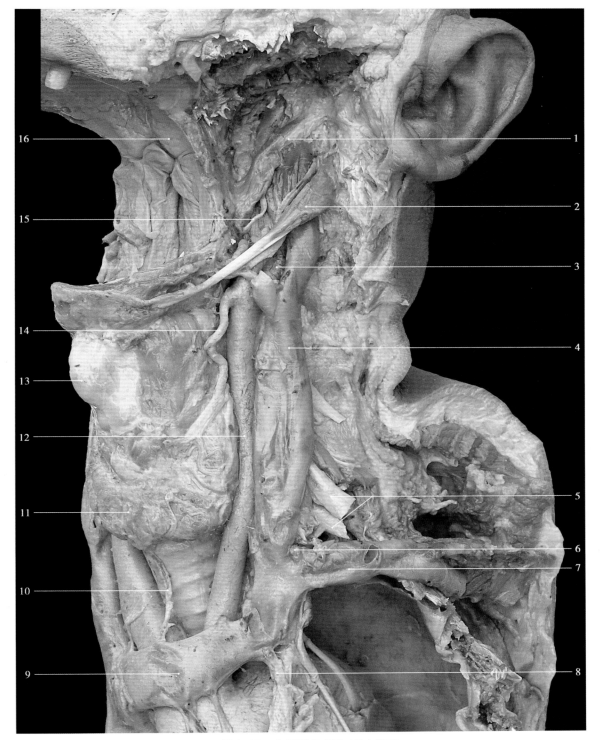

▲ 图2-47　左侧颈总动脉、颈内静脉

Fig. 2-47　Left common carotid artery and internal jugular vein

1. 茎突咽肌 stylopharyngeus
2. 二腹肌后腹 posterior belly of digastric
3. 颈内动脉 internal carotid artery
4. 颈内静脉 internal jugular vein
5. 臂丛 brachial plexus
6. 静脉角 venous angle
7. 左锁骨下静脉 left subclavian vein
8. 胸廓内静脉 internal thoracic vein

9. 左头臂静脉 left brachiocephalic vein
10. 甲状腺下静脉 inferior thyroid artery
11. 甲状腺 thyroid gland
12. 颈总动脉 common carotid artery
13. 喉结 laryngeal prominence
14. 甲状腺上动脉 superior thyroid artery
15. 舌咽神经 glossopharyngeal nerve
16. 软腭 soft palate

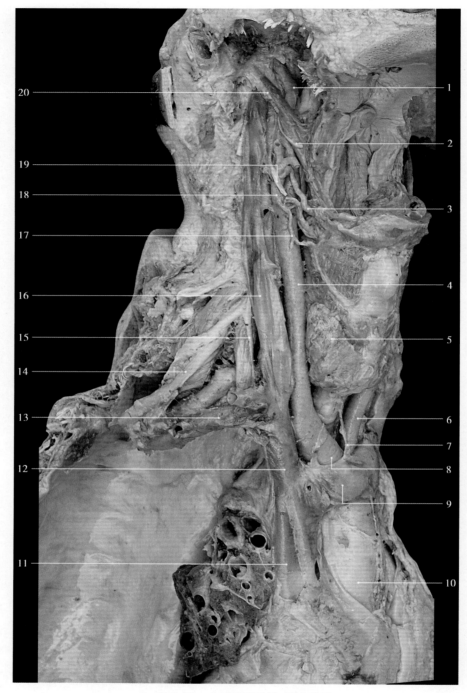

▲ 图2-48　右侧颈总动脉、颈内静脉

Fig. 2-48　Right common carotid artery and internal jugular vein

1. 颈内动脉 internal carotid artery
2. 舌咽神经 glossopharyngeal nerve
3. 舌动脉 lingual artery
4. 颈总动脉 common carotid artery
5. 甲状腺 thyroid gland
6. 左颈总动脉 left common carotid artery
7. 甲状腺下静脉 inferior thyroid vein
8. 头臂干 brachiocephalic trunk
9. 左头臂静脉 left brachiocephalic vein
10. 升主动脉 ascending aorta

11. 上腔静脉 superior vena cava
12. 右头臂静脉 right brachiocephalic vein
13. 右锁骨下静脉 right subclavian artery
14. 前斜角肌 scalenus anterior
15. 膈神经 phrenic nerve
16. 颈内静脉 internal jugular vein
17. 甲状腺上动脉 superior thyroid artery
18. 颈外动脉 external carotid artery
19. 舌下神经 hypoglossal nerve
20. 茎突咽肌 stylopharyngeus

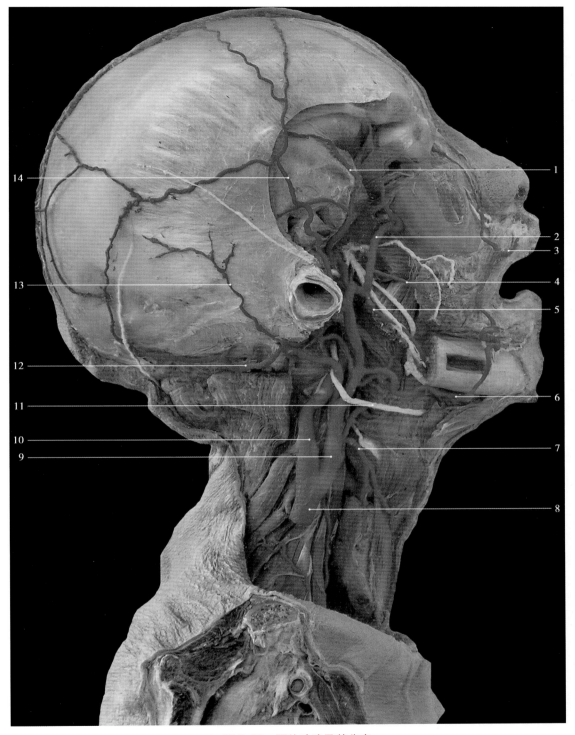

▲ 图 2-49　颈外动脉及其分支

Fig. 2-49　External carotid artery and its branches

1. 脑膜中动脉 middle meningeal artery
2. 上颌动脉 maxillary artery
3. 上唇动脉 superior labial artery
4. 面横动脉 transverse facial artery
5. 下牙槽动脉 inferior alveolar artery
6. 面动脉 facial artery
7. 甲状腺上动脉 superior thyroid artery

8. 颈总动脉 common carotid artery
9. 颈外动脉 external carotid artery
10. 颈内动脉 internal carotid artery
11. 舌下神经 hypoglossal nerve
12. 枕动脉 occipital artery
13. 耳后动脉 posterior auricular artery
14. 颞浅动脉 superficial temporal artery

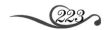

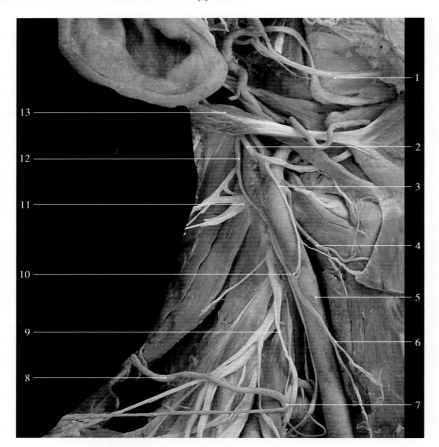

▲ 图 2-50　颈袢
Fig. 2-50　Cervical ansa

1. 下牙槽神经 inferior alveolar nerve
2. 舌下神经 hypoglossal nerve
3. 颈袢上根 superior root of cervical ansa
4. 甲状腺上动脉 superior thyroid artery
5. 颈总动脉 common carotid artery
6. 胸骨甲状肌支 branch of sternothyroid
7. 甲状颈干 thyrocervical trunk
8. 颈横动脉 transverse cervical artery
9. 膈神经 phrenic nerve
10. 颈袢 cervical ansa
11. 颈深丛 deep cervical plexus
12. 颈袢下根 inferior root of cervical ansa
13. 二腹肌后腹 posterior belly of digastric

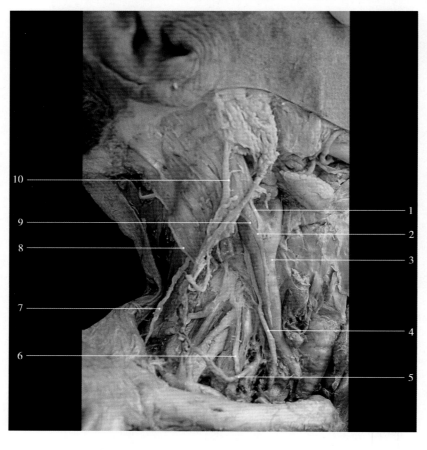

▲ 图 2-51　颈袢、膈神经
Fig. 2-51　Cervical ansa and phrenic nerve

1. 舌下神经降支 descending branch of hypoglossal nerve
2. 颈袢 cervical ansa
3. 颈总动脉 common carotid artery
4. 迷走神经 vagus nerve
5. 颈横动脉 transverse cervical artery
6. 膈神经 phrenic nerve
7. 副神经 accessory nerve
8. 枕小神经 lesser occipital nerve
9. 颈神经降支 descending branch of cervical nerve
10. 耳大神经 great auricular nerve

颈袢与膈神经吻接重建膈肌功能的应用解剖学要点

C_4以上脊髓损伤后膈和肋间肌瘫痪,患者丧失自主呼吸。可以用颈袢或胸锁乳突肌支与膈神经吻接,以重建自主呼吸功能(图2-50、图2-51)。

应用解剖要点：

颈袢由上根(舌下神经降支)和下根组成。上根80%位于颈内动脉和颈总动脉的表面;20%行于颈内动脉、静脉之间,上根长40mm,中间宽1.9mm,厚0.8mm。下根由C_2、C_3脊神经前根纤维组成,由外向内经过颈内静脉表面(59%)或深面(41%)。下根长32mm,中间宽1.6mm,厚0.6mm。

膈神经起始于$C_{3\sim5}$前根,在前斜角肌上部外侧汇合而成,沿前斜角肌表面下降,经胸廓上口入胸腔。膈神经起始端与舌下神经降支和颈神经降支形成的颈袢在颈动脉鞘前外侧,平喉结高度上下有一段两者之间并行,它们之间并行的长度为28.6mm。

颈袢上根约在甲状软骨中部至环状软骨下缘之间向内发出肌支从深面进入肩胛舌骨肌上腹、胸骨舌骨肌和胸骨甲状肌的上部。下根与上根合成袢后,向下发出肌支至胸骨舌骨肌和胸骨甲状肌的下部。甲状腺手术时如需切断舌骨下肌群,应在甲状腺峡部,即第1、2气管软骨环的高度切断,可防止因伤及入肌的神经而引起舌骨下肌群萎缩以致气管凸出。

颈袢与喉上神经、喉返神经吻接可以重建声带功能。

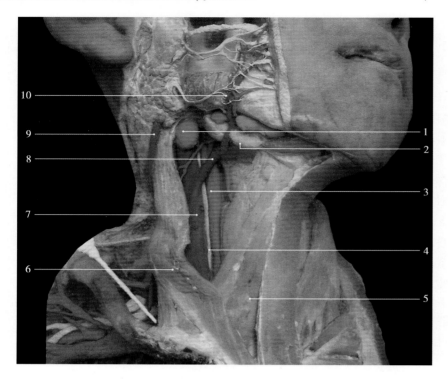

◀ 图 2-52　颈内静脉的位置
Fig. 2-52　Position of the internal jugular vein

1. 下颌下淋巴结 submandibular lymph node
2. 下颌下腺 submandibular gland
3. 颈内动脉 internal carotid artery
4. 迷走神经 vagus nerve
5. 胸骨舌骨肌 sternohyoid
6. 胸锁乳突肌 sternocleidomastoid
7. 颈内静脉 internal jugular vein
8. 面总静脉 common facial vein
9. 颈外静脉 external jugular vein
10. 面静脉 facial vein

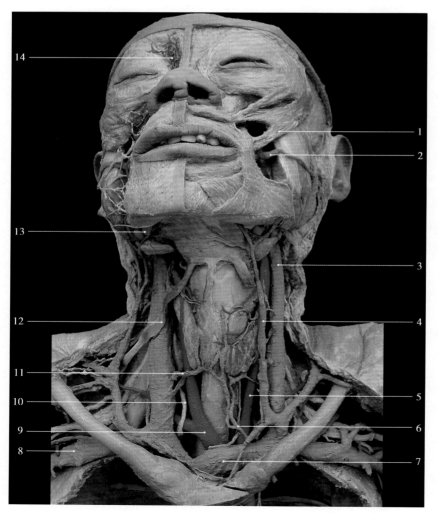

◀ 图 2-53　颈部静脉前面观
Fig. 2-53　Anterior aspect of the veins in the neck

1. 颧大肌 zygomaticus major
2. 腮腺管 parotid duct
3. 颈内静脉 internal jugular vein
4. 颈外静脉 external jugular vein
5. 颈总动脉 common carotid artery
6. 甲状腺下静脉 inferior thyroid vein
7. 左头臂静脉 left brachiocephalic vein
8. 锁骨下静脉 subclavian vein
9. 头臂干 brachiocephalic trunk
10. 膈神经 phrenic nerve
11. 甲状腺中静脉 middle thyroid vein
12. 肩胛舌骨肌 omohyoid
13. 下颌下淋巴结 submandibular lymph node
14. 眶上动脉 supraorbital artery

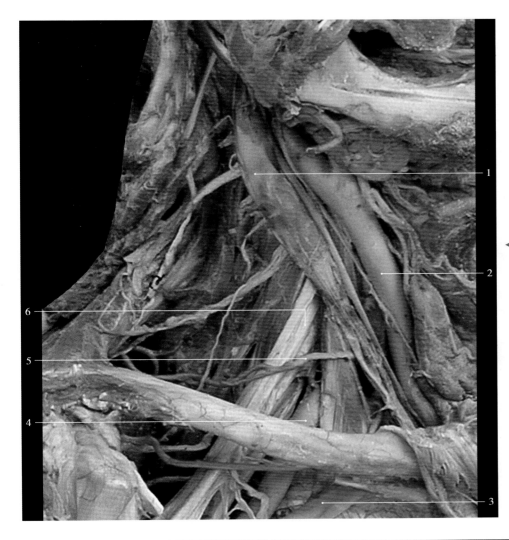

◀ 图 2-54　颈内静脉侧面观
Fig. 2-54　Lateral aspect of the internal jugular vein

1. 颈内静脉 internal jugular vein
2. 颈总动脉 common carotid artery
3. 锁骨下静脉 subclavian vein
4. 锁骨下动脉 subclavian artery
5. 颈横动脉 transverse cervical artery
6. 臂丛 brachial plexus

颈内静脉的应用解剖学要点

颈内静脉在颈动脉鞘内居于动脉的外侧,下行至胸锁关节的深面,与锁骨下静脉汇合形成头臂静脉,汇合处的夹角称颈静脉角,左侧的颈静脉角为胸导管的注入点,右侧的颈静脉角为右淋巴导管注入处。颈内静脉起始处膨大,称为颈静脉上球,右侧的上球比左侧的大,该球位于颈静脉窝内。颈内静脉的末端也有一个膨大称为颈静脉下球,位于胸锁乳突肌胸骨头与锁骨头所形成的锁骨上小窝的后方。在颈静脉下球的上方有一对瓣膜(图 2-52～图 2-54)。

应用解剖要点:

结扎一侧的颈内静脉不会影响脑部的血液回流。因此,颈内静脉可作为如肠系膜上静脉与下腔静脉搭桥术的移植体。临床上常选颈内静脉穿刺和插管通至上腔静脉,作为测定中心静脉压和输入深静脉营养的途径。

由于右侧的颈内静脉较粗,而且与头臂静脉几乎成一直线通上腔静脉。因此,颈内静脉穿刺和插管术宜在右侧施行。

穿刺和插管的部位常选在胸锁乳突肌前缘中点或稍上方,将胸锁乳突肌的前缘推向后施行,也可在胸锁乳突肌后缘中、下 1/3 交界处或在该肌的胸骨头与锁骨头之间的三角形间隙内进行。

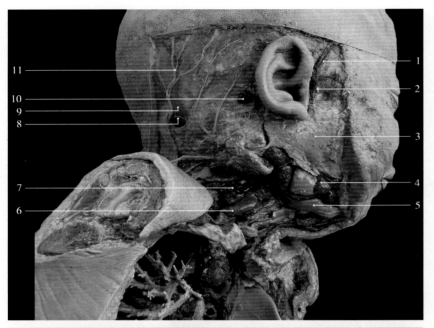

◀ 图 2-55　下颌下淋巴结
Fig. 2-55　Submandibular lymph nodes

1. 颞浅动脉 superficial temporal artery
2. 耳前淋巴结 preauricular lymph nodes
3. 腮腺 parotid gland
4. 下颌下淋巴结 submandibular lymph node
5. 下颌下腺 submandibular gland
6. 颈内静脉 internal jugular vein
7. 颈上深淋巴结 superior deep cervical lymph nodes
8. 枕淋巴结 occipital lymph nodes
9. 枕动脉 occipital artery
10. 乳突淋巴结 mastoid lymph node
11. 枕大神经 greater occipital nerve

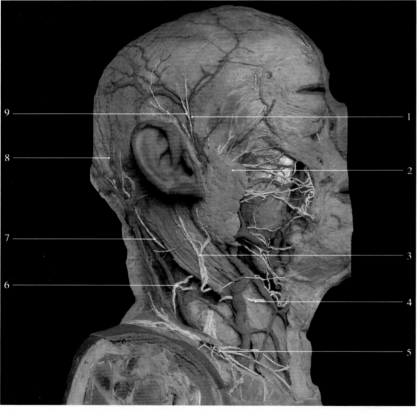

◀ 图 2-56　颈浅丛
Fig. 2-56　Superficial cervical plexus

1. 颞浅动脉 superficial temporal artery
2. 腮腺 parotid gland
3. 耳大神经 great auricular nerve
4. 颈横神经 transverse nerve of neck
5. 锁骨上神经 supraclavicular nerve
6. 副神经 accessory nerve
7. 枕小神经 lesser occipital nerve
8. 枕动脉 occipital artery
9. 颞浅神经 superficial temporal nerve

颈浅丛阻滞术的应用解剖学要点

颈浅丛自胸锁乳突肌后缘中点处浅出,位于颈阔肌深面,呈向上、下和横行向前的放射状分布于颈部皮肤,分支有枕小神经、耳大神经、颈横神经和锁骨上神经(图 2-56)。

颈浅丛阻滞术:进针点常选在患者颈部呈侧屈稍后伸位的胸锁乳突肌后缘中点处。

穿刺层次:皮肤→浅筋膜→深筋膜→颈阔肌→颈浅丛。

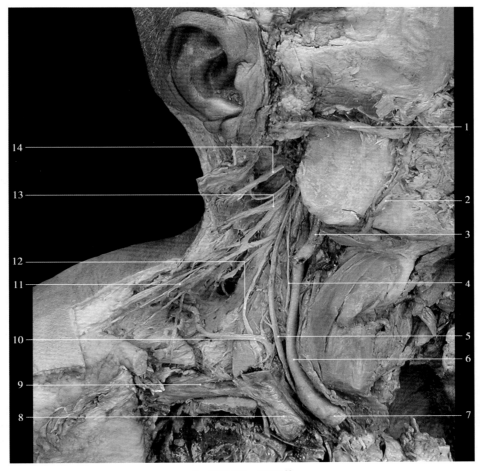

▲ 图2-57 颈深丛
Fig. 2-57 Deep cervical plexus

1. 腮腺管 parotid duct
2. 面动脉 facial artery
3. 颈内动脉 internal carotid artery
4. 颈交感干 cervical sympathetic trunk
5. 迷走神经 vagus nerve
6. 颈总动脉 common carotid artery
7. 头臂干 brachiocephalic trunk
8. 上腔静脉 superior vena cava
9. 锁骨下静脉 subclavian vein
10. 颈横动脉 transverse cervical artery
11. 锁骨上神经 supraclavicular nerve
12. 膈神经 phrenic nerve
13. 颈深丛 deep cervical plexus
14. 副神经 accessory nerve

颈深丛的应用解剖学要点

颈深丛位于$C_{1\sim4}$椎体侧面、胸锁乳突肌和颈内静脉深面、中斜角肌和肩胛提肌的前方。椎动脉和椎静脉于椎间孔处纵行于颈神经的前方(图2-57)。

应用解剖要点:

颈深丛阻滞术:进针点常选在乳突尖至颈动脉结节(C_6横突前方)的连线,从体表确定第2~4颈椎横突的位置,即乳突尖下1.5cm为C_2横突,乳突尖和锁骨中点连线的中点为C_4横突,上述两者之间为C_3横突。上述三点为进针点。

穿刺的层次为:皮肤→浅筋膜→深筋膜→胸锁乳突肌→相应颈椎的横突→颈丛根。

注意点:颈椎横突短,上下两横突间距较大,从颈外侧进针有误入颈段蛛网膜下隙或刺破椎动脉、椎静脉的危险,也有累及膈神经和喉返神经的可能。颈深丛不宜两侧同时阻滞。故在进药前一定要回抽见针内无回血或无回液方可推注药物。

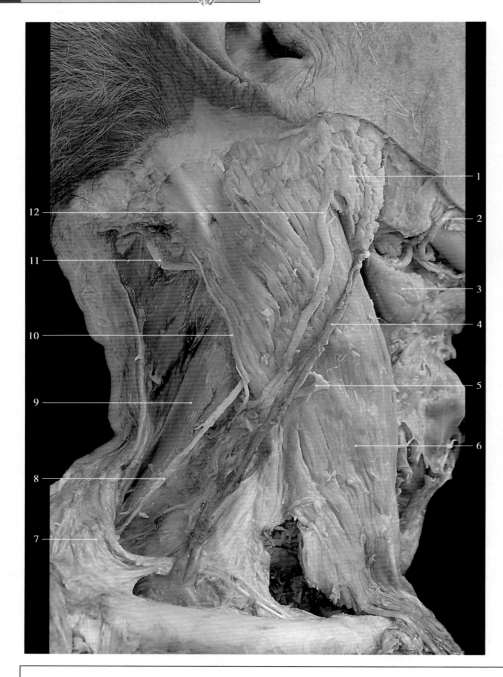

◀ 图 2-58　副神经
Fig. 2-58　Accessory nerve

1. 腮腺 parotid gland
2. 面动脉 facial artery
3. 下颌下腺 submandibular gland
4. 颈外静脉 external jugular vein
5. 颈横神经 transverse cervical nerve
6. 胸锁乳突肌 sternocleidomastoid
7. 斜方肌 trapezius
8. 副神经 accessory nerve
9. 头夹肌 splenius
10. 枕小神经 lesser occipital nerve
11. 第 3 颈神经后支 posterior branch of the 3rd cervical nerve
12. 耳大神经 greater auricular nerve

副神经在颈后三角内的应用解剖学要点

　　副神经与迷走神经伴行,穿颈静脉孔出颅后被胸锁乳突肌及二腹肌后腹所遮蔽,向后下方斜降,绕经颈内静脉前外侧,经枕动脉前侧进入胸锁乳突肌上部,并发支至胸锁乳突肌。然后至甲状软骨上缘稍上方,约平胸锁乳突肌后缘中点处穿出,继续斜向后下方,经过颈后三角,于此跨过肩胛提肌的表面。副神经在颈后三角内位置浅表,与颈浅淋巴结相邻。在临床出现的斜方肌瘫痪病例中,因在颈后三角内摘除淋巴结作活组织检查所引起的副神经受损约占 89.7%。

　　应用解剖要点:

　　副神经显露段(胸锁乳突肌后缘至斜方肌前缘之间)的长度为 50.04mm。副神经在出胸锁乳突肌后缘和入斜方肌前缘两处距乳突尖的距离分别为 63.11mm 和 83.35mm(图 2-58)。

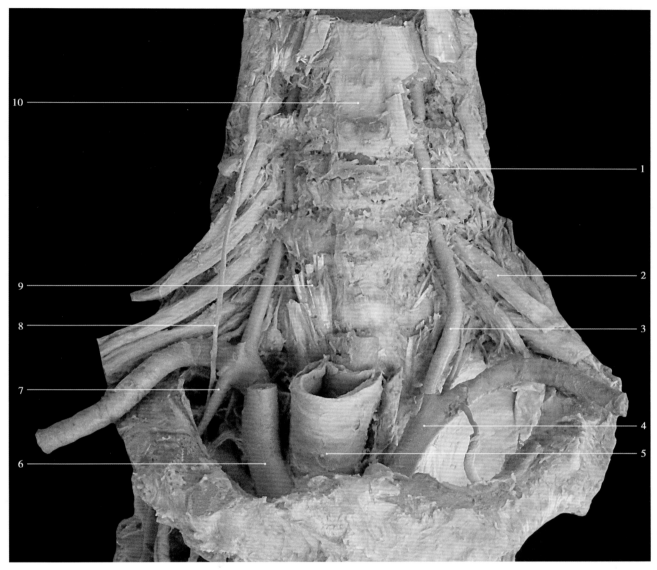

▲ 图 2-59　椎动脉的起始
Fig. 2-59　Onset of the vertebral artery

1. 椎动脉横突部 transverse part of vertebral artery
2. 臂丛 brachial plexus
3. 椎动脉颈部 cervical part of vertebral artery
4. 锁骨下动脉 subclavian artery
5. 气管 trachea
6. 头臂干 brachiocephalic trunk
7. 胸廓内动脉 internal thoracic artery
8. 膈神经 phrenic nerve
9. 颈长肌 longus colli
10. 前纵韧带 anterior longitudinal ligament

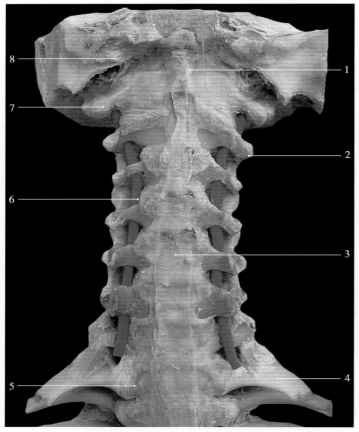

◀ 图 2-60　椎动脉与横突孔前面观
Fig. 2-60　Anterior aspect of the vertebral artery and the transverse foramen

1. 寰椎 atlas
2. 枢椎横突 transverse process of axis
3. 前纵韧带 anterior longitudinal ligament
4. 第 1 肋 the 1st rib
5. 胸肋关节 sternocostal joints
6. 椎动脉 vertebral artery
7. 寰椎横突 transverse process of atlas
8. 枕髁 occipital condyle

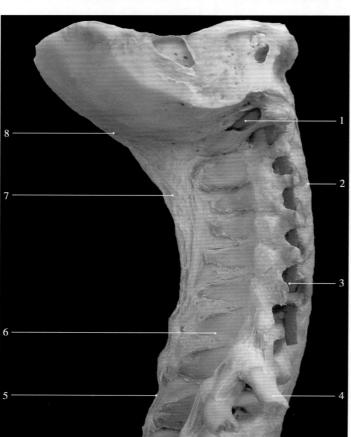

◀ 图 2-61　椎动脉颈段的走行侧面观
Fig. 2-61　Lateral aspect of the course of the cervical vertebral artery

1. 椎动脉寰椎部 atlantic part of vertebral artery
2. 前纵韧带 anterior longitudinal ligament
3. 椎动脉 vertebral artery
4. 第 1 肋 the 1st rib
5. 棘上韧带 supraspinous ligament
6. 第 7 颈椎棘突 spinous process of the 7th cervical vertebra
7. 项韧带 ligamentum nuchae
8. 枕外隆突 external occipital protuberance

第四节 颈根部结构

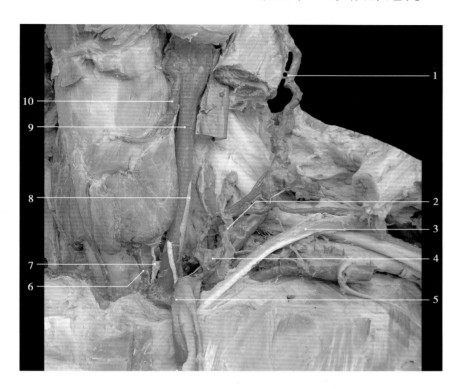

◀ 图 2-62　胸导管颈段（一）
Fig. 2-62　Cervical part of thoracic duct(1)

1. 颈外静脉 external jugular vein
2. 左颈干 left jugular trunk
3. 锁骨下肌 subclavius
4. 胸导管 thoracic duct
5. 左颈内静脉 left internal jugular vein
6. 甲状腺最下静脉 vena thyreoidea ima
7. 喉返神经 recurrent laryngeal nerve
8. 迷走神经 vagus nerve
9. 颈总动脉 common carotid artery
10. 甲状腺上动脉 superior thyroid artery

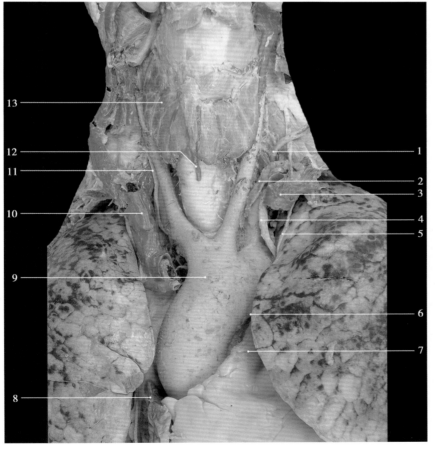

◀ 图 2-63　胸导管颈段（二）
Fig. 2-63　Cervical part of thoracic duct(2)

1. 甲状颈干 thyrocervical trunk
2. 胸导管颈段 cervical part of thoracic duct
3. 左锁骨下静脉 left subclavian vein
4. 左迷走神经 left vagus nerve
5. 左膈神经 left phrenic nerve
6. 左肺前缘 anterior margin of left lung
7. 肺动脉 pulmonary artery
8. 上腔静脉 superior vena cava
9. 升主动脉 ascending aorta
10. 右头臂静脉 right brachiocephalic vein
11. 右迷走神经 right vagus nerve
12. 甲状腺下静脉 inferior thyroid vein
13. 甲状腺 thyroid gland

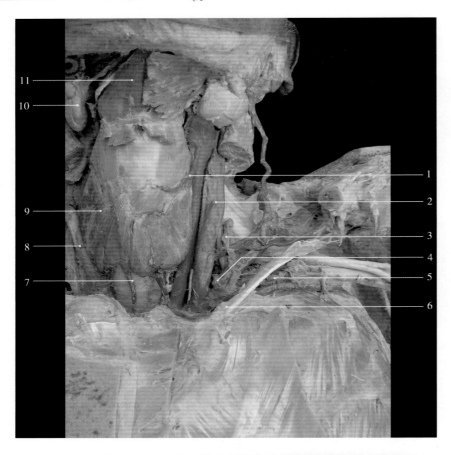

◀ 图 2-64 左锁骨下干、左颈干
Fig. 2-64 Left subclavian trunk and left jugular trunk

1. 甲状腺上动脉 superior thyroid artery
2. 颈内静脉 internal jugular vein
3. 左颈干 left jugular trunk
4. 胸导管 thoracic duct
5. 左锁骨下干 left subclavian trunk
6. 锁骨下肌 subclavius
7. 甲状腺下静脉 inferior thyroid vein
8. 右颈总动脉 right common carotid artery
9. 甲状腺 thyroid gland
10. 下颌下腺 submandibular gland
11. 舌骨舌肌 hyoglossus

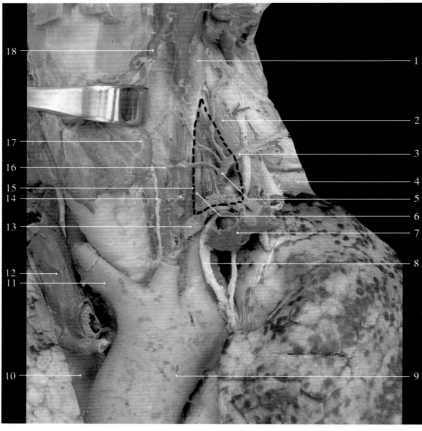

◀ 图 2-65 左侧椎动脉三角（一）
Fig. 2-65 Left triangle of vertebral artery（1）

1. 颈长肌 longus colli
2. 前斜角肌 scalenus anterior
3. 颈横动脉 transverse cervical artery
4. 锁骨下动脉 subclavian artery
5. 甲状颈干 thyrocervical trunk
6. 椎动脉 vertebral artery
7. 左锁骨下静脉 left subclavian vein
8. 左膈神经 left phrenic nerve
9. 主动脉弓 aortic arch
10. 上腔静脉 superior vena cava
11. 头臂干 brachiocephalic trunk
12. 右头臂静脉 right brachiocephalic vein
13. 胸导管 thoracic duct
14. 喉返神经 recurrent laryngeal nerve
15. 椎动脉三角 triangle of vertebral artery
16. 甲状腺下动脉 inferior thyroid artery
17. 甲状腺 thyroid gland
18. 甲状腺上动脉 superior thyroid artery

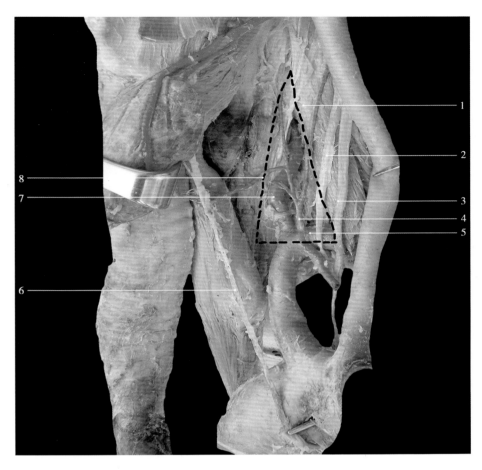

◀ 图 2-66 左侧椎动脉三角（二）
Fig. 2-66 Left triangle of vertebral artery（2）

1. 前斜角肌 scalenus anterior
2. 膈神经 phrenic nerve
3. 迷走神经 vagus nerve
4. 甲状颈干 thyrocervical trunk
5. 锁骨下动脉 subclavian artery
6. 左喉返神经 left recurrent laryngeal nerve
7. 椎动脉 vertebral artery
8. 椎动脉三角 triangle of vertebral artery

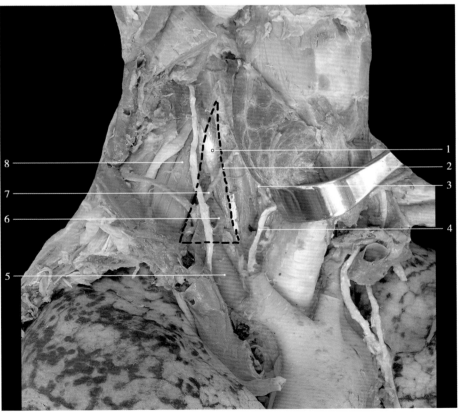

◀ 图 2-67 右侧椎动脉三角（一）
Fig. 2-67 Right triangle of vertebral artery（1）

1. 颈长肌 longus colli
2. 椎动脉三角 triangle of vertebral artery
3. 甲状腺下动脉 inferior thyroid artery
4. 左喉返神经 left recurrent laryngeal nerve
5. 锁骨下动脉 subclavian artery
6. 椎动脉 vertebral artery
7. 甲状腺下动脉 inferior thyroid artery
8. 前斜角肌 scalenus anterior

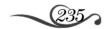

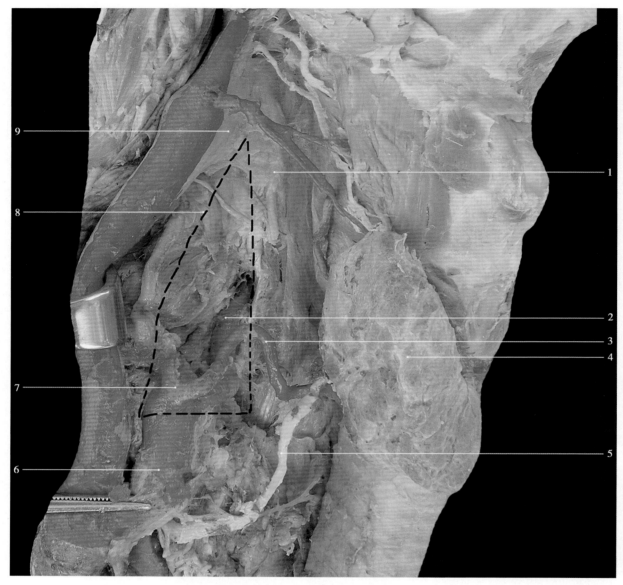

▲ 图 2-68　右侧椎动脉三角（二）
Fig. 2-68　Right triangle of vertebral artery（2）

1. 颈长肌 longus colli
2. 椎动脉 vertebral artery
3. 甲状腺下动脉 inferior thyroid artery
4. 甲状腺 thyroid gland
5. 喉返神经 recurrent laryngeal nerve
6. 锁骨下动脉 subclavian artery
7. 甲状颈干 thyrocervical trunk
8. 椎动脉三角 triangle of vertebral artery
9. 前斜角肌 scalenus anterior

椎动脉三角的应用解剖学要点

　　椎动脉三角位于颈根部的深层，椎体的两侧。三角的外侧界为前斜角肌的内侧缘，内侧界为颈长肌的外侧缘，下界为锁骨下动脉的第 1 段（即锁骨下动脉起始处至前斜角肌内侧缘），尖为第 6 颈椎横突前结节。椎动脉三角内的主要结构有：椎动脉、椎静脉、甲状腺下动脉（或甲状颈干）、颈交感干、颈胸神经节等（图 2-65 ～图 2-68）。

　　应用解剖要点：

　　椎动脉三角的后方为胸膜顶、第 7 颈椎横突、C_8 神经前支和第 1 肋颈；前方有颈动脉鞘、膈神经、甲状腺下动脉及胸导管（左）等。

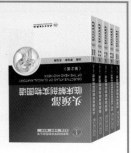
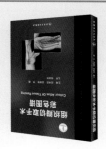
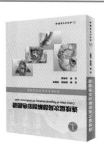
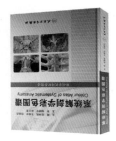
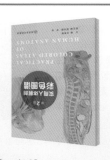
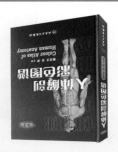

"影像"是临床医生洞察人体病理生理变化的"第三只眼"

—— 数百位"观千剑而识器"的影像专家帮你练就识破人体病理生理变化的火眼金睛

《中华影像医学丛书》
——影像科医师的"红色典藏"

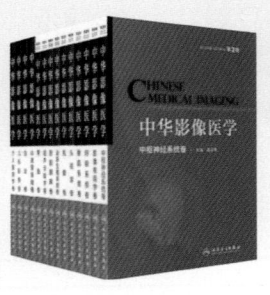

本套丛书共14卷，由医学影像学泰斗吴恩惠教授发起，是国内第一套医学影像学大型系列丛书。

《中华医学影像技术学》
——国内该领域专家理论与实践的全面展现

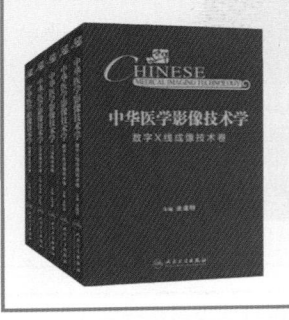

本套丛书共5卷，为中华医学会影像技术分会的倾心之作。

《实用放射学》

本书由中国医科大学附属第二医院郭启勇教授主编，内容丰富、翔实，侧重于实用，临床价值高。

《实用医学影像技术》

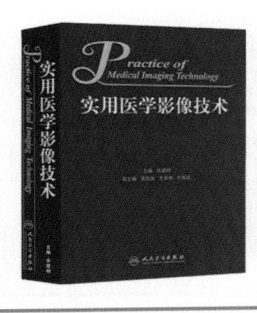

本书由中华医学会影像技术分会第七届主任委员余建明主编，为影像技师临床操作的案头必备。

《中国医师协会超声医师分会指南丛书》

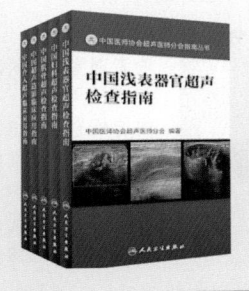

该套书为中国医师协会超声医师分会编著的用于规范临床超声实践的权威指南。

研究生规划教材·专科医师核心能力导引丛书

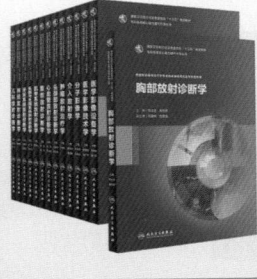

该套书以解决临床实际问题、提升临床思维能力为切入点和落脚点，回顾历史、剖析现状、展望未来。

购书请扫二维码
登录人卫智慧服务商城

了解更多图书，
请关注我们的公众号

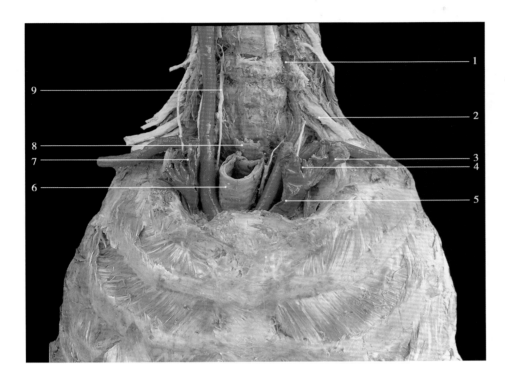

▶ 图 2-69　颈根部结构（一）
Fig. 2-69　Structures in the root of neck（1）

1. 椎动脉 vertebral artery
2. 臂丛 brachial plexus
3. 左锁骨下静脉 left subclavian vein
4. 胸导管 thoracic duct
5. 左头臂静脉 left brachiocephalic vein
6. 气管 trachea
7. 右颈内静脉 right internal jugular vein
8. 食管 esophagus
9. 喉返神经 recurrent laryngeal nerve

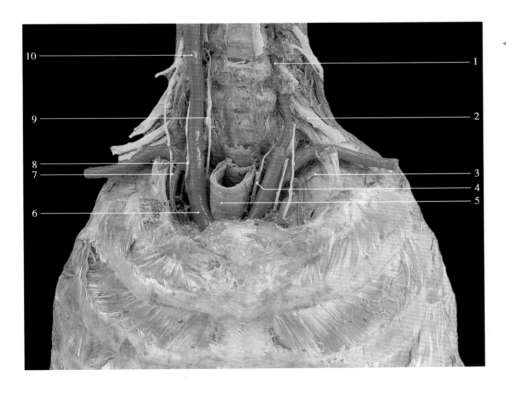

▶ 图 2-70　颈根部结构（头臂静脉已切除）（二）
Fig. 2-70　Structures in the root of neck（the brachiocephalic vein was removed）（2）

1. 椎动脉 vertebral artery
2. 臂丛 brachial plexus
3. 肺尖 apex of lung
4. 喉返神经 recurrent laryngeal nerve
5. 气管 trachea
6. 头臂干 brachiocephalic trunk
7. 膈神经 phrenic nerve
8. 迷走神经 vagus nerve
9. 右喉返神经 right recurrent laryngeal nerve
10. 颈总动脉 common carotid artery

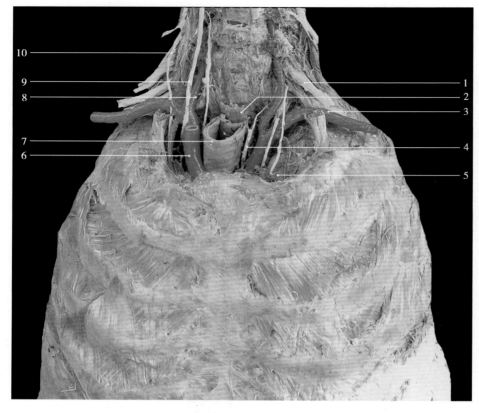

◀ 图 2-71 颈根部结构（颈总动脉已切除）（三）
Fig. 2-71 Structures in the root of neck (the common carotid artery was removed) (3)

1. 臂丛 brachial plexus
2. 食管 esophagus
3. 锁骨下动脉 subclavian artery
4. 喉返神经 recurrent laryngeal nerve
5. 肺尖 apex of lung
6. 头臂干 brachiocephalic trunk
7. 气管 trachea
8. 椎动脉 vertebral artery
9. 迷走神经 vagus nerve
10. 膈神经 phrenic nerve

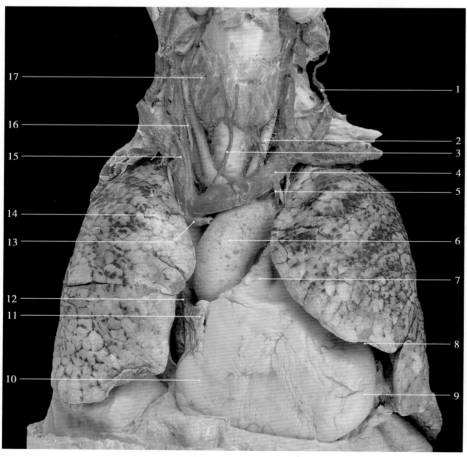

◀ 图 2-72 颈根部结构（胸前壁已打开）（四）
Fig. 2-72 Structures in the root of neck (the anterior thoracic wall was opened) (4)

1. 颈外静脉 external jugular vein
2. 左颈总动脉 left common carotid artery
3. 甲状腺下静脉 inferior thyroid vein
4. 左头臂静脉 left brachiocephalic vein
5. 左胸腺静脉 left thymic veins
6. 主动脉弓 aortic arch
7. 肺动脉 pulmonary artery
8. 心切迹 cardiac notch
9. 心尖 cardiac apex
10. 右心室 right ventricle
11. 右心耳 right auricle
12. 上腔静脉 superior vena cava
13. 右胸腺静脉 right thymic veins
14. 右肺 right lung
15. 右头臂静脉 right brachiocephalic vein
16. 膈神经 phrenic nerve
17. 甲状腺 thyroid gland

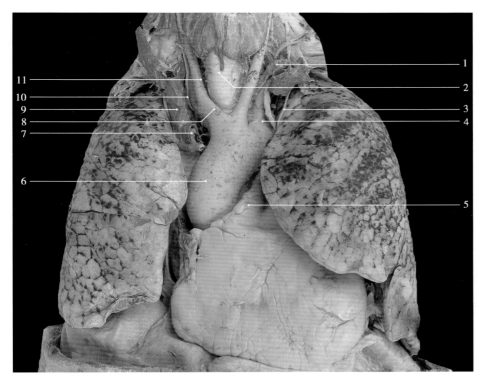

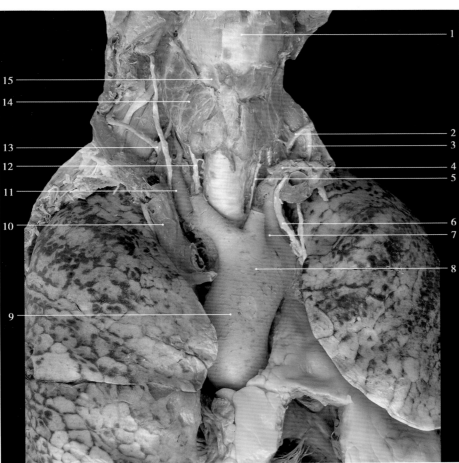

◀ 图2-73　颈根部结构（胸前壁已打开）（五）
Fig. 2-73　Structures in the root of neck（the anterior thoracic wall was opened）（5）

1. 胸导管 thoracic duct
2. 气管 trachea
3. 左膈神经 left phrenic nerve
4. 左锁骨下动脉 left subclavian artery
5. 肺动脉 pulmonary artery
6. 升主动脉 ascending aorta
7. 上腔静脉 superior vena cava
8. 头臂干 brachiocephalic trunk
9. 右头臂静脉 right brachiocephalic vein
10. 右膈神经 right phrenic nerve
11. 右颈总动脉 right common carotid artery

◀ 图2-74　颈根部结构（胸前壁已打开）（六）
Fig. 2-74　Structures in the root of neck（the anterior thoracic wall was opened）（6）

1. 喉结 laryngeal prominence
2. 颈横动脉 transverse cervical artery
3. 膈神经 phrenic nerve
4. 胸导管 thoracic duct
5. 左喉返神经 left recurrent laryngeal nerve
6. 迷走神经 vagus nerve
7. 锁骨下动脉 subclavian artery
8. 主动脉弓 aortic arch
9. 升主动脉 ascending aorta
10. 头臂静脉 brachiocephalic vein
11. 颈总动脉 common carotid artery
12. 喉返神经 recurrent laryngeal nerve
13. 甲状颈干 thyrocervical trunk
14. 甲状腺 thyroid gland
15. 环状软骨 cricoid cartilage

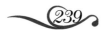

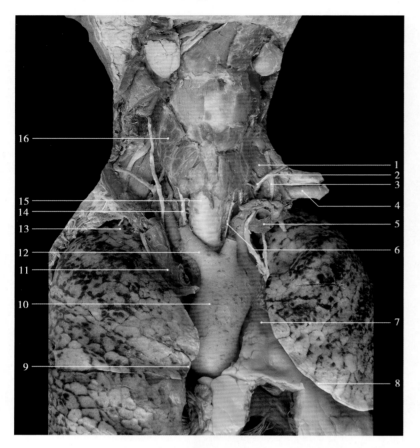

◀ 图 2-75 颈根部结构（胸前壁已打开）
（七）
Fig. 2-75 Structures in the root of neck
(the anterior thoracic wall was opened)
(7)

1. 前斜角肌 scalenus anterior
2. 甲状颈干 thyrocervical trunk
3. 膈神经 phrenic nerve
4. 左锁骨下动脉 left subclavian artery
5. 左锁骨下静脉 left subclavian vein
6. 左喉返神经 left recurrent laryngeal nerve
7. 肺动脉 pulmonary artery
8. 左肺前缘 anterior margin of left lung
9. 右肺前缘 anterior margin of right lung
10. 升主动脉 ascending aorta
11. 右头臂静脉 right brachiocephalic vein
12. 头臂干 brachiocephalic trunk
13. 右肺尖 apex of right lung
14. 右喉返神经 right recurrent laryngeal nerve
15. 气管颈段 cervical part of trachea
16. 甲状腺侧叶 lateral lobe of thyroid gland

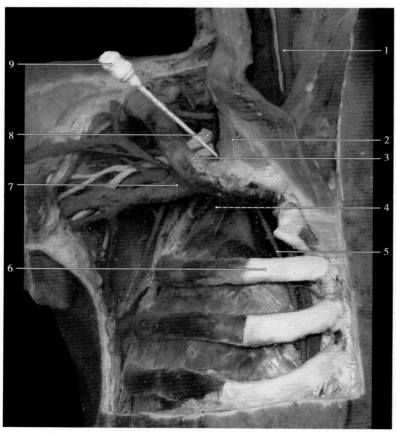

◀ 图 2-76 锁骨下静脉穿刺术进针点
Fig. 2-76 Needling point of the subclavian vein puncture

1. 颈总动脉 common carotid artery
2. 胸锁乳突肌锁骨头 clavicular head of sternocleidomastoid
3. 锁骨 clavicle
4. 肺尖 apex of lung
5. 胸廓内动脉 internal thoracic artery
6. 第 2 肋软骨 the 2nd costal cartilage
7. 锁骨下静脉 subclavian vein
8. 臂丛 brachial plexus
9. 穿刺针 transfixion pin

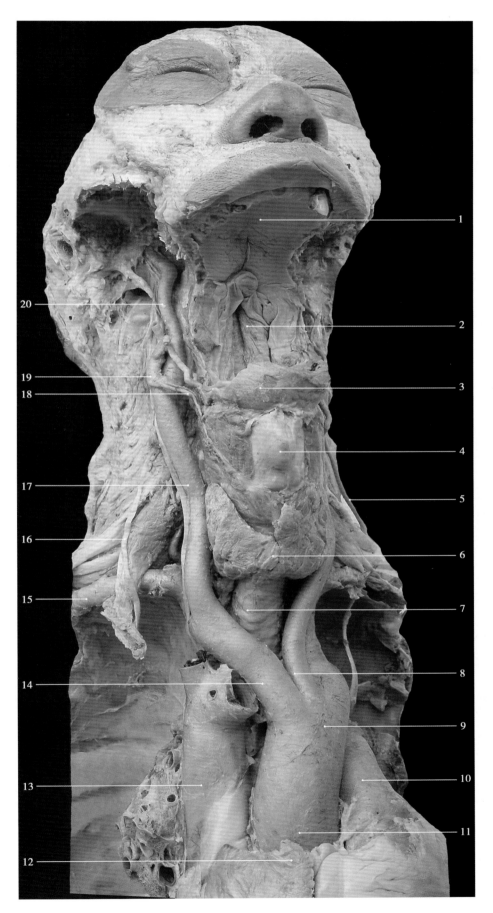

◀ 图 2-77 头臂干
Fig. 2-77 Brachiocephalic trunk

1. 硬腭 hard palate
2. 咽后壁 retropharyngeal wall
3. 舌骨体 body of hyoid bone
4. 喉结 laryngeal prominence
5. 迷走神经 vagus nerve
6. 甲状腺 thyroid gland
7. 气管 trachea
8. 左颈总动脉 left common carotid artery
9. 主动脉弓 aortic arch
10. 肺动脉 pulmonary artery
11. 升主动脉 ascending aorta
12. 右心耳 right auricle
13. 上腔静脉 superior vena cava
14. 头臂干 brachiocephalic trunk
15. 锁骨下动脉 subclavian artery
16. 膈神经 phrenic nerve
17. 右颈总动脉 right common carotid artery
18. 甲状腺上动脉 superior thyroid artery
19. 颈外动脉 external carotid artery
20. 颈内动脉 internal carotid artery

 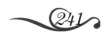

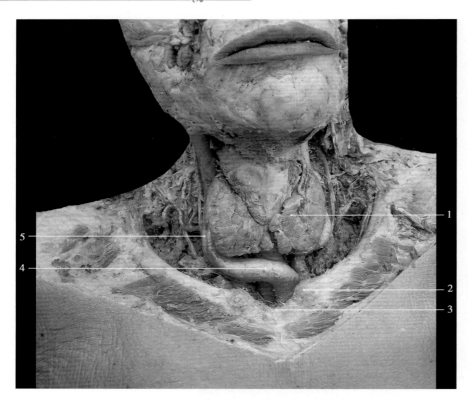

◀ 图 2-78　头臂干位置变异
（一）
Fig. 2-78　Location variation
of the brachiocephalic trunk
(1)

1. 甲状腺 thyroid gland
2. 左胸锁关节 left sternocla-
vicular joint
3. 颈静脉切迹 jugular notch
4. 变异头臂干 variation of brachiocephalic trunk
5. 右颈总动脉 right common
carotid artery

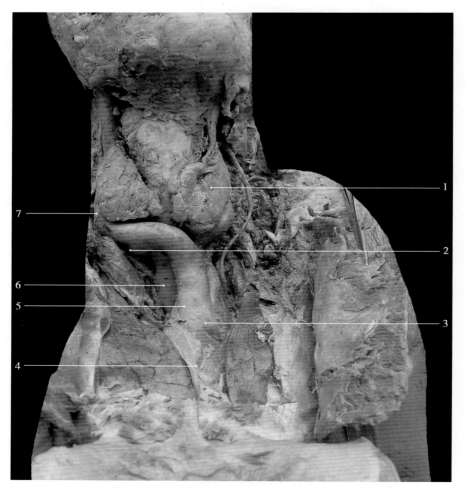

◀ 图 2-79　头臂干位置变异
（二）
Fig. 2-79　Location variation
of the brachiocephalic trunk
(2)

1. 甲状腺 thyroid gland
2. 右锁骨下动脉 right subcla-
vian artery
3. 主动脉弓 aortic arch
4. 升主动脉 ascending aorta
5. 头臂干 brachiocephalic trunk
6. 气管 trachea
7. 右颈总动脉 right common
carotid artery

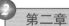

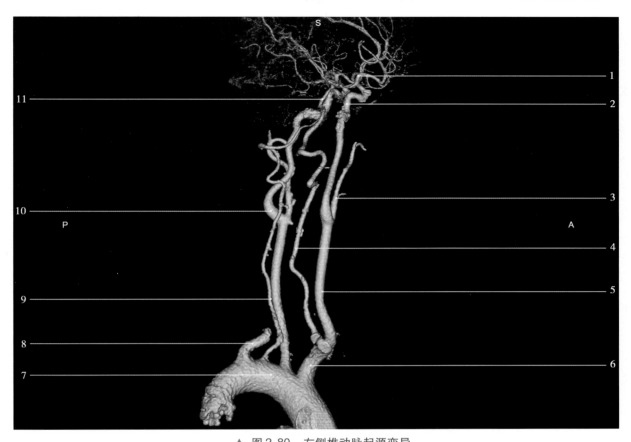

▲ 图2-80 左侧椎动脉起源变异

Fig. 2-80 Origin variation of the left vertebral artery

1. 大脑中动脉 middle cerebral artery
2. 颈内动脉海绵窦部 cavernous part of internal carotid artery
3. 颈外动脉 external carotid artery
4. 右侧椎动脉 right vertebral artery
5. 颈总动脉 common carotid artery
6. 头臂干 brachiocephalic trunk

7. 主动脉弓 aortic arch
8. 左锁骨下动脉 left subclavian artery
9. 左侧椎动脉 left vertebral artery
10. 颈动脉窦 carotid sinus
11. 基底动脉 basilar artery

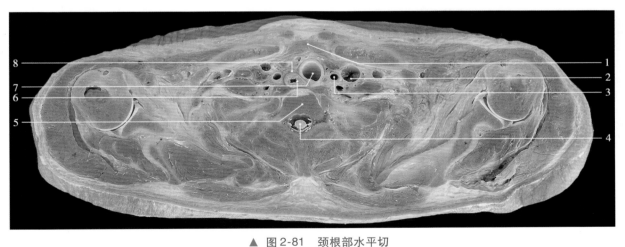

▲ 图2-81 颈根部水平切

Fig. 2-81 Horizontal section of the root of neck

1. 舌骨下肌群 infrahyoid muscles
2. 颈内静脉 internal jugular vein
3. 颈内动脉 internal carotid artery
4. 颈段脊髓 cervical part of spinal cord

5. 椎体 vertebral body
6. 食管 esophagus
7. 气管 trachea
8. 甲状腺侧叶 lateral lobe of thyroid gland

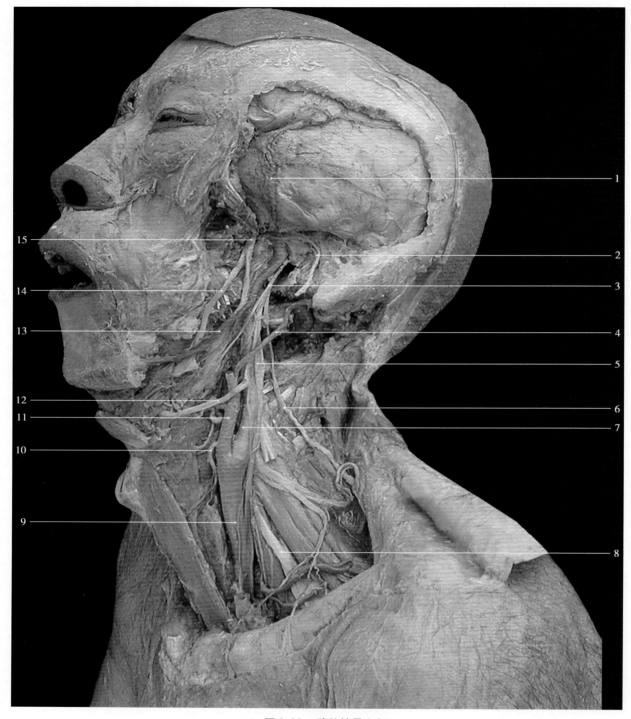

▲ 图 2-82 臂丛锁骨上部
Fig. 2-82 Supraclavicular part of brachial plexus

1. 脑膜中动脉 middle meningeal artery
2. 面神经 facial nerve
3. 舌咽神经 glossopharyngeal nerve
4. 枕动脉 occipital artery
5. 迷走神经 vagus nerve
6. 副神经 accessory nerve
7. 颈内动脉 internal carotid artery
8. 臂丛 brachial plexus

9. 颈总动脉 common carotid artery
10. 甲状腺上动脉 superior thyroid artery
11. 颈外动脉 external carotid artery
12. 舌下神经 hypoglossal nerve
13. 下牙槽动脉 inferior alveolar artery
14. 舌神经 lingual nerve
15. 下颌神经 mandibular nerve

臂丛锁骨上部阻滞术的应用解剖学要点

臂丛锁骨上部主要是臂丛的根和干。

1. $C_{5\sim8}$ 和 T_1 前支分别从相应的椎间孔行向外侧，$C_{5\sim7}$ 脊神经前支通过椎动脉的后方外行，臂丛各根在锁骨下动脉第 2 段的上方经过斜角肌间隙，在此处 $C_{5,6}$ 合成上干，C_7 延续为中干，C_8 和 T_1 的大部纤维合成下干。

2. 臂丛的上、中、下干行于颈侧区下部，与锁骨下动脉第 1 段一同跨越第 1 肋的上面，上、中干在此处位于锁骨下动脉的上方，而下干则位于动脉的后方。臂丛的三干进行中，与斜角肌和锁骨下血管共同被椎前筋膜所包绕（图 2-82）。

应用解剖要点：

1. 斜角肌间沟入路（胸锁乳突肌锁骨头后缘平环状软骨摸到前斜角肌肌腹后稍向外即为斜角肌间沟）。

穿刺层次：皮肤→浅筋膜→深筋膜→颈阔肌→斜角肌间沟→臂丛锁骨上部。

该点入路易误穿入颈段硬膜外隙刺伤脊髓颈段或椎动脉等。药物也可侵及颈段交感干、星状神经节和膈神经等。

2. 锁骨中点上方 1.0cm 处进针。

穿刺层次：皮肤→浅筋膜→深筋膜→颈阔肌→臂丛。

该点穿刺有刺破胸膜顶而引发气胸的可能，也可引起膈神经和星状神经节被阻滞的症状。

前臂尺侧的神经分布主要来自于 C_8 和 T_1 组成的臂丛下干，行该点阻滞时，因要防止穿刺过度靠内刺破胸膜顶，易引起进针深度不够和药物不及下干，是臂丛锁骨上阻滞术引起前臂尺侧效果不佳的解剖学原因。

第五节 甲 状 腺

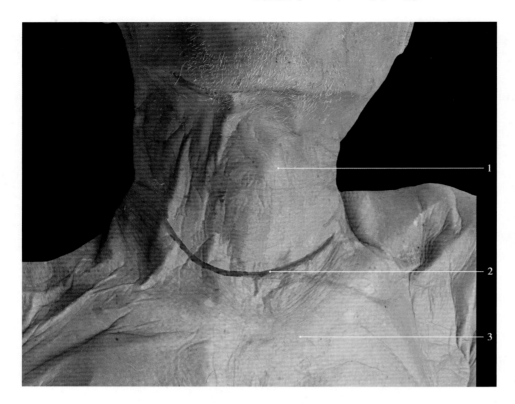

◀ 图 2-83 甲状腺手术切口（一）

Fig. 2-83 Incision of the thyroid operation (1)

1. 喉结 laryngeal prominence
2. 切口划线 incision line
3. 胸锁关节 sternoclavicular joint

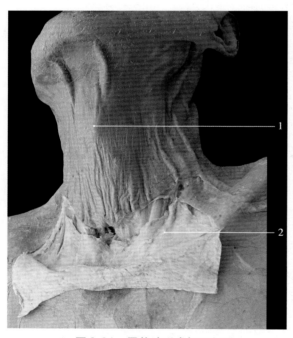

▲ 图 2-84 甲状腺手术切口（二）

Fig. 2-84 Incision of the thyroid operation (2)

1. 喉结 laryngeal prominence
2. 颈阔肌 platysma

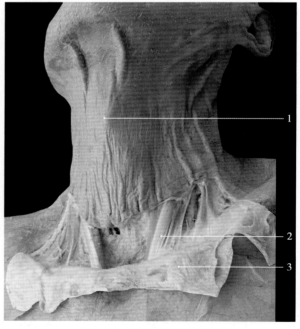

▲ 图 2-85 甲状腺手术切口（三）

Fig. 2-85 Incision of the thyroid operation (3)

1. 喉结 laryngeal prominence
2. 胸锁乳突肌胸骨头 sternal head of sternocleidomastoid
3. 颈阔肌（翻向下）platysma（it was turned down）

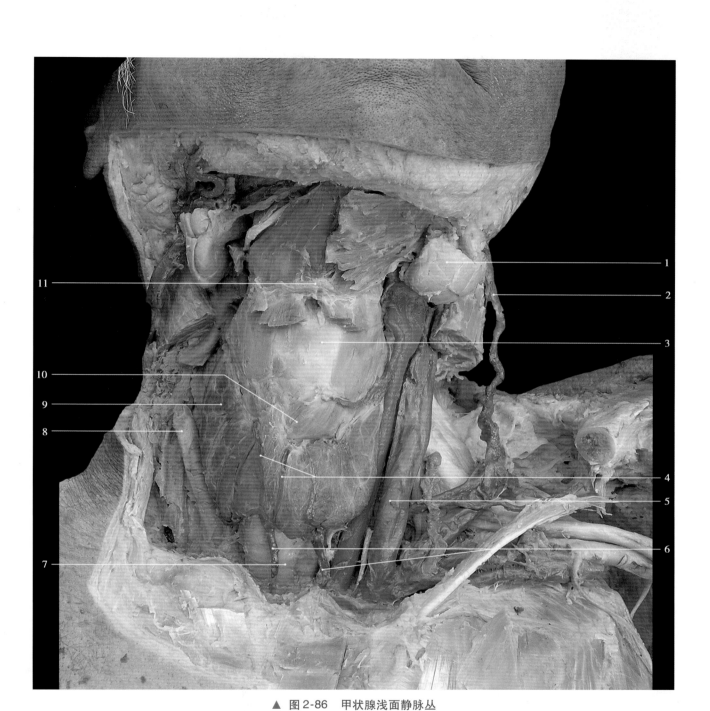

▲ 图 2-86 甲状腺浅面静脉丛
Fig. 2-86 Superficial venous plexus of the thyroid gland

1. 下颌下腺 submandibular gland
2. 颈外静脉 external jugular vein
3. 喉结 laryngeal prominence
4. 静脉丛 venous plexus
5. 左颈内静脉 left internal jugular vein
6. 甲状腺下静脉 inferior thyroid veins
7. 气管颈段 cervical part of trachea
8. 右颈总动脉 right common carotid artery
9. 甲状腺 thyroid gland
10. 环状软骨 cricoid cartilage
11. 舌骨 hyoid bone

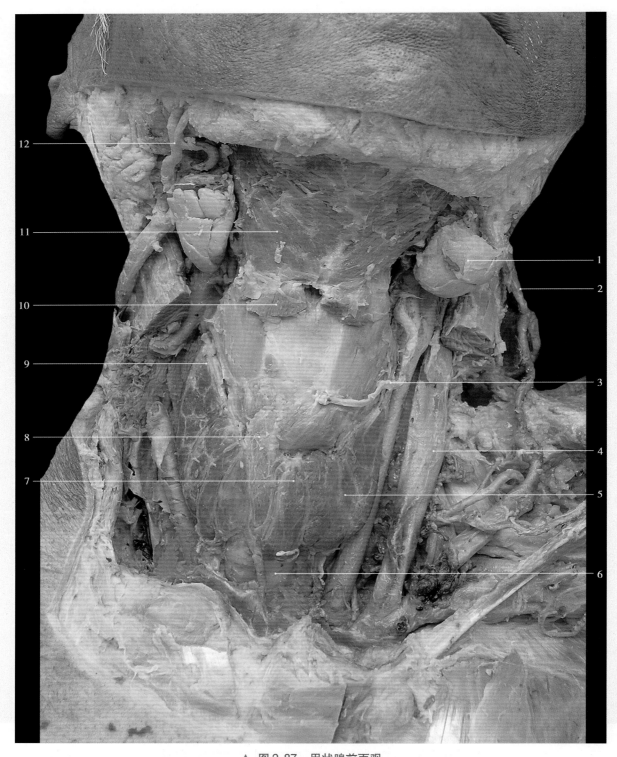

▲ 图 2-87 甲状腺前面观

Fig. 2-87 Anterior aspect of the thyroid gland

1. 下颌下腺 submandibular gland   7. 甲状腺峡部 isthmus of thyroid gland
2. 颈外静脉 external jugular vein   8. 锥状叶 pyramidal lobe
3. 甲状腺上动脉 superior thyroid artery   9. 甲状腺上极 upper pole of thyroid gland
4. 颈内静脉 internal jugular vein   10. 胸骨舌骨肌 sternohyoid
5. 甲状腺 thyroid gland   11. 下颌舌骨肌 mylohyoid
6. 气管颈段 cervical part of trachea   12. 面动脉 facial artery

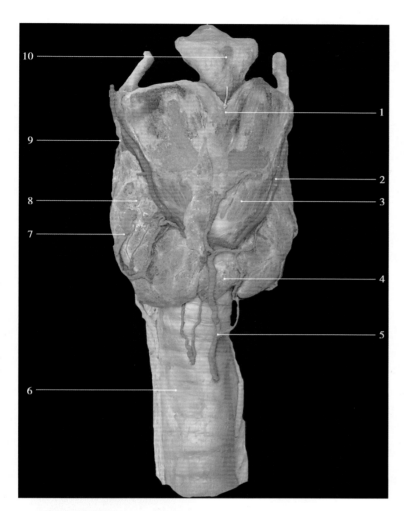

▲ 图 2-88 甲状腺血管前面观
Fig. 2-88 Anterior aspect of the thyroid vessels

1. 喉结 laryngeal prominence
2. 甲状腺上动脉 superior thyroid artery
3. 环甲肌 cricothyroid
4. 甲状腺峡部 isthmus of thyroid gland
5. 甲状腺下静脉 inferior thyroid vein
6. 气管 trachea
7. 甲状腺中静脉 middle thyroid vein
8. 甲状腺 thyroid gland
9. 甲状腺上静脉 superior thyroid vein
10. 会厌 epiglottis

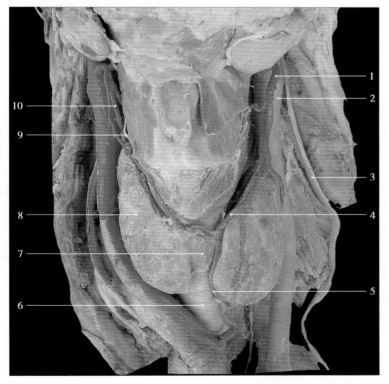

▲ 图 2-89 甲状腺上动脉
Fig. 2-89 Superior thyroid artery

1. 甲状腺上动脉 superior thyroid artery
2. 颈外动脉 external carotid artery
3. 迷走神经 vagus nerve
4. 腺前支 anterior glandular branch
5. 甲状腺下静脉 inferior thyroid vein
6. 气管 trachea
7. 甲状腺峡部 isthmus of thyroid gland
8. 甲状腺侧叶 lateral lobe of thyroid gland
9. 喉上神经内支 internal branch of superior laryngeal nerve
10. 喉上动脉 superior laryngeal artery

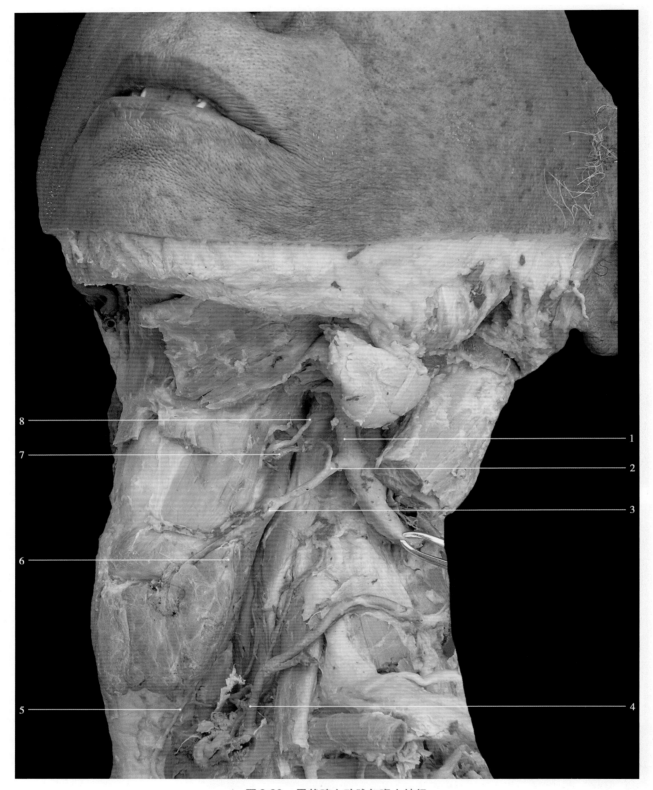

▲ 图 2-90　甲状腺上动脉与喉上神经

Fig. 2-90　Superior thyroid artery and superior laryngeal nerve

1. 颈外动脉 external carotid artery
2. 甲状腺上动脉 superior thyroid artery
3. 腺体支 glandular branch
4. 甲状颈干 thyrocervical trunk
5. 喉返神经 recurrent laryngeal nerve
6. 甲状腺上极 upper pole of thyroid gland
7. 喉上动脉内支 internal branch of superior laryngeal artery
8. 喉上神经内支 internal branch of superior laryngeal nerve

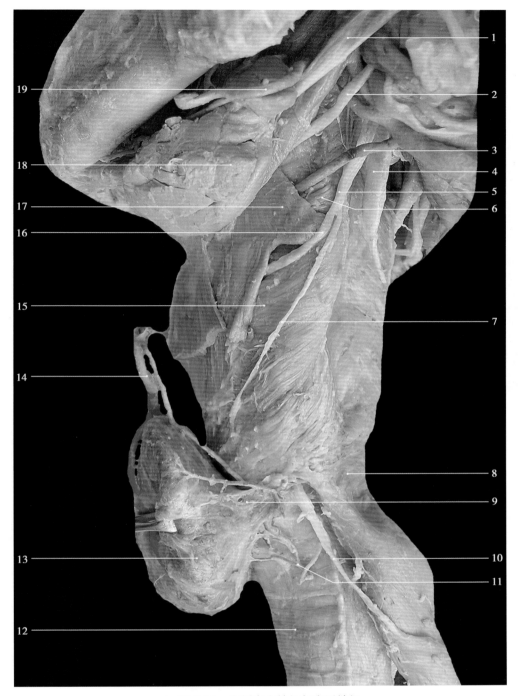

▲ 图 2-91　左侧喉上神经与喉返神经

Fig. 2-91　Left superior laryngeal nerve and recurrent laryngeal nerve

1. 二腹肌后腹 posterior belly of digastric muscle
2. 舌下神经 hypoglossal nerve
3. 舌动脉 lingual artery
4. 颈上神经节 superior cervical ganglion
5. 喉上神经 superior laryngeal nerve
6. 咽上缩肌 superior constrictor of pharynx
7. 喉上神经外支 external branch of superior laryngeal nerve
8. 食管第1狭窄 the 1st stenosis of esophagus
9. 甲状腺悬韧带 suspensory ligament of thyroid gland
10. 喉返神经 recurrent laryngeal nerve

11. 甲状腺下动脉 inferior thyroid artery
12. 气管 trachea
13. 甲状腺 thyroid gland
14. 甲状腺上动脉 superior thyroid artery
15. 咽中缩肌 middle constrictor of pharynx
16. 喉上神经内支 internal branch of superior laryngeal nerve
17. 下颌舌骨肌 mylohyoid
18. 下颌下腺 submandibular gland
19. 面动脉 facial artery

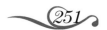

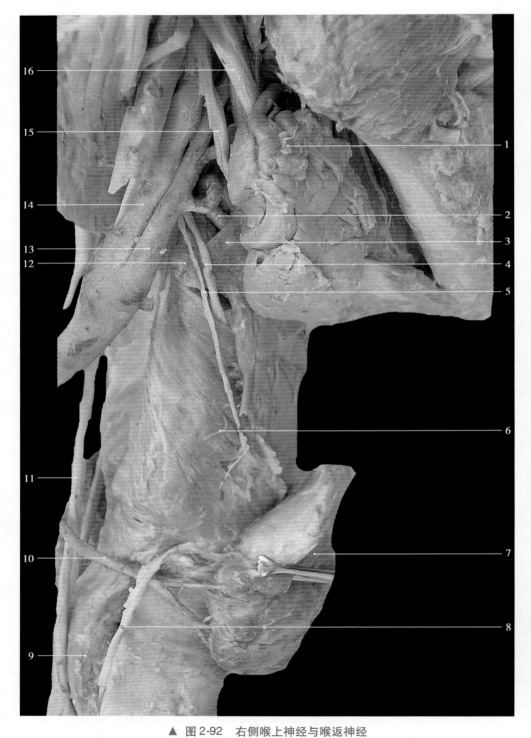

▲ 图 2-92　右侧喉上神经与喉返神经

Fig. 2-92　Right superior laryngeal nerve and recurrent laryngeal nerve

1. 下颌下腺 submandibular gland
2. 舌动脉 lingual artery
3. 下颌舌骨肌 mylohyoid
4. 喉上神经内支 internal branch of superior laryngeal nerve
5. 喉上神经外支 external branch of superior laryngeal nerve
6. 咽中缩肌 middle constrictor of pharynx
7. 甲状腺 thyroid gland
8. 喉返神经 recurrent laryngeal nerve

9. 食管 esophagus
10. 甲状腺下动脉 inferior thyroid artery
11. 迷走神经 vagus nerve
12. 舌骨大角 greater cornu of hyoid bone
13. 颈外动脉 external carotid artery
14. 颈内动脉 internal carotid artery
15. 舌下神经 hypoglossal nerve
16. 二腹肌后腹 posterior belly of digastric

甲状腺上动脉与喉上神经关系的应用解剖学要点

　　甲状腺手术并发喉上神经损伤的发生率为 0.4%～1.0%,引起喉上神经损伤的重要原因之一就是对甲状腺侧叶和喉上部及喉上动脉与喉上神经有关的应用解剖知识了解不足(图 2-89、图 2-90)。

　　应用解剖要点：

　　为了便于描述甲状腺上动脉与喉上神经的位置关系,通常以舌骨大角至环状软骨中点作一连线,在此线的上、中、下三段记录其相互关系；

　　1. 连线上段　89.2% 的甲状腺上动脉与喉上神经外支紧密伴行,神经在动脉的内侧者为 80.4%；后方者为 8.8%；10.8% 因甲状腺上动脉起点较低而未与神经伴行。

　　2. 连线中段　在该段全部动脉与神经紧密伴行,85.3% 的神经位于动脉的内侧,13.7% 的喉上神经外支位于甲状腺上动脉的后方,在动脉的两分支之间仅为 1.0%。

　　3. 连线下段　在此段内,神经与动脉很快分离,神经向内前下方斜行入环甲肌,动脉向外下入腺体上极。

　　当喉上神经外支入环甲肌点平甲状腺上极上方时,神经与动脉距离约 7.0mm；若入肌点平上极下方时,神经距动脉约 11.0mm。因此,结扎甲状腺上血管的位置,越靠近腺体安全系数越大,结扎位置过高,可能牵涉喉上神经外支。施行手术时,应慎重分离紧靠血管内后方的喉上神经外支。当甲状腺肿大时,应向上内推动血管,使其靠近神经,故此时紧贴腺体表面结扎血管非常重要。

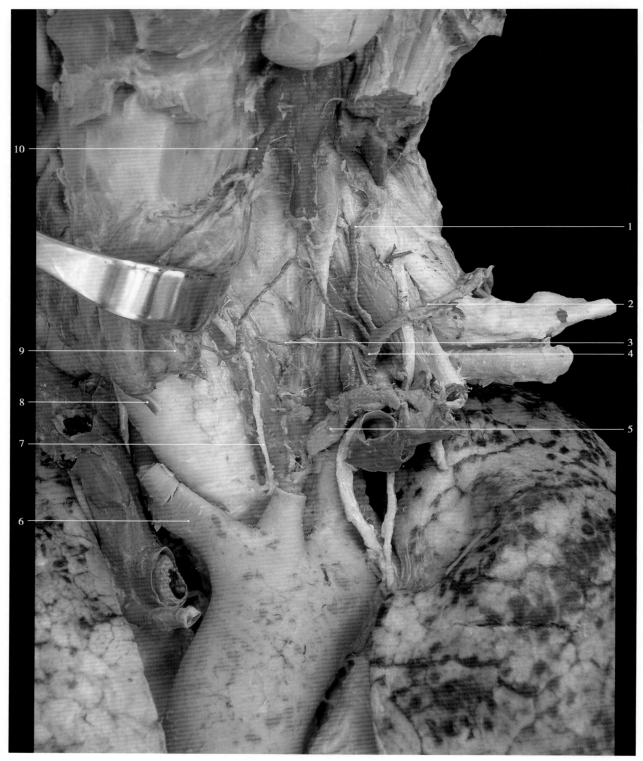

▲ 图 2-93　左甲状腺下动脉与喉返神经的关系

Fig. 2-93　Relationship between the left inferior thyroid artery and the recurrent laryngeal nerve

1. 颈升动脉 ascending cervical artery
2. 颈横动脉 transverse cervical artery
3. 甲状腺下动脉 inferior thyroid artery
4. 甲状颈干 thyrocervical trunk
5. 胸导管 thoracic duct

6. 头臂干 brachiocephalic trunk
7. 喉返神经 recurrent laryngeal nerve
8. 甲状腺下静脉 inferior thyroid vein
9. 甲状腺 thyroid gland
10. 甲状腺上动脉 superior thyroid artery

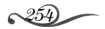

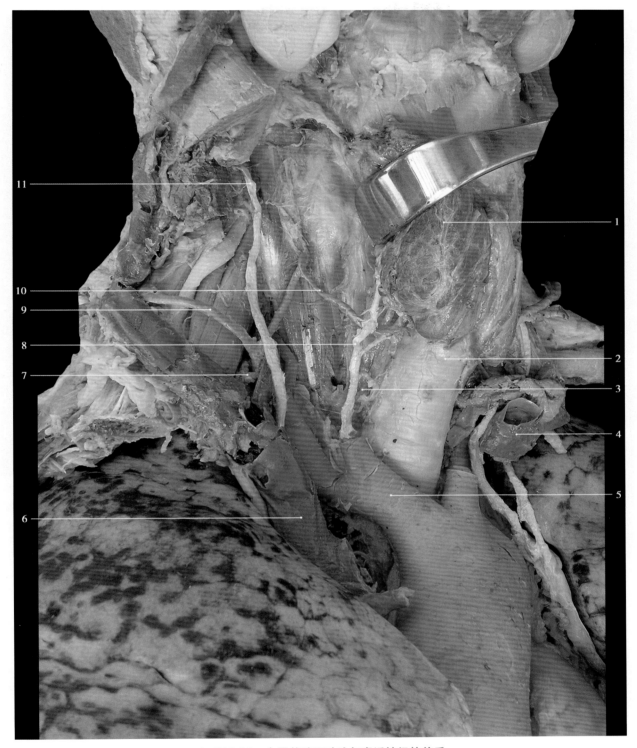

▲ 图2-94　右甲状腺下动脉与喉返神经的关系

Fig. 2-94　Relationship between the right inferior thyroid artery and the recurrent laryngeal nerve

1. 甲状腺 thyroid gland
2. 气管颈段 cervical part of trachea
3. 食管 esophagus
4. 左锁骨下静脉 left subclavian vein
5. 头臂干 brachiocephalic trunk
6. 右头臂静脉 right brachiocephalic vein
7. 甲状颈干 thyrocervical trunk
8. 喉返神经 recurrent laryngeal nerve
9. 颈横动脉 transverse cervical artery
10. 甲状腺下动脉 inferior thyroid artery
11. 膈神经 phrenic nerve

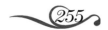

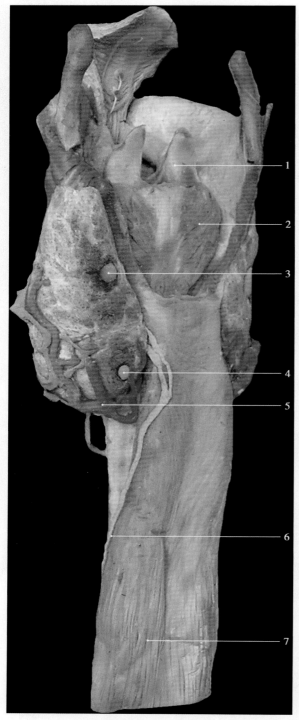

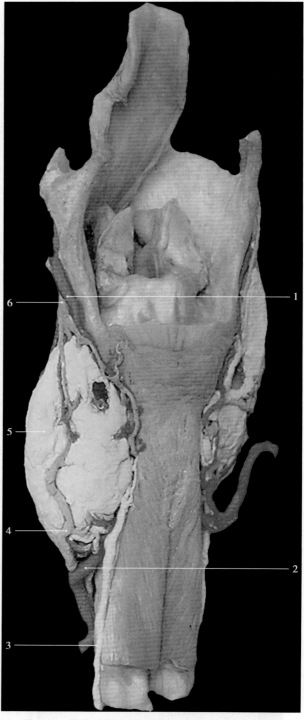

▲ 图 2-95　甲状腺下动脉与喉返神经的关系左侧面观(一)
Fig. 2-95　Left aspect of the relationship between the inferior thyroid artery and the recurrent laryngeal nerve (1)

1. 杓状软骨 arytenoid cartilage
2. 环杓后肌 posterior cricoarytenoid
3. 上甲状旁腺 superior parathyroid gland
4. 下甲状旁腺 inferior parathyroid gland
5. 甲状腺下动脉 inferior thyroid artery
6. 喉返神经 recurrent laryngeal nerve
7. 食管 esophagus

▲ 图 2-96　甲状腺下动脉与喉返神经的关系左侧面观(二)
Fig. 2-96　Left aspect of the relationship between the inferior thyroid artery and the recurrent laryngeal nerve (2)

1. 甲状腺上动脉 superior thyroid artery
2. 甲状腺下动脉 inferior thyroid artery
3. 喉返神经 recurrent laryngeal nerve
4. 甲状腺下静脉 inferior thyroid vein
5. 甲状腺 thyroid gland
6. 甲状腺上静脉 superior thyroid vein

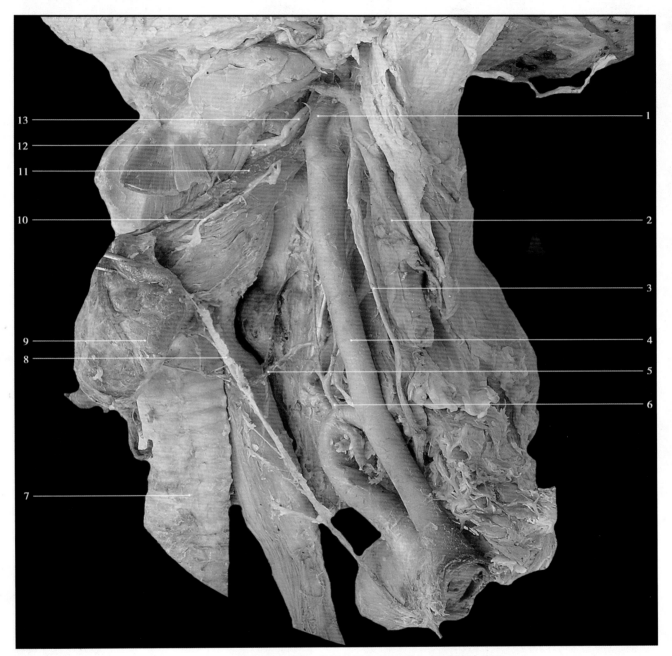

▲ 图2-97 左侧喉上神经、喉返神经与甲状腺上、下动脉的关系

Fig. 2-97　Relationship of the left superior laryngeal nerve，the recurrent laryngeal nerve，
the superior thyroid artery and the inferior thyroid artery

1. 颈外动脉 external carotid artery
2. 颈内静脉 internal jugular vein
3. 迷走神经 vagus nerve
4. 颈总动脉 common carotid artery
5. 甲状腺下动脉 inferior thyroid artery
6. 甲状颈干 thyrocervical trunk
7. 气管 trachea
8. 喉返神经 recurrent laryngeal nerve
9. 甲状腺 thyroid gland
10. 喉上神经外支 external branch of superior laryngeal nerve
11. 甲状腺上动脉 superior thyroid artery
12. 喉上神经内侧支 internal branch of superior laryngeal nerve
13. 喉上神经 superior laryngeal nerve

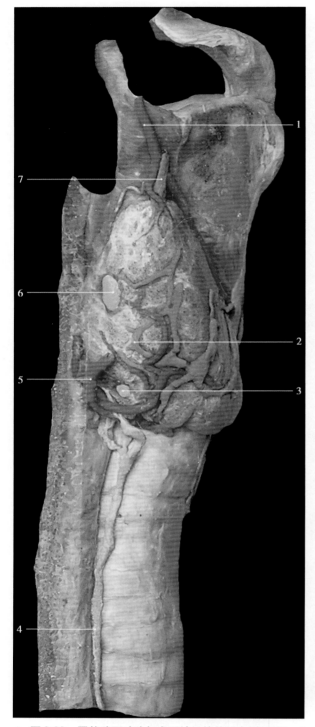

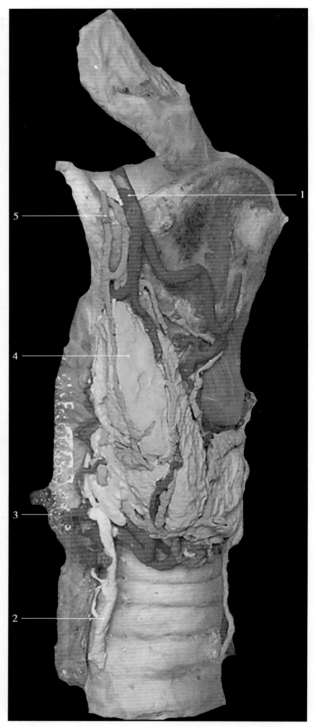

▲ 图 2-98　甲状腺下动脉与喉返神经的关系右侧面观（一）
Fig. 2-98　Right aspect of the relationship between the inferior thyroid artery and the recurrent laryngeal nerve（1）

1. 甲状腺上动脉 superior thyroid artery
2. 甲状腺静脉丛 thyroid venous plexus
3. 下甲状旁腺 inferior parathyroid gland
4. 喉返神经 recurrent laryngeal nerve
5. 甲状腺下动脉 inferior thyroid artery
6. 上甲状旁腺 superior parathyroid gland
7. 甲状腺上静脉 superior thyroid vein

▲ 图 2-99　甲状腺下动脉与喉返神经的关系右侧面观（二）
Fig. 2-99　Right aspect of the relationship between the inferior thyroid artery and the recurrent laryngeal nerve（2）

1. 甲状腺上动脉 superior thyroid artery
2. 喉返神经 recurrent laryngeal nerve
3. 甲状腺下动脉 inferior thyroid artery
4. 甲状腺 thyroid gland
5. 甲状腺上静脉 superior thyroid vein

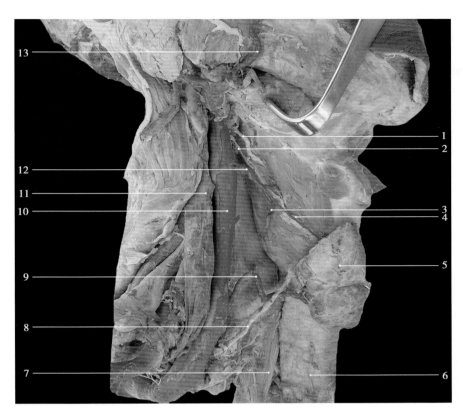

◀ 图 2-100　右侧喉上神经、喉返神经与甲状腺上、下动脉的关系

Fig. 2-100　Relationship between the right superior laryngeal nerve, the recurrent laryngeal nerve, the superior thyroid artery and the inferior thyroid artery

1. 喉上神经内支 internal branch of superior laryngeal nerve
2. 喉上神经外支 external branch of superior laryngeal nerve
3. 喉上动脉 superior laryngeal artery
4. 腺前支 anterior glandular branch
5. 甲状腺 thyroid gland
6. 气管 trachea
7. 食管 esophagus
8. 喉返神经 recurrent laryngeal nerve
9. 甲状腺下动脉 inferior thyroid artery
10. 颈总动脉 common carotid artery
11. 颈内静脉 internal jugular vein
12. 甲状腺上动脉 superior thyroid artery
13. 面动脉 facial artery

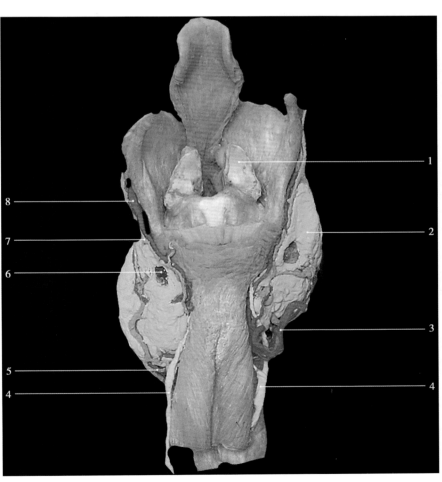

◀ 图 2-101　甲状腺下动脉与喉返神经的关系后面观

Fig. 2-101　Posterior aspect of the relationship between the inferior thyroid artery and the recurrent laryngeal nerve

1. 杓状软骨 arytenoid cartilage
2. 甲状腺 thyroid gland
3. 右甲状腺下动脉 right inferior thyroid artery
4. 喉返神经 recurrent laryngeal nerve
5. 左甲状腺下动脉 left inferior thyroid artery
6. 甲状旁腺 parathyroid gland
7. 甲状腺上静脉 superior thyroid vein
8. 甲状腺上动脉 superior thyroid artery

甲状腺下动脉与喉返神经关系的应用解剖学要点

甲状腺下动脉93.6%起于甲状颈干,2%者直接起于锁骨下动脉,或起于椎动脉和胸廓内动脉,一侧的甲状腺下动脉缺如为3%。甲状腺下动脉自甲状颈干发出后,越过颈交感干的前方者为53.2%,后方者为46.8%,然后在环状软骨或第1、2气管软骨环高度转向内下方,在颈动脉鞘后方呈一明显的向上凸的弓状,最后在接近甲状腺侧叶后缘中点或稍下方穿入甲状腺假被膜。甲状腺下动脉进入甲状腺实质之前分为两大支者为76.4%;不分支入腺体者为6.1%;分3支或4支入腺体者为14.7%和2.8%。甲状腺下动脉一般无静脉伴行(图2-91～图2-101)。

应用解剖要点:

甲状腺下动脉是甲状腺次全切除术需结扎的动脉,因其位置较深,操作较甲状腺上动脉结扎困难。在结扎该动脉时,重要的是不能损伤喉返神经。为了避免手术误伤喉返神经,根据动脉与喉返神经的位置关系,结合临床应用意义,可将其分为安全型和危险型。

安全型为甲状腺下动脉在未分支之前其主干与喉返神经呈交叉关系,动脉不是位于喉返神经的前方,就是经神经的后方进入腺体,或一侧的甲状腺下动脉缺如者。安全型右侧的出现率为46.4%,左侧为66.1%。该型分离结扎动脉时,因动脉与神经的位置关系简单,稍加小心,一般不会伤及神经。

危险型是指甲状腺下动脉入腺体之前的分支与喉返神经之间存在交叉横越,或喉返神经的分支与动脉之间的交叉情况。此型右侧的出现率为53.6%,左侧为33.9%。因该型在分离动脉时,需将甲状腺侧叶拉向前,会引起神经向前移位,是神经损伤的常见原因。

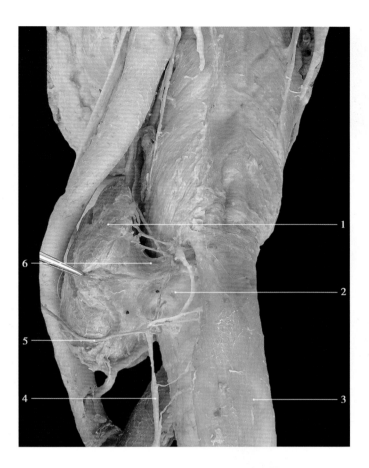

◀ 图 2-102 甲状腺悬韧带左侧观
Fig. 2-102 Left aspect of the suspensory ligament of thyroid gland

1. 甲状腺 thyroid gland
2. 气管 trachea
3. 食管 esophagus
4. 喉返神经 recurrent laryngeal nerve
5. 甲状腺下动脉 inferior thyroid artery
6. 甲状腺悬韧带 suspensory ligament of thyroid gland

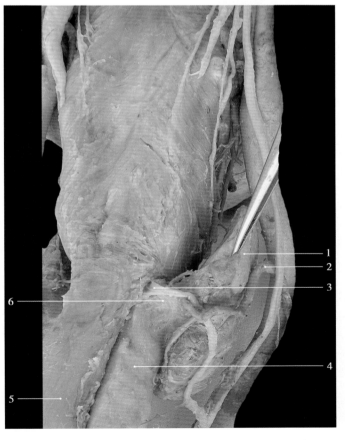

◀ 图 2-103 甲状腺悬韧带右侧观
Fig. 2-103 Right aspect of the suspensory ligament of thyroid gland

1. 甲状腺 thyroid gland
2. 甲状腺上动脉 superior thyroid artery
3. 喉返神经 recurrent laryngeal nerve
4. 气管 trachea
5. 食管 esophagus
6. 甲状腺悬韧带 thyroid suspensory ligament

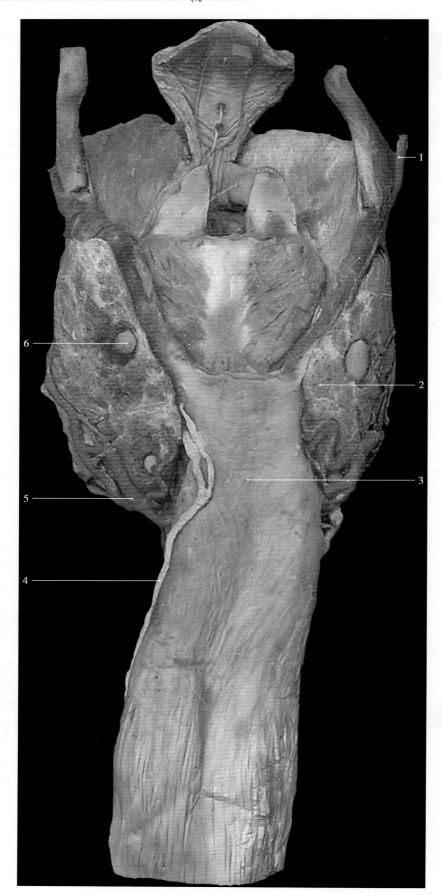

◀ 图 2-104　甲状旁腺
Fig. 2-104　Parathyroid gland

1. 甲状腺上动脉 superior thyroid artery
2. 甲状腺 thyroid gland
3. 食管第 1 狭窄 the 1st stenosis of esophagus
4. 喉返神经 recurrent laryngeal nerve
5. 甲状腺下动脉 inferior thyroid artery
6. 上甲状旁腺 superior parathyroid gland

甲状旁腺的应用解剖学要点

甲状旁腺在活体上为棕黄色的长椭圆形小体,呈米粒状或扁圆形黄豆状。一般为上、下两对,位于甲状腺两侧叶的后方。甲状旁腺有薄层的结缔组织膜包裹。上一对甲状旁腺95%位于甲状腺侧叶后缘中点以上,即在环状软骨下缘高度附近,位置隐蔽,是一般不宜招致损伤的位置。下一对甲状旁腺62.2%位于甲状腺侧叶后缘中1/3与下1/3交界处以下至下端的后下方,也是正常的较为隐蔽的、不宜招致损伤的位置(图2-104)。甲状旁腺分泌甲状旁腺素,其主要作用是使骨钙释放入血,维持血钙平衡。甲状腺手术中,如不慎将甲状旁腺摘除或损伤,可引起血钙降低,出现暂时性或持久性的手足搐搦症状,甚至可危及生命。

应用解剖要点:

甲状腺手术中如何鉴别变异的甲状旁腺与淋巴结或副甲状腺有一定困难。避免损伤或误摘甲状旁腺的最关键是:手术者应了解80%以上甲状旁腺的正常位置,即上一对甲状旁腺位于甲状腺侧叶后缘中点以上到上1/4与3/4交界处;下一对甲状旁腺位于甲状腺侧叶后缘下1/3段,它们均在甲状腺假被膜与真被膜之间。甲状腺的次全切除术一般是保留甲状腺的侧叶后部,这就是保护甲状旁腺免遭切除并防止损伤喉返神经的良好措施(图2-95、图2-96、图2-98、图2-99、图2-101)。

此外,手术者还应了解约有16%位置变异的甲状旁腺易遭受损伤,手术中应注意甲状腺侧叶前面或侧面靠近外侧缘下部有无甲状旁腺的存在。更重要的是,要严格紧靠甲状腺真被膜处,清理并完整地保留真被膜以外的侧叶上、下端附近的脂肪组织和疏松结缔组织。用此方法处理甲状腺残端,能有效地防止甲状旁腺被误摘或损伤。

第六节　喉 与 气 管

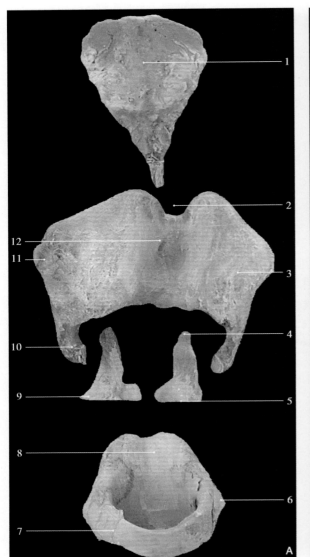

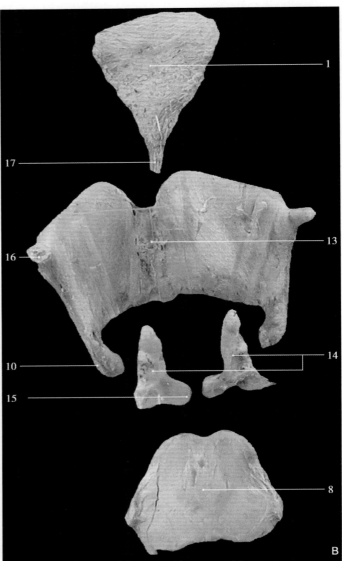

▲ 图 2-105　喉软骨

Fig. 2-105　Laryngeal cartilages

A：前面观　B：后面观

1. 会厌软骨 epiglottic cartilage
2. 上切迹 superior thyroid notch
3. 左板 left lamina
4. 杓状软骨尖 apex of arytenoid cartilage
5. 杓状软骨底 base of arytenoid cartilage
6. 甲关节面 thyroid articular surface
7. 环状软骨弓 arch of cricoid cartilage
8. 环状软骨板 lamina of cricoid cartilage
9. 肌突 muscular process

10. 下角 inferior cornu
11. 右板 right lamina
12. 喉结 laryngeal prominence
13. 甲状软骨 thyroid cartilage
14. 杓状软骨 arytenoid cartilage
15. 声带突 vocal process
16. 上角 superior cornu
17. 会厌软骨茎 stalk of epiglottis

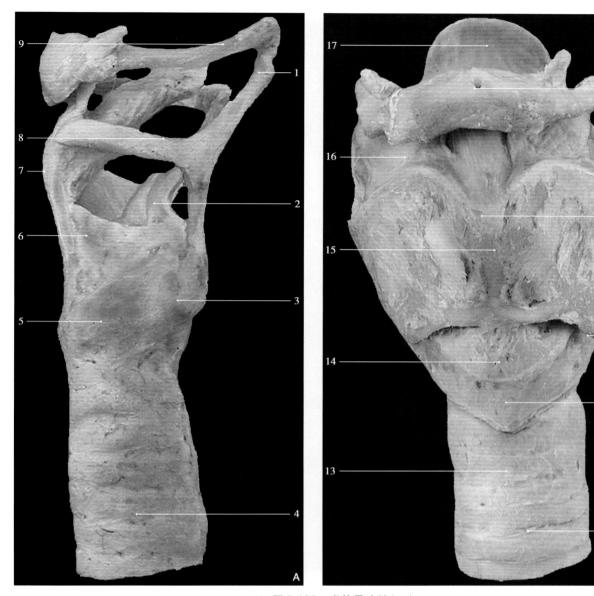

▲ 图 2-106　喉软骨连结（一）

Fig. 2-106　Joints of the laryngeal cartilages（1）

A：侧面观　B：前面观

1. 上角 superior cornu
2. 杓状软骨 arytenoid cartilage
3. 环甲关节 cricothyroid joint
4. 气管 trachea
5. 环状软骨 cricoid cartilage
6. 弹性圆锥 conus elasticus
7. 喉结 laryngeal prominence
8. 甲状软骨上缘 superior margin of thyroid cartilage
9. 舌骨大角 greater cornu of hyoid bone

10. 舌骨 hyoid bone
11. 环状软骨弓 arch of cricoid cartilage
12. 环状韧带 anular ligament
13. 气管软骨 tracheal cartilages
14. 环甲正中韧带 median cricothyroid ligament
15. 甲状软骨 thyroid cartilage
16. 甲状舌骨膜 thyrohyoid membrane
17. 会厌软骨 epiglottic cartilage

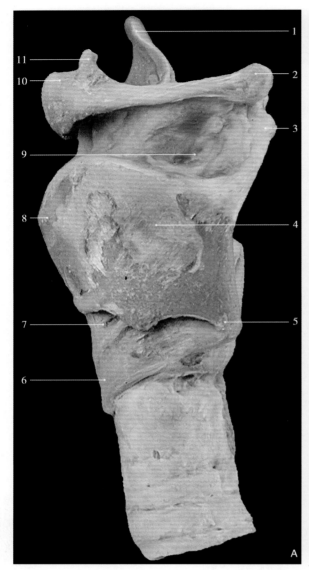
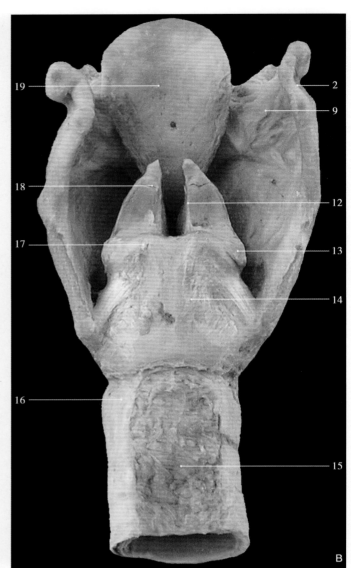

▲ 图 2-107　喉软骨连结（二）

Fig. 2-107　Joints of the laryngeal cartilages（2）

A：侧面观　B：后面观

1. 会厌 epiglottis
2. 舌骨大角 greater cornu of hyoid bone
3. 上角 superior cornu
4. 甲状软骨 thyroid cartilage
5. 环甲关节 cricothyroid joint
6. 环状软骨 cricoid cartilage
7. 弹性圆锥 conus elasticus
8. 喉结 laryngeal prominence
9. 甲状舌骨膜 thyrohyoid membrane
10. 舌骨体 body of hyoid bone
11. 舌骨小角 lesser cornu of hyoid bone
12. 声带突 vocal process
13. 肌突 muscular process
14. 环状软骨板 lamina of cricoid cartilage
15. 膜壁 membranous wall
16. 气管软骨 tracheal cartilages
17. 环杓关节 cricoarytenoid joint
18. 杓状软骨 arytenoid cartilage
19. 会厌软骨 epiglottic cartilage

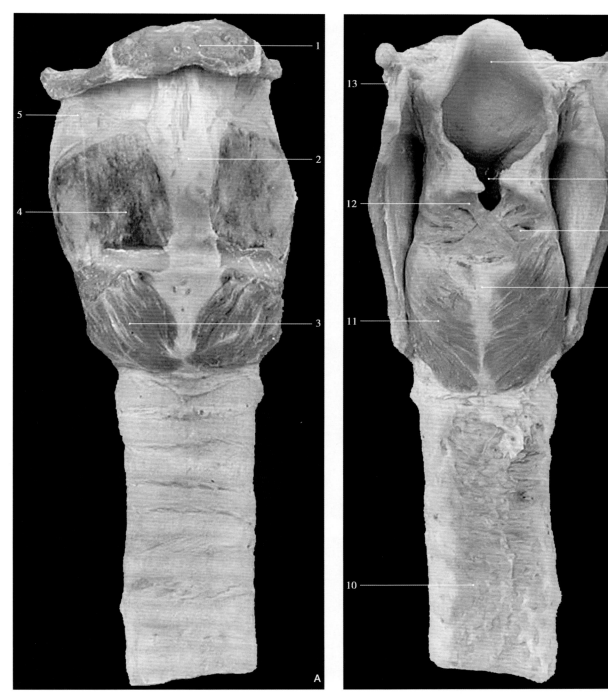

▲ 图 2-108　喉肌(一)

Fig. 2-108　Muscles of the larynx(1)

A:前面观　B:后面观

1. 舌骨 hyoid bone
2. 喉结 laryngeal prominence
3. 环甲肌 cricothyroid
4. 甲状软骨 thyroid cartilage
5. 甲状舌骨膜 thyrohyoid membrane
6. 会厌软骨 epiglottic cartilage
7. 杓间切迹 interarytenoid notch

8. 杓横肌 transverse arytenoid
9. 环状软骨板 lamina of cricoid cartilage
10. 膜壁 membranous wall
11. 环杓后肌 posterior cricoarytenoid
12. 杓斜肌 oblique arytenoid
13. 甲状舌骨外侧韧带 lateral thyrohyoid ligament

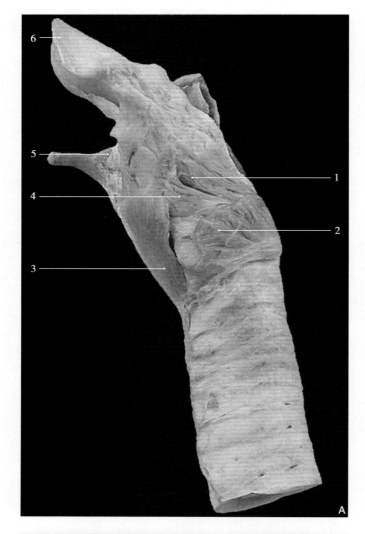

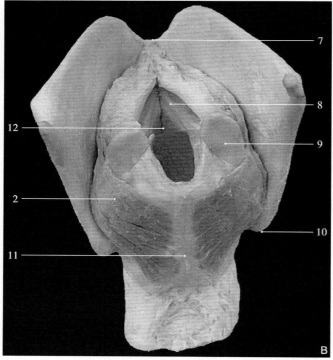

◀ 图 2-109　喉肌（二）
Fig. 2-109　Muscles of the larynx（2）

A：侧面观　B：上面观
1. 甲状会厌肌 thyroepiglottic muscle
2. 环杓后肌 posterior cricoarytenoid
3. 环杓侧肌 lateral cricoarytenoid
4. 甲杓肌 thyroarytehoid
5. 杓会厌肌 aryepiglottic muscle
6. 会厌 epiglottis
7. 上切迹 superior thyroid notch
8. 声带肌 vocalis
9. 杓状软骨 arytenoid cartilage
10. 下角 inferior cornu
11. 环状软骨 cricoid cartilage
12. 声门裂 fissure of glottis

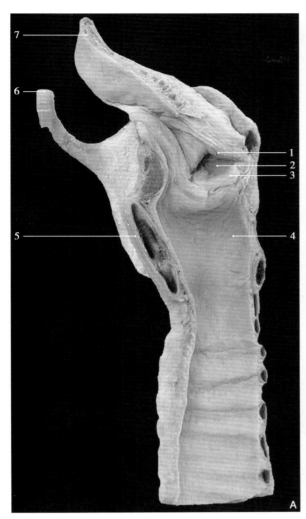
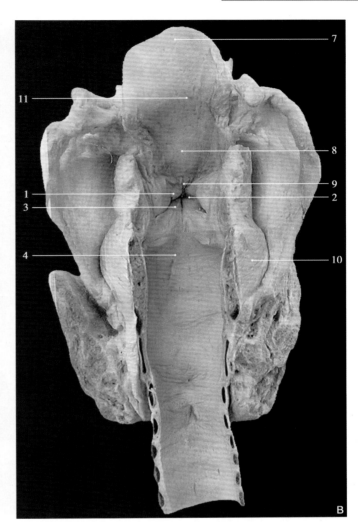

▲ 图 2-110 喉腔矢状切面

Fig. 2-110 Sagittal section of the laryngeal cavity

A:正中矢状切面 B:喉腔冠状切面

1. 前庭襞 vestibular fold
2. 喉室 ventricle of larynx
3. 声襞 vocal fold
4. 声门下腔 infraglottic cavity
5. 环状软骨板 lamina of cricoid cartilage
6. 上角 superior cornu of thyroid cartilage

7. 会厌 epiglottis
8. 会厌结节 tubercle of epiglottis
9. 前庭裂 vestibular fissure
10. 环状软骨 cricoid cartilage
11. 喉前庭 vestibule of larynx

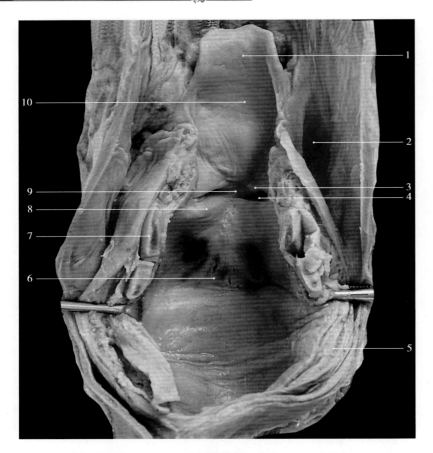

◀ 图2-111　喉腔内结构后面观
Fig. 2-111　Posterior aspect of the structures in the laryngeal cavity

1. 会厌 epiglottis
2. 梨状隐窝 piriform recess
3. 前庭襞 vestibular fold
4. 喉室 ventricle of larynx
5. 第1气管软骨 the 1st tracheal cartilage
6. 声门下腔 infraglottic cavity
7. 环状软骨 cricoid cartilage
8. 声襞 vocal fold
9. 喉中间腔 intermedial cavity of larynx
10. 喉前庭 vestibule of larynx

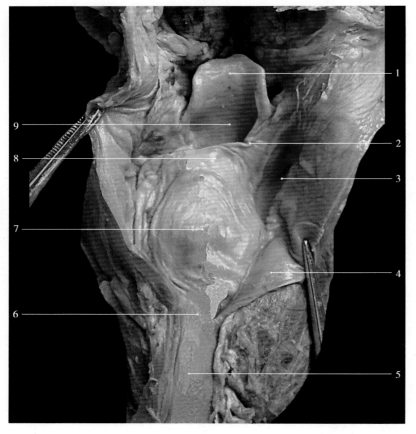

◀ 图2-112　梨状隐窝
Fig. 2-112　Piriform recess

1. 会厌 epiglottis
2. 杓会厌襞 aryepiglottic fold
3. 梨状隐窝 piriform recess
4. 咽后壁（向后翻）retropharyngeal wall（turned back）
5. 食管 esophagus
6. 食管第1狭窄 the 1st stenosis of esophagus
7. 环状软骨板 lamina of cricoid cartilage
8. 杓状软骨 arytenoid cartilage
9. 喉口 aperture of larynx

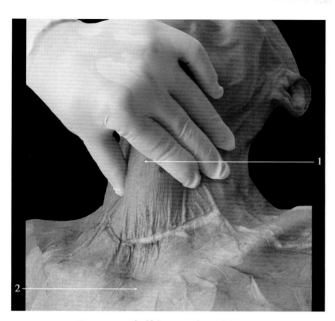

▲ 图2-113　气管切开手术入路切口（一）
Fig. 2-113　Surgical approach of the tracheotomy（1）

1. 喉结 laryngeal prominence
2. 颈静脉切迹 jugular notch

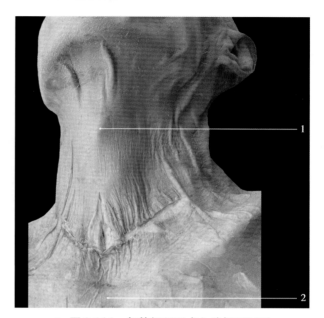

▲ 图2-114　气管切开手术入路切口（二）
Fig. 2-114　Surgical approach of the tracheotomy（2）

1. 喉结 laryngeal prominence
2. 颈静脉切迹 jugular notch

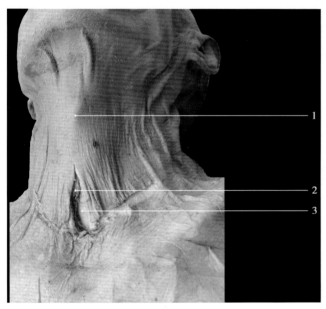

▲ 图2-115　气管切开手术入路切口（三）
Fig. 2-115　Surgical approach of the tracheotomy（3）

1. 喉结 laryngeal prominence
2. 皮下组织 subcutaneous tissue
3. 第3气管软骨环 the third ring of tracheal cartilage

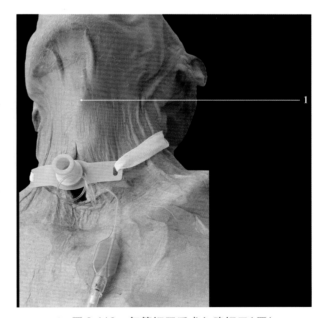

▲ 图2-116　气管切开手术入路切口（四）
Fig. 2-116　Surgical approach of the tracheotomy（4）

1. 喉结 laryngeal prominence

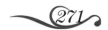

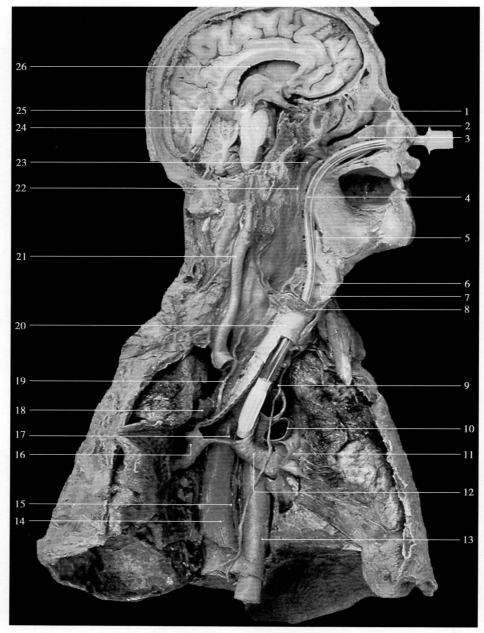

▲ 图 2-117 气管插管径路
Fig. 2-117 Approach of the tracheal intubation

1. 中鼻甲 middle nasal concha
2. 中鼻道 middle nasal meatus
3. 下鼻甲 inferior nasal concha
4. 气管插管 tracheal intubation
5. 会厌 epiglottis
6. 前庭襞 vestibular fold
7. 喉室 ventricle of larynx
8. 环状软骨 cricoid cartilage
9. 左迷走神经 left vagus nerve
10. 左肺动脉 left pulmonary artery
11. 左上肺静脉 left superior pulmonary vein
12. 左主支气管 left principle bronchus
13. 降主动脉 descending aorta
14. 食管 esophagus
15. 胸导管 thoracic duct
16. 右主支气管 right principle bronchus
17. 气管隆嵴 carina of trachea
18. 奇静脉 azygos vein
19. 右迷走神经 right vagus nerve
20. 气管 trachea
21. 颈总动脉 common carotid artery
22. 鼻咽部 nasal part of pharynx
23. 咽鼓管圆枕 tubal torus
24. 脑桥 pons
25. 中脑 midbrain
26. 侧脑室 lateral ventricle

第七节 咽 与 食 管

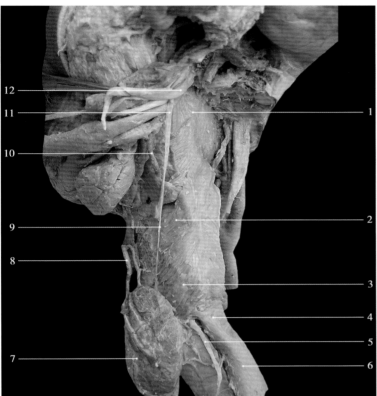

◀ 图 2-118　咽肌侧面观
Fig. 2-118　Lateral aspect of the pharyngeal muscle

1. 咽上缩肌 superior constrictor of pharynx
2. 咽中缩肌 middle constrictor of pharynx
3. 咽下缩肌 inferior constrictor of pharynx
4. 食管第1狭窄 the 1st stenosis of esophagus
5. 喉返神经 recurrent laryngeal nerve
6. 食管 esophagus
7. 甲状腺 thyroid gland
8. 甲状腺上动脉 superior thyroid artery
9. 喉上神经外支 external branch of superior laryngeal nerve
10. 喉上动脉 superior laryngeal artery
11. 喉上神经 superior laryngeal nerve
12. 迷走神经 vagus nerve

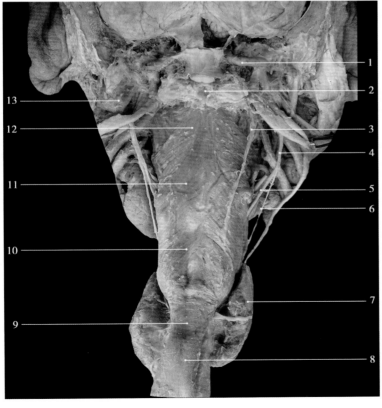

◀ 图 2-119　咽肌后面观
Fig. 2-119　Posterior aspect of the pharyngeal muscle

1. 椎动脉 vertebral artery
2. 咽结节 pharyngeal tubercle
3. 舌咽神经咽支 pharyngeal branch of glossopharyngeal nerve
4. 喉上神经 superior laryngeal nerve
5. 喉上神经内支 internal branch of superior laryngeal nerve
6. 喉上神经外支 external branch of superior laryngeal nerve
7. 甲状腺 thyroid gland
8. 食管 esophagus
9. 食管第1狭窄 the 1st stenosis of esophagus
10. 咽下缩肌 inferior constrictor of pharynx
11. 咽中缩肌 middle constrictor of pharynx
12. 咽上缩肌 superior constrictor of pharynx
13. 颈内静脉 internal jugular vein

273

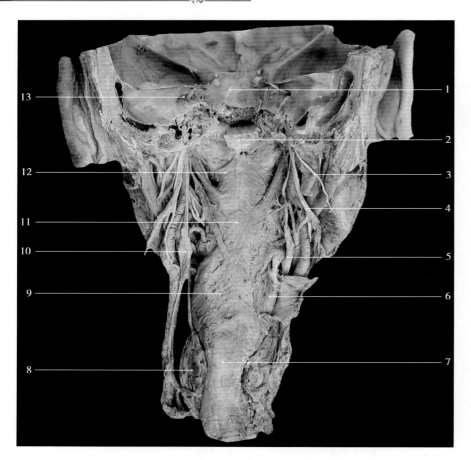

◀ 图 2-120　咽的后面观
Fig. 2-120　Posterior aspect of the pharynx

1. 斜坡 clivus
2. 咽结节 pharyngeal tubercle
3. 副神经 accessory nerve
4. 舌下神经 hypoglossal nerve
5. 迷走神经 vagus nerve
6. 腭咽肌 palatopharyngeus
7. 食管 esophagus
8. 甲状腺 thyroid gland
9. 咽下缩肌 inferior constrictor of pharynx
10. 颈上神经节 superior cervical ganglion
11. 咽中缩肌 middle constrictor of pharynx
12. 咽上缩肌 superior constrictor of pharynx
13. 内耳门 internal acoustic pore

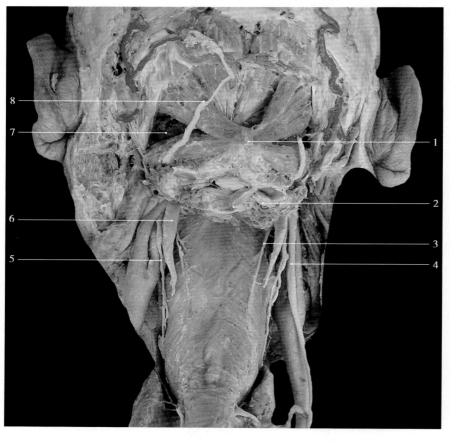

◀ 图 2-121　舌咽神经咽支
Fig. 2-121　Pharyngeal branch of glossopharyngeal nerve

1. 枢椎棘突 spinous process of axis
2. 椎动脉 vertebral artery
3. 舌咽神经咽支 pharyngeal branch of glossopharyngeal nerve
4. 迷走神经 vagus nerve
5. 喉上神经 superior laryngeal nerve
6. 颈上神经节 superior cervical ganglion
7. 枕下三角 suboccipital triangle
8. 枕大神经 greater occipital nerve

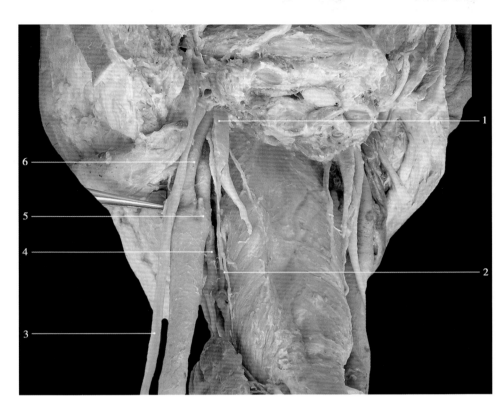

◀ 图 2-122　左侧颈动脉小球
Fig. 2-122　Left carotid glomus

1. 颈上神经节 superior cervical ganglion
2. 喉上神经外支 external branch of superior laryngeal nerve
3. 迷走神经 vagus nerve
4. 甲状腺上动脉 superior thyroid artery
5. 颈动脉小球 carotid glomus
6. 颈内动脉 internal carotid artery

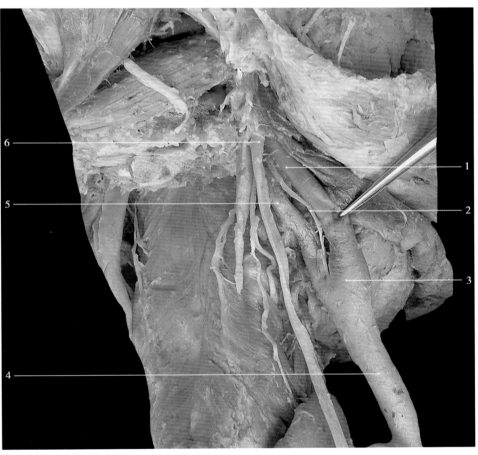

◀ 图 2-123　右侧颈动脉小球
Fig. 2-123　Right carotid glomus

1. 颈内动脉 internal carotid artery
2. 舌咽神经颈动脉窦支 carotid sinus branch of glossopharyngeal nerve
3. 颈动脉小球 carotid glomus
4. 颈总动脉 common carotid artery
5. 颈外动脉 external carotid artery
6. 迷走神经 vagus nerve

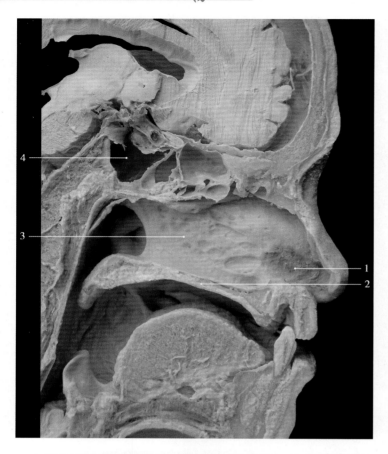

◀ 图 2-124 鼻中隔
Fig. 2-124 Nasal septum

1. 鼻中隔软骨部 cartilaginous part of nasal septum
2. 硬腭 hard palate
3. 鼻中隔 nasal septum
4. 蝶窦 sphenoidal sinus

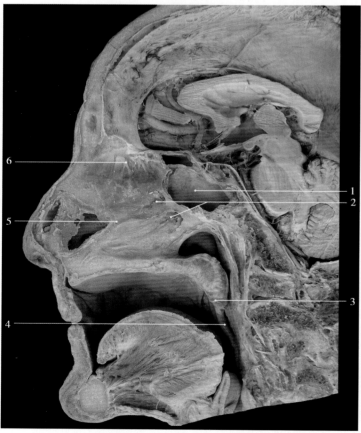

◀ 图 2-125 鼻中隔的动脉
Fig. 2-125 Artery of the nasal septum

1. 蝶窦 sphenoidal sinus
2. 上唇动脉鼻中隔支 nasal septal branch of superior labial artery
3. 腭垂 uvula
4. 腭咽弓 palatopharyngeal arch
5. 鼻中隔 nasal septum
6. 嗅丝 fila olfactoria

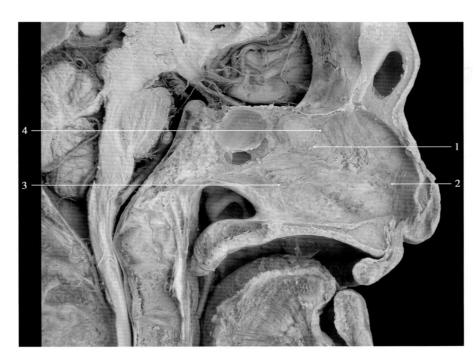

◀ 图 2-126　筛前、后动脉
Fig. 2-126　Anterior and posterior ethmoidal artery

1. 鼻中隔 nasal septum
2. 鼻中隔软骨部 cartilaginous part of nasal septum
3. 筛后动脉 posterior ethmoidal artery
4. 筛前动脉 anterior ethmoidal artery

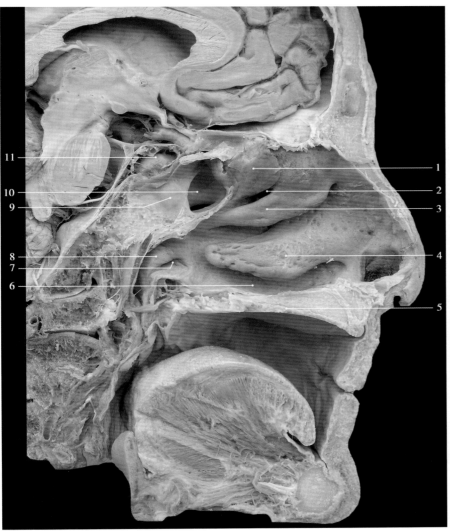

◀ 图 2-127　鼻腔外侧壁结构
Fig. 2-127　Structures of the lateral wall of nasal cavity

1. 上鼻甲 superior nasal concha
2. 上鼻道 superior nasal meatus
3. 中鼻甲 middle nasal concha
4. 下鼻甲 inferior nasal concha
5. 硬腭 hard palate
6. 下鼻道 inferior nasal meatus
7. 咽鼓管咽口 pharyngeal opening of auditory tube
8. 咽鼓管圆枕 tubal torus
9. 上颌窦中隔 median septum of maxillary sinus
10. 上颌窦 maxillary sinus
11. 颈内动脉海绵窦部 cavernous part of internal carotid artery

 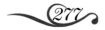

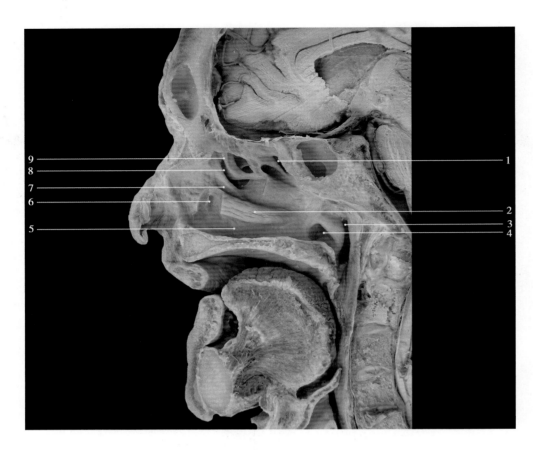

◀ 图 2-128 钩突、半月裂孔
Fig. 2-128 Uncinate process and semilunar hiatus

1. 蝶筛隐窝 spheno-ethmoidal recess
2. 下鼻甲 inferior nasal concha
3. 咽隐窝 pharyngeal recess
4. 咽鼓管咽口 pharyngeal opening of auditory tube
5. 下鼻道 inferior nasal meatus
6. 鼻泪管开口 opening of nasolacrimal canal
7. 上鼻道 superior nasal meatus
8. 半月裂孔 semilunar hiatus
9. 钩突 uncinate process

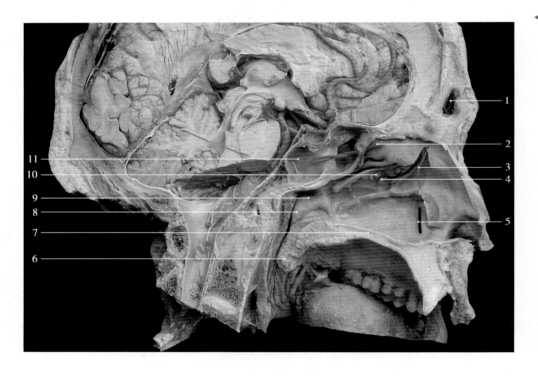

◀ 图 2-129 鼻旁窦开口
Fig. 2-129 Opening of the paranasal sinuses

1. 额窦 frontal sinus
2. 蝶窦开口引线 indicatrix of opening of sphenoidal sinus
3. 额窦开口引线 indicatrix of opening of frontal sinus
4. 筛窦开口引线 indicatrix of opening of ethmoidal sinus
5. 鼻泪管开口引线 indicatrix of opening of nasolacrimal canal
6. 腭垂 uvula
7. 硬腭 hard palate
8. 咽鼓管圆枕 tubal torus
9. 咽隐窝 pharyngeal recess
10. 上颌窦开口引线 indicatrix of opening of maxillary sinus
11. 蝶窦 sphenoidal sinus

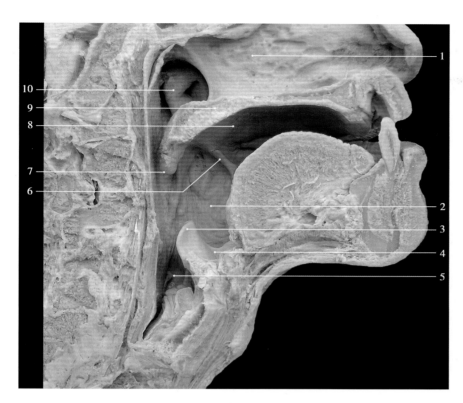

◀ 图 2-130　口咽侧面观
Fig. 2-130　Lateral aspect of the oropharynx

1. 鼻中隔 nasal septum
2. 口咽 oropharynx
3. 会厌 epiglottis
4. 舌会厌正中襞 median glossoepiglottic fold
5. 喉咽 laryngopharynx
6. 腭舌弓 palatoglossal arch
7. 腭垂 uvula
8. 口腔 oral cavity
9. 硬腭 hard palate
10. 咽鼓管圆枕 tubal torus

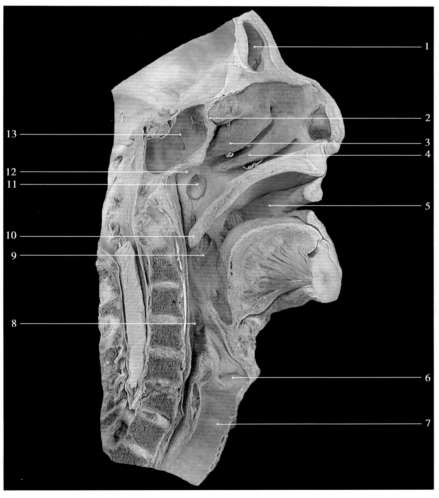

◀ 图 2-131　咽正中矢状面观
Fig. 2-131　Median sagittal aspect of the pharynx

1. 额窦 frontal sinus
2. 蝶筛隐窝 sphenoethmoidal recess
3. 中鼻甲 middle concha
4. 下鼻甲 inferior concha
5. 口腔 oral cavity
6. 喉室 ventricle of larynx
7. 气管 trachea
8. 喉咽 laryngopharynx
9. 口咽 oropharynx
10. 腭垂 uvula
11. 咽鼓管咽口 pharyngeal opening of auditory tube
12. 鼻咽 nasopharynx
13. 蝶窦 sphenoidal sinus

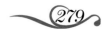

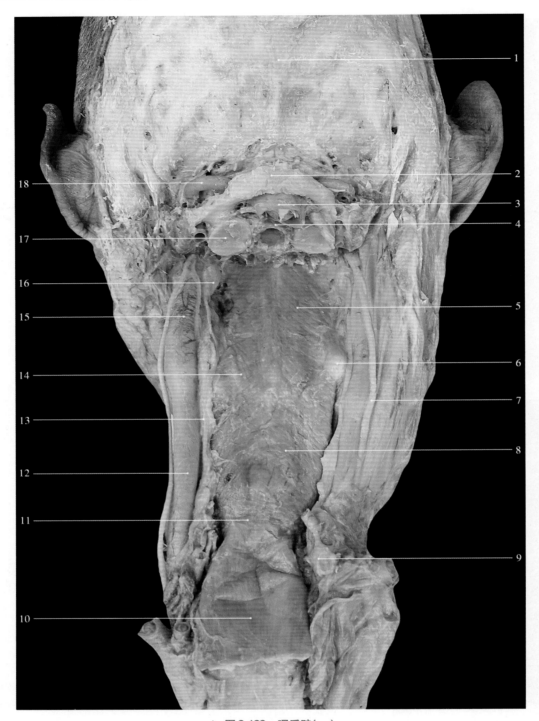

▲ 图 2-132　咽后壁（一）
Fig. 2-132　Posterior wall of the pharynx（1）

1. 枕外隆凸 external occipital protuberance
2. 寰椎后结节 posterior tubercle of atlas
3. 硬脊膜 spinal dura mater
4. 寰椎横韧带 transvers ligament of atlas
5. 咽上缩肌 superior constrictor of pharynx
6. 舌骨大角 greater cornu of hyoid bone
7. 迷走神经 vagus nerve
8. 咽下缩肌 inferior constrictor of pharynx
9. 星状神经节 stellate ganglion
10. 食管 esophagus
11. 食管第 1 狭窄 the 1st stenosis of esophagus
12. 颈总动脉 common carotid artery
13. 颈交感干 cervical sympathetic trunk
14. 咽中缩肌 middle constrictor of pharynx
15. 颈内动脉 internal carotid artery
16. 颈上神经节 superior cervical ganglion
17. 寰椎下关节面 inferior articular surface of atlas
18. 椎动脉寰椎部 atlantic part of vertebral artery

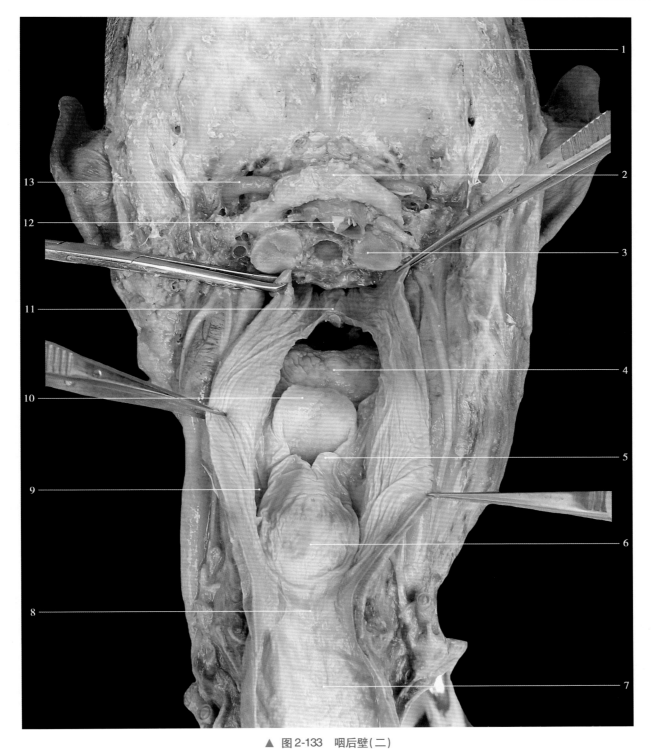

▲ 图 2-133 咽后壁（二）

Fig. 2-133 Posterior wall of the pharynx（2）

1. 枕外隆凸 external occipital protuberance
2. 寰椎后结节 posterior tubercle of atlas
3. 寰椎下关节面 inferior articular surface of atlas
4. 舌根 root of tongue
5. 杓状软骨 arytenoid cartilage
6. 环状软骨板 lamina of cricoid cartilage
7. 食管 esophagus

8. 食管第 1 狭窄 the 1st stenosis of esophagus
9. 梨状隐窝 piriform recess
10. 会厌 epiglottis
11. 软腭 soft palate
12. 脊髓 spinal cord
13. 椎动脉寰椎部 atlantic part of vertebral artery

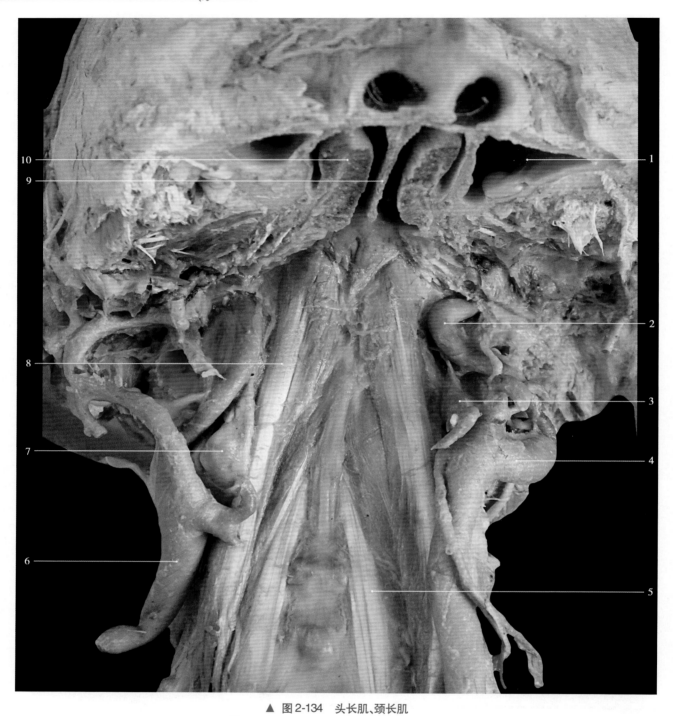

▲ 图2-134 头长肌、颈长肌
Fig. 2-134 Longus capitis and longus colli

1. 上颌窦 maxillary sinus
2. 颈内动脉 internal carotid artery
3. 左侧颈上神经节 left superior cervical ganglion
4. 颈动脉窦 carotid sinus
5. 颈长肌 longus colli
6. 颈总动脉 common carotid artery
7. 右侧颈上神经节 right superior cervical ganglion
8. 头长肌 longus capitis
9. 鼻中隔 nasal septum
10. 下鼻甲 inferior nasal concha

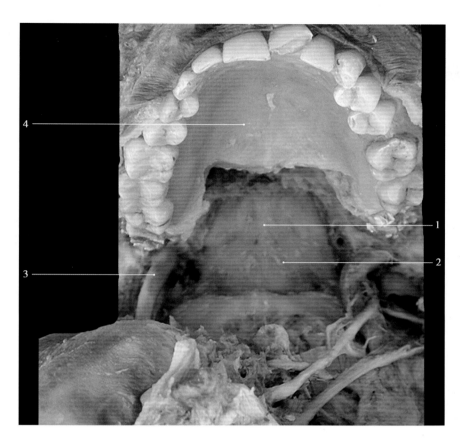

◀ 图 2-135 咽结节（一）
Fig. 2-135 Pharyngeal tubercle (1)

1. 咽结节 pharyngeal tubercle
2. 枕骨基底部 basilar part of occipital bone
3. 颈外动脉 external carotid artery
4. 硬腭 hard palate

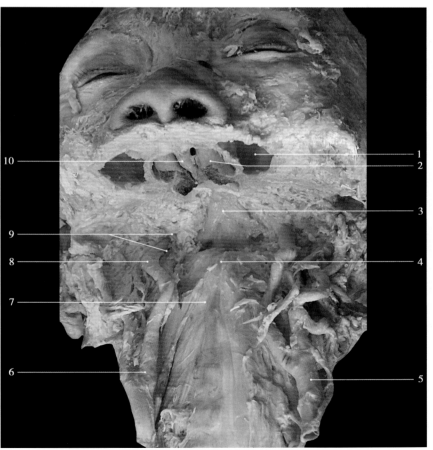

◀ 图 2-136 咽结节（二）
Fig. 2-136 Pharyngeal tubercle (2)

1. 上颌窦 maxillary sinus
2. 下鼻甲 inferior nasal concha
3. 咽结节 pharyngeal tubercle
4. 寰椎前弓 anterior arch of atlas
5. 颈总动脉 common carotid artery
6. 颈动脉窦 carotid sinus
7. 头长肌 longus capitis
8. 颈内动脉 internal carotid artery
9. 颈动脉管外口 external opening of carotid canal
10. 鼻中隔 nasal septum

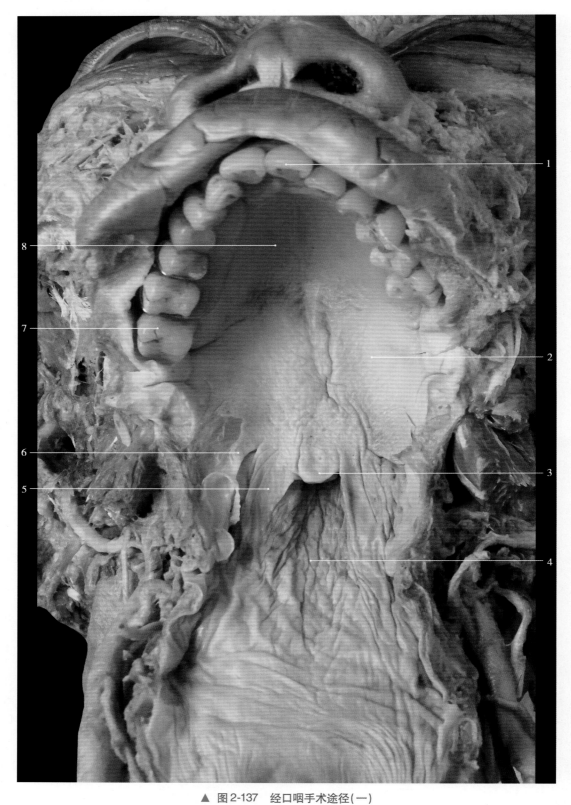

▲ 图2-137　经口咽手术途径（一）

Fig. 2-137　Surgical approach through the oropharynx（1）

1. 切牙 incisor
2. 软腭 soft palate
3. 腭垂 uvula
4. 咽后壁 retropharyngeal wall
5. 腭咽弓 palatopharyngeal arch
6. 腭舌弓 palatoglossal arch
7. 磨牙 molar
8. 硬腭 hard palate

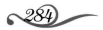

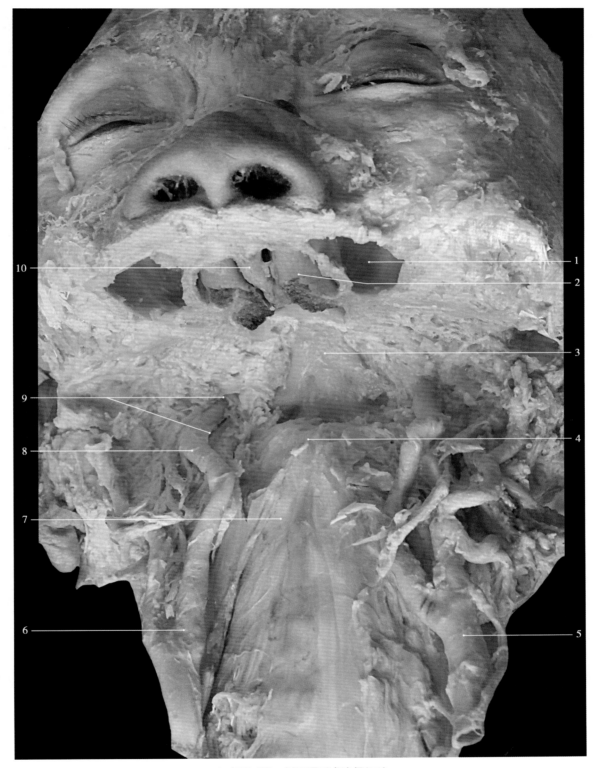

▲ 图 2-138 经口咽手术途径（二）

Fig. 2-138 Surgical approach through the oropharynx（2）

1. 上颌窦 maxillary sinus
2. 下鼻甲 inferior nasal concha
3. 咽结节 pharyngeal tuberecle
4. 寰椎前弓 anterior arch of atlas
5. 颈总动脉 common carotid artery
6. 颈动脉窦 carotid sinus
7. 头长肌 longus capitis
8. 颈内动脉 internal carotid artery
9. 颈动脉管外口 external opening of carotid canal
10. 鼻中隔 nasal septum

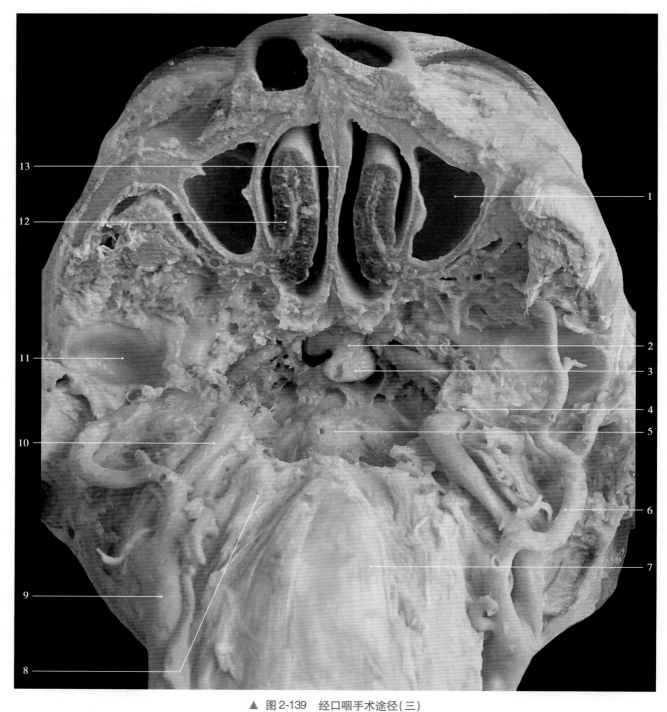

▲ 图2-139 经口咽手术途径(三)

Fig. 2-139 Surgical approach through the oropharynx(3)

1. 上颌窦 maxillary sinus
2. 垂体柄 pituitary stalk
3. 垂体 hypophysis
4. 颈动脉管外口 external opening of carotid canal
5. 斜坡区硬膜 dura mater in clivus region
6. 颈外动脉 external carotid artery
7. 头长肌 longus capitis
8. 颈上神经节 superior cervical ganglion
9. 颈总动脉 common carotid artery
10. 颈内动脉 internal carotid artery
11. 关节盘 articular disc of temporomandibular joint
12. 下鼻甲 inferior nasal concha
13. 鼻中隔 nasal septum

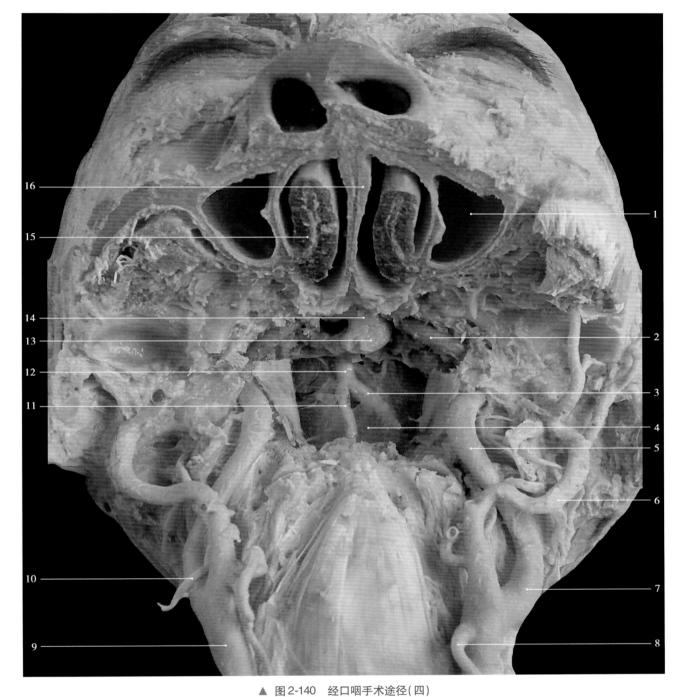

▲ 图2-140 经口咽手术途径(四)

Fig. 2-140 Surgical approach through the oropharynx(4)

1. 上颌窦 maxillary sinus
2. 颈内动脉岩部 petrosal part of internal carotid artery
3. 左侧椎动脉 left vertebral artery
4. 蛛网膜 arachnoid mater
5. 颈内动脉 internal carotid artery
6. 颈外动脉 external carotid artery
7. 颈动脉窦 carotid sinus
8. 甲状腺上动脉 superior thyroid artery
9. 颈总动脉 common carotid artery
10. 舌下神经 hypoglossal nerve
11. 右侧椎动脉 right vertebral artery
12. 基底动脉 basilar artery
13. 垂体 hypophysis
14. 垂体柄 pituitary stalk
15. 下鼻甲 inferior nasal concha
16. 鼻中隔 nasal septum

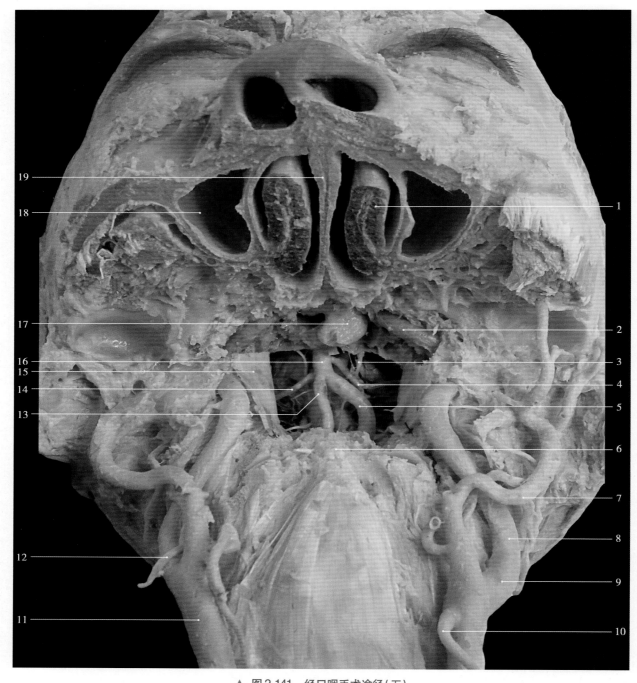

▲ 图2-141　经口咽手术途径(五)
Fig. 2-141　Surgical approach through the oropharynx(5)

1. 下鼻甲 inferior nasal concha
2. 颈内动脉岩部 petrosal part of internal carotid artery
3. 展神经 abducent nerve
4. 左侧小脑下前动脉 left anterior inferior cerebellar artery
5. 左侧椎动脉 left vertebral artery
6. 齿突 dens
7. 颈外动脉 external carotid artery
8. 颈内动脉 internal carotid artery
9. 颈动脉窦 carotid sinus
10. 甲状腺上动脉 superior thyroid artery

11. 颈总动脉 common carotid artery
12. 舌下神经 hypoglossal nerve
13. 右侧椎动脉 right vertebral artery
14. 右侧小脑下前动脉 right anterior inferior cerebellar artery
15. 硬膜(翻向外) dura mater(turned laterally)
16. 基底动脉 basilar artery
17. 垂体 hypophysis
18. 上颌窦 maxillary sinus
19. 鼻中隔 nasal septum

经口咽至斜坡区手术入路的应用解剖学要点

斜坡区肿瘤(脑膜瘤、神经鞘瘤、脊索瘤、表皮样瘤等)因其深居颅底中线部位,毗邻脑干、椎-基底动脉等重要结构,对颅底中线处硬膜外的下斜坡区和枕骨大孔腹侧肿瘤等病变,选用经口咽至斜坡的手术入路的优点有:①手术入路途径短;②对病变区显露较充分;③从脑干腹侧入路可减少对脑组织和脑神经等的牵拉。缺点为:①经口咽至颅底入路手术感染概率高;②无法进行麻醉插管。

应用解剖要点:

1. 手术入路 张大口腔,在软腭下方正中线切开咽后壁,分离颅底的咽结节,以咽结节为圆心,以 20mm 为半径在斜坡的颅底外面凿开骨窗,切开寰椎前弓和寰枕关节的前半部以扩大手术视野。从颅底的外侧面显示硬脑膜,纵向切开硬膜,显示基底动脉、大脑后动脉、展神经等(图 2-132 ~ 图 2-141)。

2. 舌下神经管外口内侧缘、颈动脉管外口内侧缘、破裂孔内侧缘距正中线的距离分别为 17.18mm、25.24mm、10.54mm。

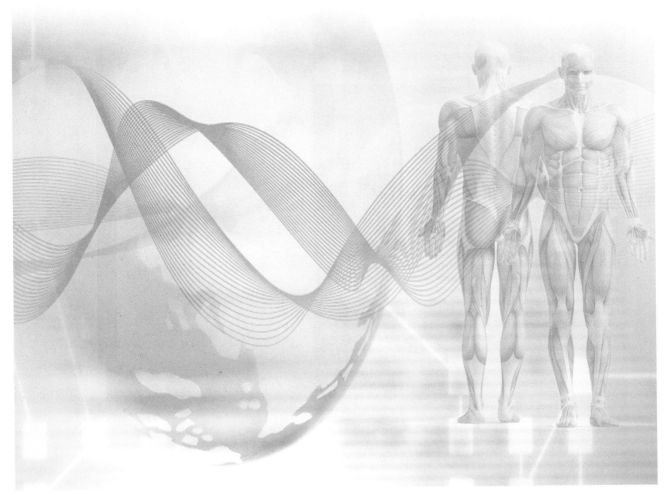

第八节 项区和颈后区

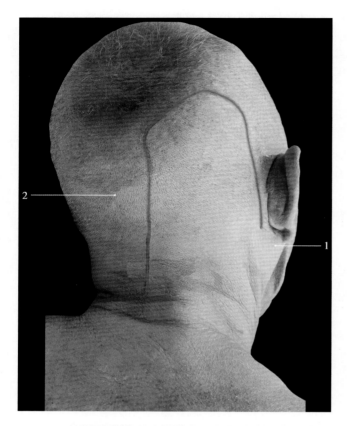

◀ 图2-142 枕区切口（一）
Fig. 2-142 Incision of the occipital region（1）

1. 乳突 mastoid process
2. 枕外隆凸 external occipital protuberance

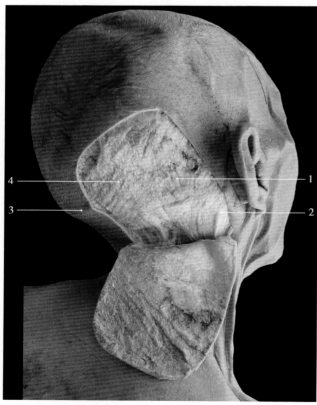

◀ 图2-143 枕区切口（二）
Fig. 2-143 Incision of the occipital region（2）

1. 枕额肌枕腹 occipital belly of occipitofrontalis
2. 乳突 mastoid process
3. 枕外隆凸 external occipital protuberance
4. 浅筋膜 superficial fascia

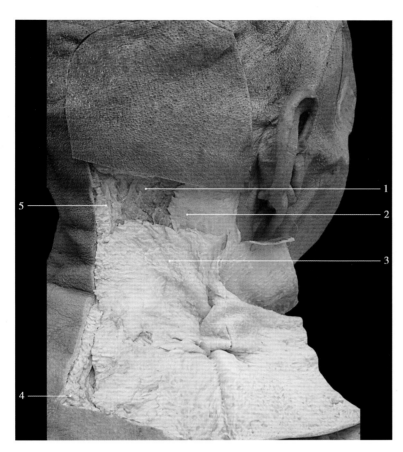

◀ 图 2-144　颈后区结构-浅筋膜
Fig. 2-144　Structures in the posterior region of neck-the superficial fascia

1. 头夹肌 splenius capitis
2. 深筋膜 deep fascia
3. 浅筋膜 superficial fascia
4. 隆椎棘突 spinous process of vertebra prominens
5. 项韧带 ligamentum nuchae

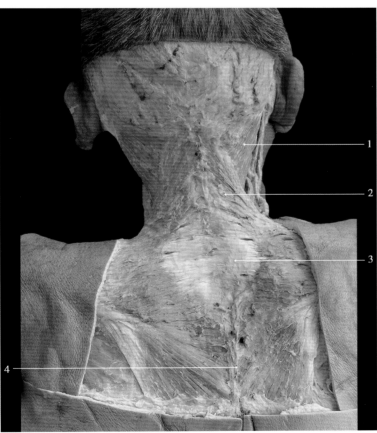

◀ 图 2-145　颈后区浅层结构
Fig. 2-145　Superficial structures in the posterior region of neck

1. 夹肌 splenius
2. 斜方肌 trapezius
3. 斜方肌腱膜 aponeurosis of trapezius
4. 棘上韧带 supraspinous ligament

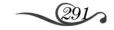

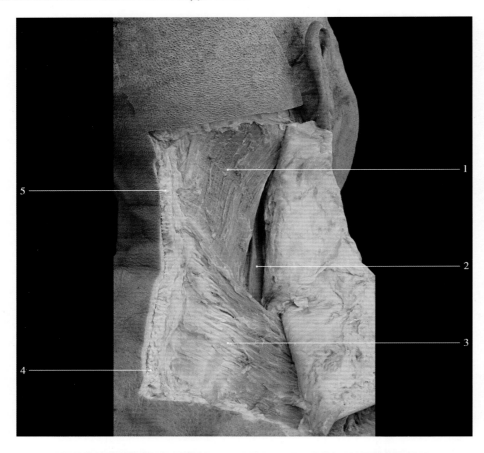

◀ 图 2-146　颈后区结构-
斜方肌、夹肌
Fig. 2-146　Structures
in the posterior region of
neck-the trapezius and
splenius

1. 夹肌 splenius
2. 肩胛提肌 levator sca-
pulae
3. 斜方肌 trapezius
4. 棘上韧带 supraspinous
ligament
5. 项韧带 ligamentum nu-
chae

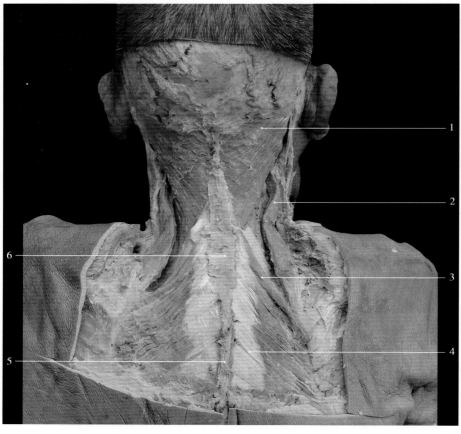

◀ 图 2-147　颈后区结构-
夹肌、菱形肌
Fig. 2-147　Structures
in the posterior region of
neck-the splenius and
rhomboideus

1. 夹肌 splenius
2. 肩胛提肌 levator sca-
pulae
3. 小菱形肌 rhomboideus
minor
4. 大菱形肌 rhomboideus
major
5. 棘上韧带 supraspinous
ligament
6. 项韧带 ligamentum nu-
chae

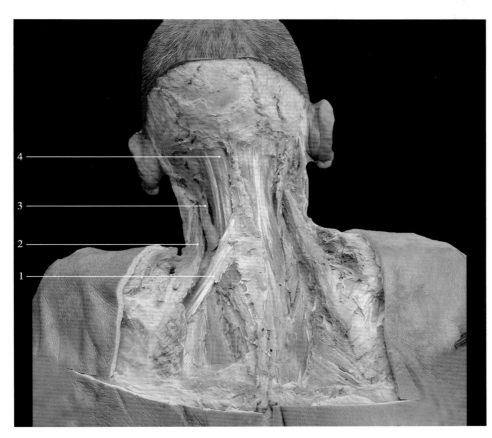

◀ 图 2-148 颈后区结构-半棘肌、上后锯肌
Fig. 2-148 Structures in the posterior region of neck-the semispinalis and serratus posterior superior

1. 上后锯肌 serratus posterior superior
2. 肩胛提肌 levator scapulae
3. 颈夹肌 splenius cervicis
4. 半棘肌 semispinalis

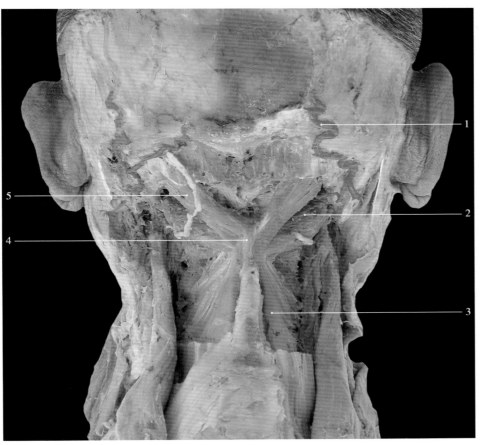

◀ 图 2-149 枕下三角
Fig. 2-149 Suboccipital triangle

1. 枕动脉 occipital artery
2. 枕下三角 suboccipital triangle
3. 颈半棘肌 semispinalis cervicis
4. 枢椎棘突 spinous process of axis
5. 头后大直肌 rectus capitis posterior major

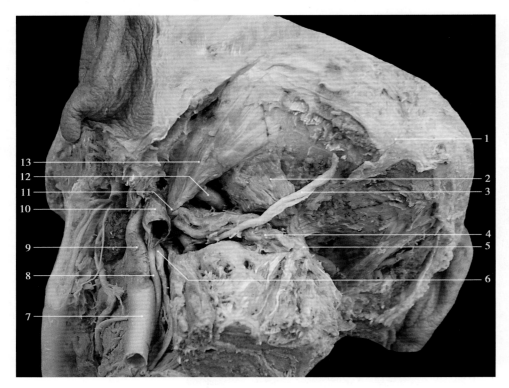

◀ 图 2-150　左侧枕下三角
Fig. 2-150　Left sub-occipital triangle

1. 枕外隆凸 external occipital protuberance
2. 头后大直肌 rectus capitis posterior major
3. 枕大神经 greater occipital nerve
4. 头下斜肌 obliquus capitis inferior
5. 枢椎棘突 spinous process of axis
6. 颈上神经节 superior cervical ganglion
7. 颈总动脉 common carotid artery
8. 迷走神经 vagus nerve
9. 颈内动脉 internal carotid artery
10. 颈内静脉 internal jugular vein
11. 寰椎横突 transverse process of atlas
12. 椎动脉寰椎部 atlantic part of vertebral artery
13. 头上斜肌 obliquus capitis superior

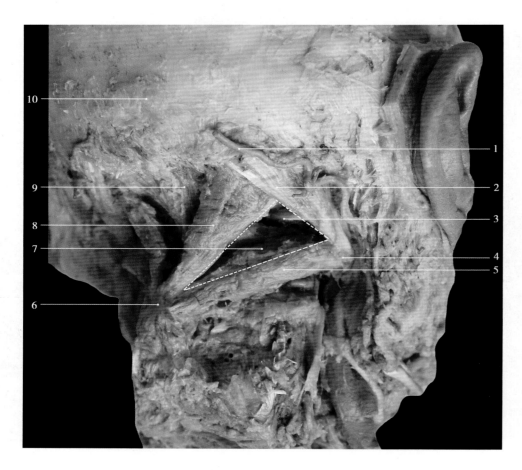

◀ 图 2-151　右侧枕下三角
Fig. 2-151　Right sub-occipital triangle

1. 枕动脉 occipital artery
2. 头上斜肌 obliquus capitis superior
3. 椎动脉寰椎部 atlantic part of vertebral artery
4. 寰椎横突 transverse process of atlas
5. 头下斜肌 obliquus capitis inferior
6. 枢椎棘突 spinous process of axis
7. 枕下三角 suboccipital triangle
8. 头后大直肌 rectus capitis posterior major
9. 头后小直肌 rectus capitis posterior minor
10. 枕外隆凸 external occipital protuberance

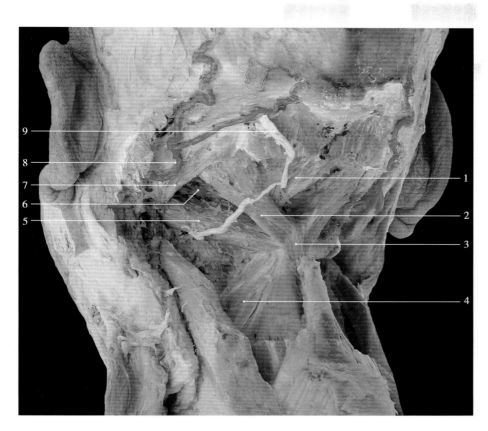

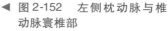

图 2-152 左侧枕动脉与椎动脉寰椎部

Fig. 2-152 Left occipital artery and atlantic part of vertebral artery

1. 头后小直肌 rectus capitis posterior minor
2. 头后大直肌 rectus capitis posterior major
3. 枢椎棘突 spinous process of axis
4. 颈棘肌 spinalis cervicis
5. 头下斜肌 obliquus capitis inferior
6. 椎动脉寰椎部 atlantic part of vertebral artery
7. 头上斜肌 obliquus capitis superior
8. 枕动脉 occipital artery
9. 枕大神经 greater occipital nerve

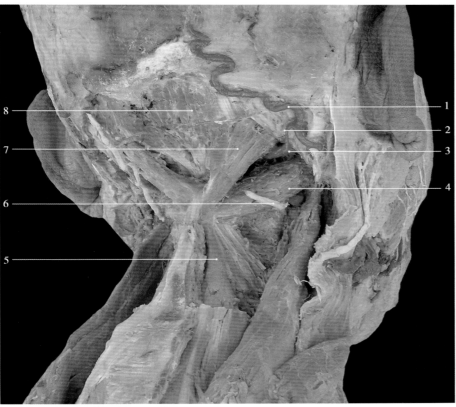

图 2-153 右侧枕动脉与椎动脉寰椎部

Fig. 2-153 Right occipital artery and atlantic part of vertebral artery

1. 枕动脉 occipital artery
2. 枕动脉椎动脉交通支 communicating branch between occipital artery and vertebral artery
3. 椎动脉寰椎部 atlantic part of vertebral artery
4. 头下斜肌 obliquus capitis inferior
5. 颈半棘肌 semispinalis cervicis
6. 枕大神经 greater occipital nerve
7. 头后大直肌 rectus capitis posterior major
8. 头半棘肌(已切断) semispinalis capitis(severed)

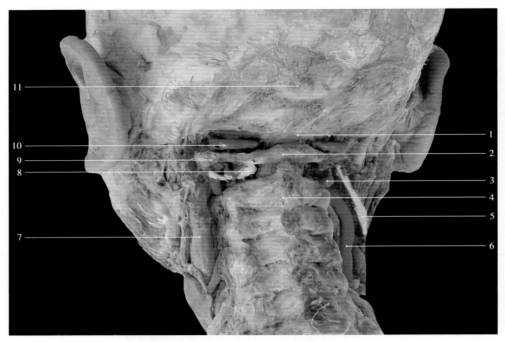

▲ 图 2-154　左侧椎动脉寰椎部
Fig. 2-154　Left atlantic part of vertebral artery

1. 寰枕后膜 posterior atlantooccipital membrane
2. 寰椎后结节 posterior tubercle of atlas
3. 椎动脉横突部 transverse part of vertebral artery
4. 枢椎棘突 spinous process of axis
5. 迷走神经 vagus nerve
6. 颈内动脉 internal carotid artery
7. 颈内静脉 internal jugular vein
8. 第 2 脊神经节 the 2nd spinal ganglion
9. 寰椎横突 transverse process of atlas
10. 椎动脉寰椎部 atlantic part of vertebral artery
11. 枕骨 occipital bone

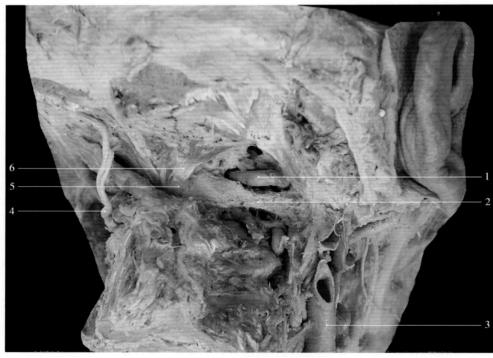

▲ 图 2-155　右侧椎动脉寰椎部
Fig. 2-155　Right atlantic part of vertebral artery

1. 椎动脉寰椎部 atlantic part of vertebral artery
2. 寰椎后弓 posterior arch of atlas
3. 颈总动脉 common carotid artery
4. 左侧枕大神经 left greater occipital nerve
5. 寰椎后结节 posterior tubercle of atlas
6. 头后小直肌 rectus capitis posterior minor

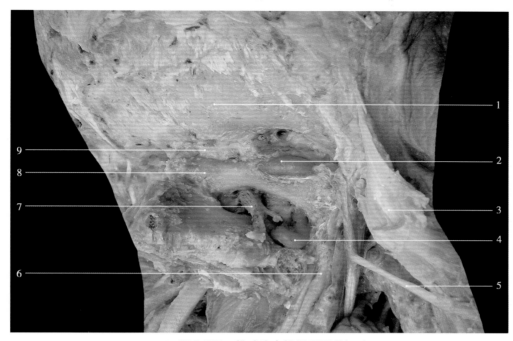

▲ 图2-156　椎动脉寰椎部后面观（一）
Fig. 2-156　Posterior aspect of the atlantic part of vertebral artery（1）

1. 枕骨 occipital bone
2. 椎动脉寰椎部 atlantic part of vertebral artery
3. 胸锁乳突肌 sternocleidomastoid
4. 椎动脉横突部 transverse part of vertebral artery
5. 副神经 accessory nerve
6. 迷走神经 vagus nerve
7. 第2脊神经节 the 2nd spinal ganglion
8. 寰椎横突 transverse process of atlas
9. 寰枕后膜 posterior atlantooccipital membrane

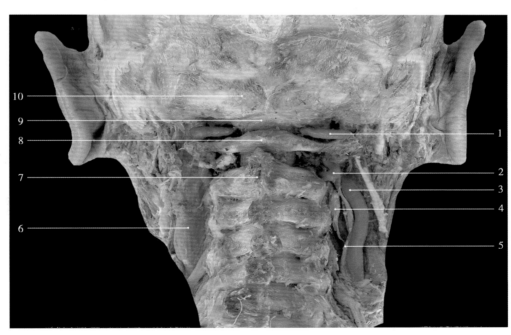

▲ 图2-157　椎动脉寰椎部后面观（二）
Fig. 2-157　Posterior aspect of the atlantic part of vertebral artery（2）

1. 椎动脉寰椎部 atlantic part of vertebral artery
2. 椎动脉横突部 transverse part of vertebral artery
3. 颈内动脉 internal carotid artery
4. 颈上神经节 superior cervical ganglion
5. 迷走神经 vagus nerve
6. 颈内静脉 internal jugular vein
7. 枢椎棘突 spinous process of axis
8. 寰枕后结节 posterior atlantooccipital tubercle
9. 寰枕后膜 posterior atlantooccipital membrane
10. 枕骨 occipital bone

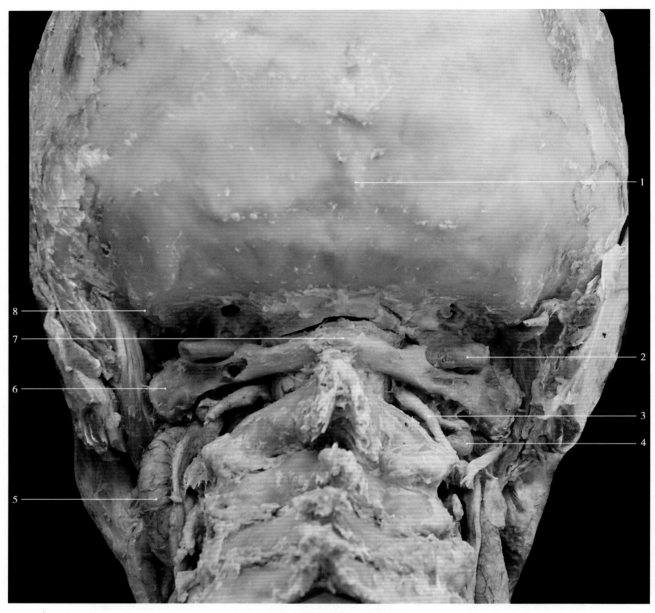

▲ 图 2-158　椎动脉寰椎部后面观（三）

Fig. 2-158　Posterior aspect of the atlantic part of vertebral artery（3）

1. 枕外隆凸 external occipital protuberance
2. 椎动脉寰椎部 atlantic part of vertebral artery
3. 枕大神经 greater occipital nerve
4. 椎动脉横突部 transverse part of vertebral artery
5. 颈总动脉 common carotid artery
6. 寰椎横突 transverse process of atlas
7. 寰椎后结节 posterior tubercle of atlas
8. 颞骨乳突 mastoid process of temporal bone

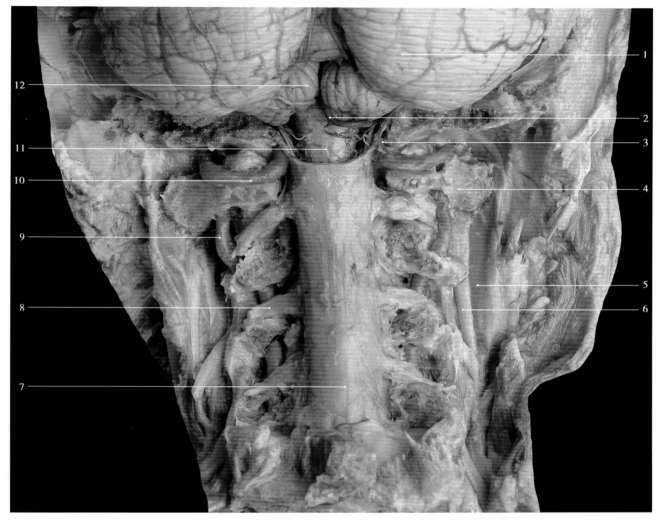

▲ 图 2-159　椎动脉寰椎部和横突部后面观

Fig. 2-159　Posterior aspect of the atlantic part and transverse part of vertebral artery

1. 小脑 cerebellum
2. 小脑下后动脉 posterior inferior cerebellar artery
3. 枕骨大孔 foramen magnum
4. 寰椎横突 transverse process of atlas
5. 颈内静脉 internal jugular vein
6. 迷走神经 vagus nerve
7. 硬脊膜 spinal dura mater
8. 第 3 脊神经 the 3rd spinal nerve
9. 椎动脉 vertebral artery
10. 椎动脉寰椎部 atlantic part of vertebral artery
11. 延髓 medulla oblongata
12. 小脑扁桃体 tonsil of cerebellum

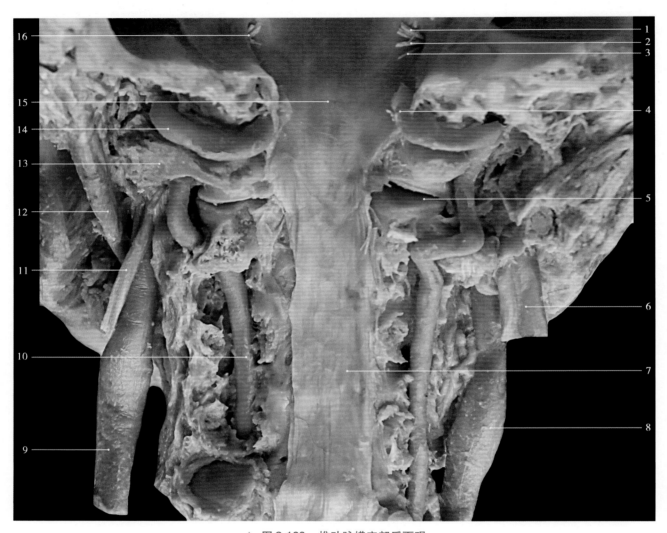

▲ 图2-160 椎动脉横突部后面观

Fig. 2-160 Posterior aspect of the transverse part of vertebral artery

1. 舌咽神经 glossopharyngeal nerve
2. 迷走神经 vagus nerve
3. 副神经 accessory nerve
4. 椎动脉颅内部 intracranial part of vertebral artery
5. 寰枢关节 atlanto axial joint
6. 颈内静脉 internal jugular vein
7. 椎管前壁 anterior wall of verterbral canal
8. 颈动脉窦 carotid sinus

9. 颈总动脉 common carotid artery
10. 椎动脉横突部 transverse part of vertebral artery
11. 迷走神经 vagus nerve
12. 茎突 styloid process of temporal bone
13. 寰椎横突 transverse process of atlas
14. 椎动脉寰椎部 atlantic part of vertebral artery
15. 枕骨大孔前壁 anterior wall of foramen magnum
16. 颈静脉孔 jugular foramen

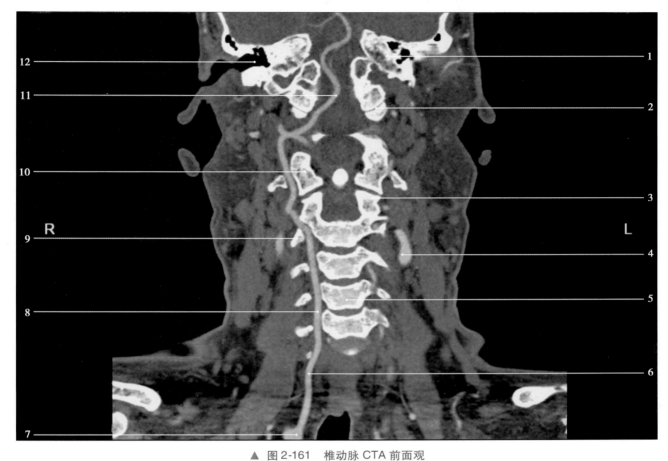

▲ 图 2-161 椎动脉 CTA 前面观

Fig. 2-161 Anterior aspect of the vertebral artery by CTA

1. 颞骨 temporal bone
2. 寰枕关节 atlantooccipital joint
3. 上关节突 superior articular process
4. 颈总动脉分叉部 furcation of common carotid artery
5. 第 5 颈椎椎体 vertebral body of the 5th cervical vertebra
6. 椎动脉 vertebral artery

7. 锁骨下动脉 subclavian artery
8. 椎动脉横突部 transverse part of vertebral artery
9. 颈椎横突 transverse process of cervical vertebra
10. 寰椎 atlas
11. 椎动脉颅内部 intracranial part of vertebral artery
12. 外耳道 external acoustic meatus

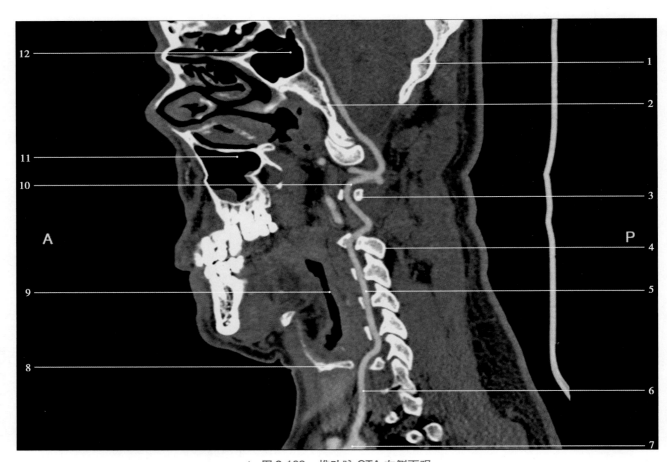

▲ 图 2-162　椎动脉 CTA 左侧面观
Fig. 2-162　Left aspect of the vertebral artery by CTA

1. 枕骨 occipital bone
2. 斜坡 clivus
3. 寰椎侧块 lateral mass of atlas
4. 颈椎椎体 vertebral body of axis
5. 椎动脉横突部 transverse part of vertebral artery
6. 椎动脉颈部 cervical part of vertebral artery
7. 锁骨下动脉 subclavian artery
8. 甲状软骨 thyroid cartilage
9. 口咽腔 oral part of pharynx
10. 椎动脉寰椎部 atlantic part of vertebral artery
11. 上颌窦 maxillary sinus
12. 蝶窦 sphenoidal sinus

椎动脉寰椎部与枕动脉端-侧吻合治疗基底动脉供血不足的应用解剖学要点

因颈椎的骨质增生使椎间孔变小而挤压椎动脉或枕下肌痉挛压迫椎动脉的寰椎部而使脑干和小脑供血不足。临床上常用颈前路侧前方椎动脉减压术,也可用枕动脉与椎动脉的寰椎部吻接以增加基底动脉的血流量(图 2-149 ~ 图 2-158)。

应用解剖要点:

椎动脉寰椎部(或第 3 段)位于枕下三角内,为椎动脉出寰椎横突孔绕寰椎侧块的后方,再经椎动脉沟向后向内走行至穿寰枕后膜的一段。全程呈水平位,其中部突向后,形成凹向前突向后的弯曲。椎动脉寰椎部长度(后壁)为 22.9mm,中部外径为 4.09mm(右侧为 3.94mm,左侧为 4.25mm),中部的体表投影在两侧乳突尖连线下 3.54mm,正中线外 32.46mm。椎动脉寰椎部由浅至深为皮肤→浅筋膜→斜方肌→头夹肌→头半棘肌→枕下三角。

枕动脉在枕部浅出的位置是在两侧乳突尖连线上方 31.35mm,距后正中线 28.58mm。枕动脉在乳突后缘至浅出点的自然长度为 49.03mm,拉直后的长度为 60.05mm,枕动脉在乳突后缘处的外径为 2.60mm,枕动脉与椎动脉寰椎部相距 16.23mm。

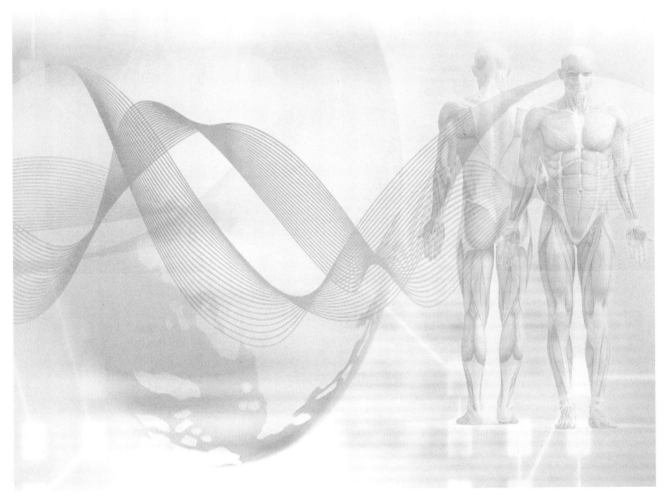

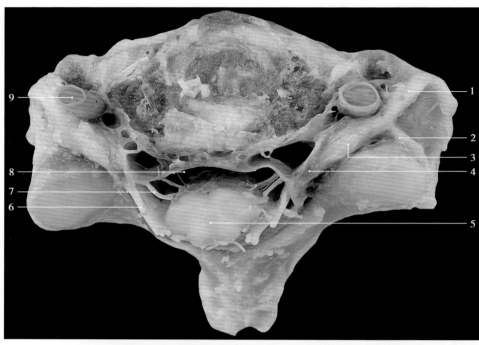

◀ 图 2-163 颈段脊髓、脊神经前后根、脊神经节上面观
Fig. 2-163 Superior aspect of the cervical part of spinal cord, the anterior and posterior roots of spinal nerve, and the spinal ganglion

1. 脊神经前支 anterior branch of spinal nerve
2. 脊神经后支 posterior branch of spinal nerve
3. 脊神经节 spinal ganglion
4. 脊神经 spinal nerve
5. 脊髓 spinal cord
6. 脊神经后根 posterior root of spinal nerve
7. 脊神经前根 anterior root of spinal nerve
8. 蛛网膜下隙 subarachnoid space
9. 椎动脉 vertebral artery

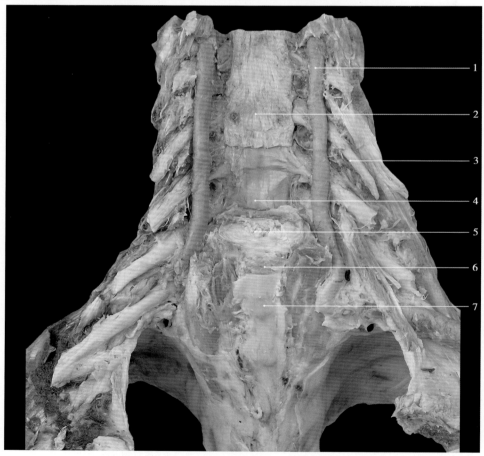

▲ 图 2-164 颈段前纵韧带、后纵韧带（椎体已切除）
Fig. 2-164 Anterior and posterior cervical longitudinal ligaments（the vertebral body was excised）

1. 椎动脉 vertebral artery
2. 后纵韧带 posterior longitudinal ligament
3. 脊神经前支 anterior branch of spinal nerve
4. 颈段硬脊膜 cervical spinal dura mater
5. 髓核 nucleus pulposus
6. 椎体 vertebral body
7. 前纵韧带 anterior longitudinal ligament

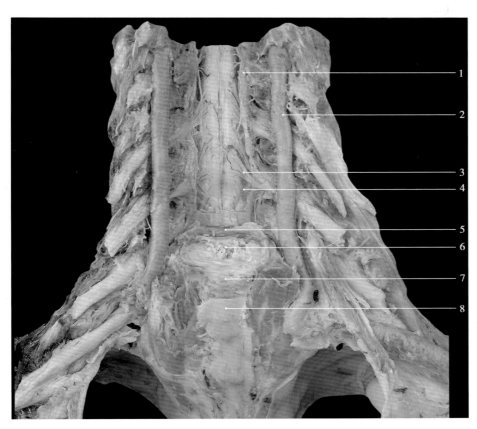

◀ 图 2-165 颈段蛛网膜前面观

Fig. 2-165 Anterior aspect of the cervical arachnoid mater

1. 硬脊膜 spinal dura mater
2. 椎动脉 vertebral artery
3. 脊神经前根 anterior root of spinal nerve
4. 蛛网膜 spinal arachnoid mater
5. 后纵韧带 posterior longitudinal ligament
6. 髓核 nucleus pulposus
7. 椎体 vertebral body
8. 前纵韧带 anterior longitudinal ligament

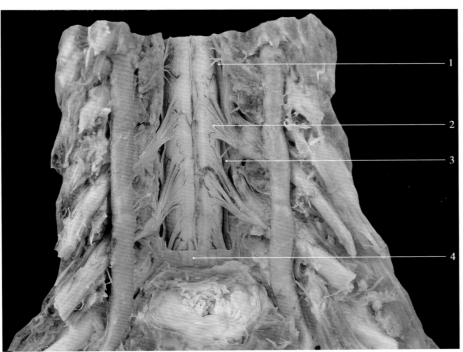

◀ 图 2-166 齿状韧带前面观

Fig. 2-166 Anterior aspect of the denticulate ligament

1. 硬脊膜 spinal dura mater
2. 脊神经前根 anterior root of spinal nerve
3. 齿状韧带 denticulate ligament
4. 蛛网膜 spinal arachnoid mater

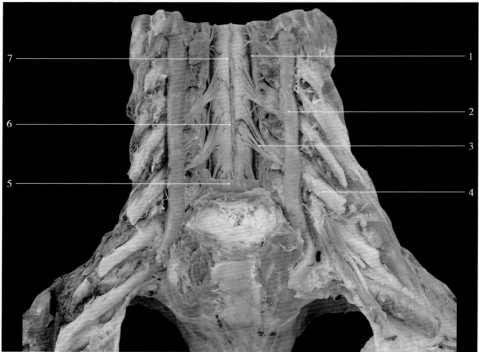

◀ 图 2-167　颈段脊神经前根（椎体已切除）

Fig. 2-167　Anterior root of the cervical spinal nerves (the vertebral body was excised)

1. 硬脊膜 spinal dura mater
2. 椎动脉 vertebral artery
3. 脊神经前根 anterior root of spinal nerve
4. 脊神经前支 anterior branch of spinal nerve
5. 蛛网膜 spinal arachnoid mater
6. 前正中沟 anterior median groove
7. 脊髓前动脉 anterior spinal artery

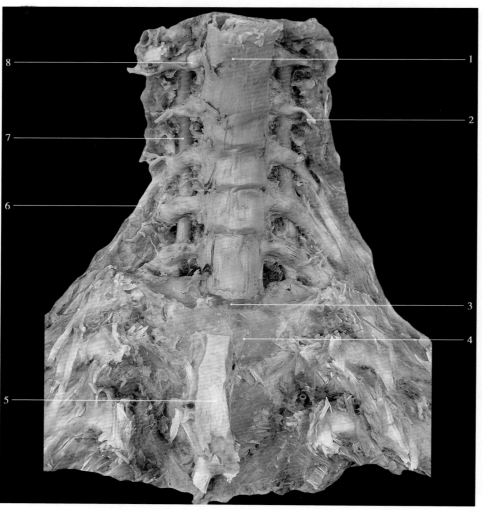

◀ 图 2-168　颈段脊神经节、脊神经与椎动脉关系后面观

Fig. 2-168　Posterior aspect of the relationship among the spinal ganglion, spinal nerves and vertebral artery

1. 颈段硬脊膜 cervical spinal dura mater
2. 脊神经后支 posterior branch of spinal nerve
3. 黄韧带 ligamenta flava
4. 椎板 lamina of vertebra
5. 棘上韧带 supraspinous ligament
6. 脊神经前支 anterior branch of spinal nerve
7. 椎动脉 vertebral artery
8. 脊神经节 spinal ganglion

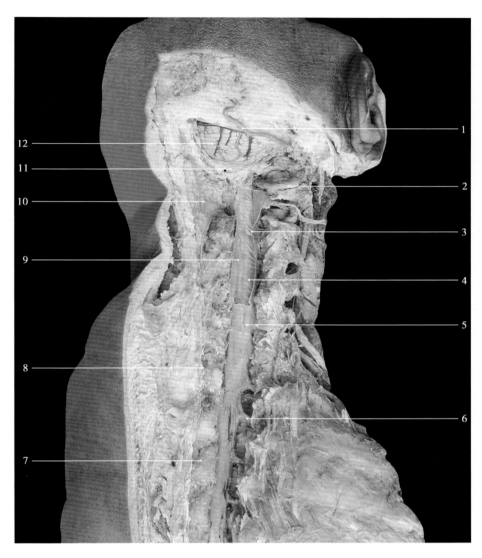

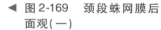

◀ 图 2-169 颈段蛛网膜后面观(一)
Fig. 2-169 Posterior aspect of the cervical spinal arachnoid mater(1)

1. 枕动脉 occipital artery
2. 椎动脉 vetebral artery
3. 颈 3 脊神经后根 posterior root of the 3rd cervical spinal nerve
4. 脊髓颈膨大 cervical enlargement of spinal cord
5. 硬脊膜 spinal dura mater
6. 胸 1 脊神经 the 1st thoracic spinal nerve
7. 棘间韧带 interspinal ligaments
8. 棘上韧带 supraspinal ligaments
9. 脊髓蛛网膜 spinal arachnoid mater
10. 项韧带 ligamentum nuchae
11. 小脑延髓池 cisterna cerebellomedullaris
12. 小脑 cerebellum

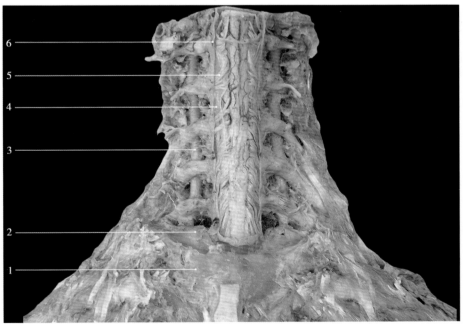

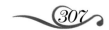

◀ 图 2-170 颈段蛛网膜后面观(二)
Fig. 2-170 Posterior aspect of the cervical spinal arachnoid mater(2)

1. 椎板 lamina of vertebra
2. 上关节突 superior articular process
3. 椎动脉 vertebral artery
4. 蛛网膜 spinal arachnoid mater
5. 脊神经后根 posterior root of spinal nerve
6. 硬脊膜 spinal dura mater

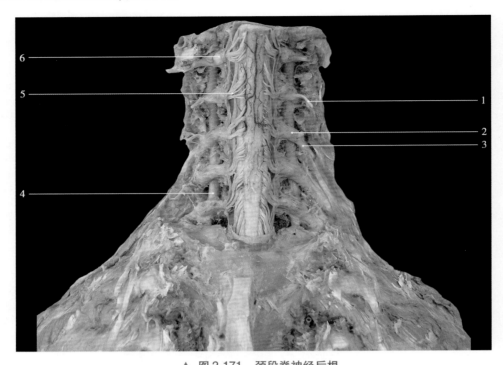

▲ 图 2-171　颈段脊神经后根

Fig. 2-171　Posterior root of the cervical spinal nerves

1. 脊神经后支 posterior branch of spinal nerve
2. 脊神经 spinal nerve
3. 脊神经前支 anterior branch of spinal nerve
4. 椎动脉 vertebral artery
5. 脊神经后根 posterior root of spinal nerves
6. 脊神经节 spinal ganglion

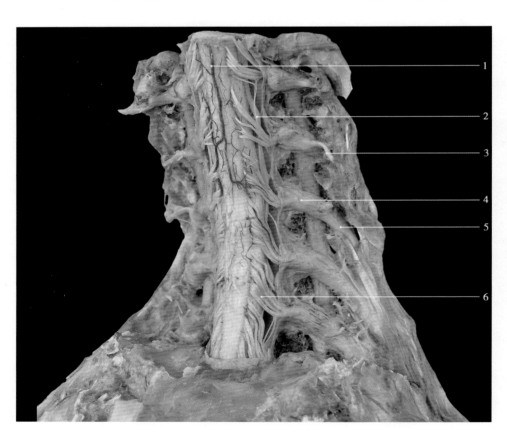

◀ 图 2-172　齿状韧带后面观

Fig. 2-172　Posterior aspect of the denticulate ligament

1. 脊髓后静脉 posterior spinal vein
2. 齿状韧带 denticulate ligament
3. 脊神经后支 posterior branch of spinal nerve
4. 脊神经 spinal nerve
5. 脊神经前支 anterior branch of spinal nerve
6. 脊神经后根 posterior root of spinal nerves

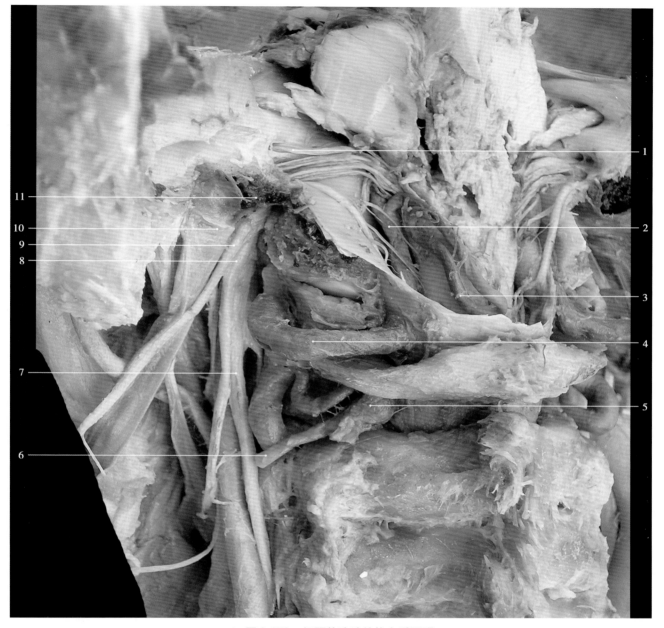

▲ 图 2-173 经颈静脉孔结构左后面观

Fig. 2-173 Left posterior aspect of the structures through the jugular foramen

1. 舌咽迷走颅内段 intracranial part of glossopharyngeal and vagus nerve
2. 椎动脉 vertebral artery
3. 小脑下后动脉尾袢 loop of inferior posterior cerebellar artery
4. 椎动脉寰椎部 atlantic part of vertebral artery
5. 第 2 脊神经节 the 2nd spinal ganglion
6. 枕大神经 greater occipital nerve

7. 迷走神经 vagus nerve
8. 舌下神经 hypoglossal nerve
9. 副神经 accessory nerve
10. 颈内静脉 internal jugular vein
11. 颈静脉孔 jugular foramen

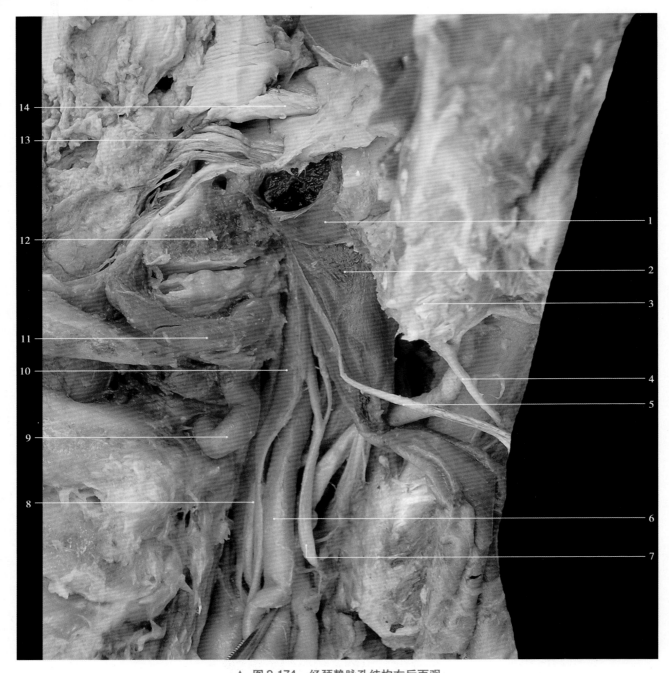

▲ 图2-174 经颈静脉孔结构右后面观

Fig. 2-174 Right posterior aspect of the structures through the jugular foramen

1. 颈静脉孔 jugular foramen
2. 颈内静脉 internal jugular vein
3. 乳突 mastoid process
4. 面神经 facial nerve
5. 副神经 accessory nerve
6. 颈内动脉 internal carotid artery
7. 迷走神经 vagus nerve

8. 颈段交感干 cervical sympathetic trunk
9. 椎动脉 vertebral artery
10. 颈上神经节 superior cervical ganglion
11. 椎动脉寰椎部 atlantic part of vertebral artery
12. 枕髁 occipital condyle
13. 迷走神经颅内部 intracranial part of vagus nerve
14. 三叉神经 trigeminal nerve

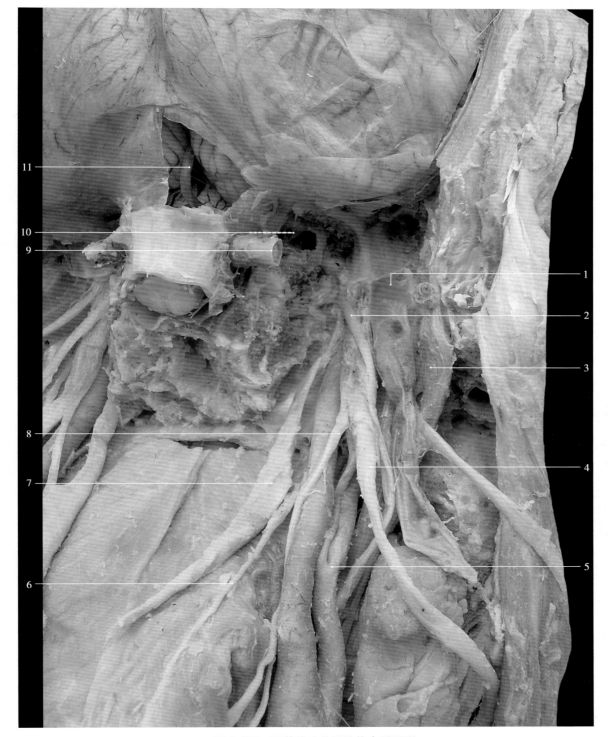

▲ 图 2-175　颈静脉孔外侧结构右后面观

Fig. 2-175　Right posterior aspect of the structures outside the jugular foramen

1. 颈内静脉 internal jugular vein
2. 舌下神经 hypoglossal nerve
3. 茎突咽肌 stylopharyngeus
4. 迷走神经 vagus nerve
5. 颈外动脉 external carotid artery
6. 舌咽神经咽支 pharyngeal branch of glossopharyngeal nerve

7. 颈上神经节 superior cervical ganglione
8. 喉上神经 superior laryngeal nerve
9. 椎动脉 vertebral artery
10. 颈静脉孔 jugular foramen
11. 小脑下后动脉 posterior inferior cerebellar artery

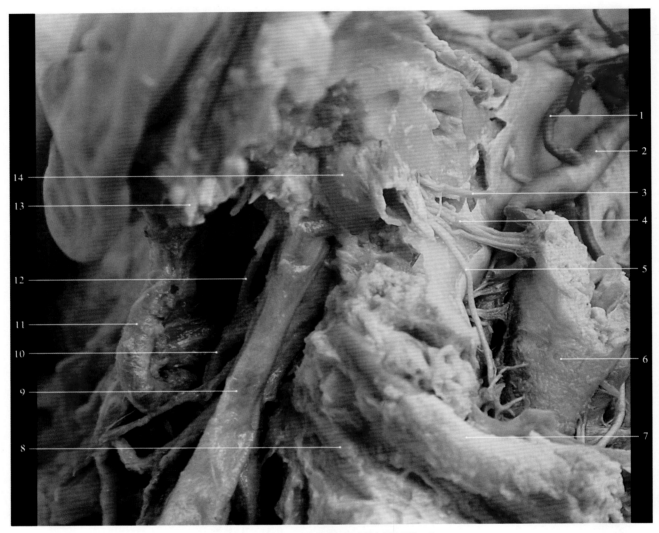

▲ 图 2-176　颈静脉球后外侧面观（一）
Fig. 2-176　Posterior lateral aspect of the jugular bulb（1）

1. 小脑下后动脉 posterior inferior cerebellar artery
2. 基底动脉 basilar artery
3. 舌咽神经颅内段 intracranial part of glossopharyngeal nerve
4. 迷走神经颅内段 intracranial part of vagus nerve
5. 副神经颅内段 intracranial part of accessory nerve
6. 延髓 medulla oblongata
7. 寰椎后弓 posterior arch of atlas

8. 椎动脉横突部 transverse part of vertebral artery
9. 颈内静脉 internal jugular vein
10. 迷走神经 vagus nerve
11. 面总静脉 common facial vein
12. 舌咽神经 glossopharyngeal nerve
13. 乳突 mastoid process of temporal bone
14. 颈静脉球 jugular bulb

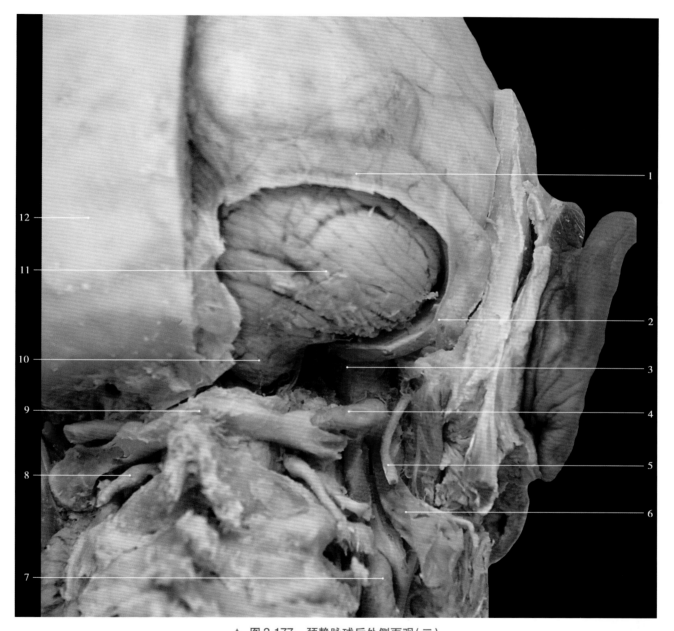

▲ 图2-177 颈静脉球后外侧面观(二)

Fig. 2-177 Posterior lateral aspect of the jugular bulb(2)

1. 横窦 transverse sinus
2. 乙状窦 sigmoid sinus
3. 颈静脉球 jugular bulb
4. 椎动脉寰椎部 atlantic part of vertebral artery
5. 枕动脉 occipital artery
6. 颈内静脉 jugular vein

7. 椎动脉横突孔部 transverse part of vertebral artery
8. 枕大神经 greater occipital nerve
9. 寰椎后结节 posterior tubercle of atlas
10. 小脑扁桃体 tonsil of cerebellum
11. 小脑 cerebellum
12. 枕骨 occipital bone

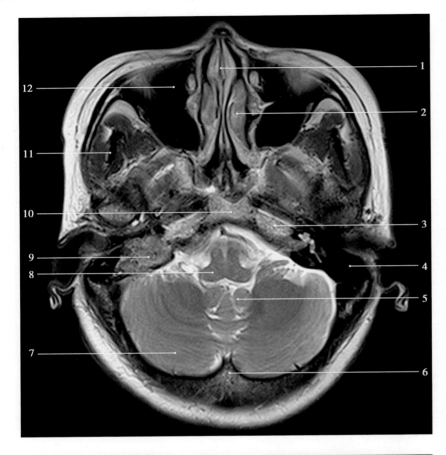

◀ 图2-178　颈静脉球瘤（一）
Fig. 2-178　Glomus jugulare tumor (1)

1. 鼻中隔 nasal septum
2. 中鼻甲 middle nasal concha
3. 颞骨岩部 petrous part of temporal bone
4. 颞骨乳突 mastoid process of temporal bone
5. 小脑扁桃体 tonsil of cerebellum
6. 窦汇 confluence of sinus
7. 小脑半球 cerebellar hemisphere
8. 延髓 medulla oblongata
9. 颈静脉球瘤 glomus jugulare tumor
10. 斜坡 clivus
11. 颞肌 temporalis
12. 上颌窦 maxillary sinus

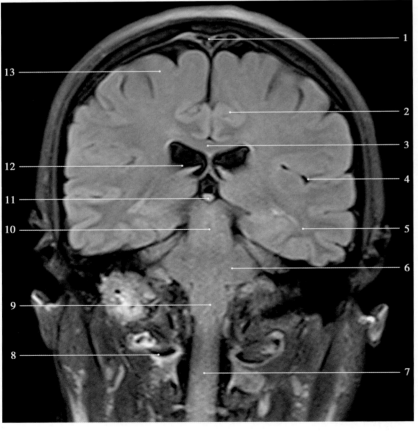

◀ 图2-179　颈静脉球瘤（二）
Fig. 2-179　Glomus jugulare tumor (2)

1. 上矢状窦 superior sagittal sinus
2. 扣带回 cingulate gyrus
3. 胼胝体 corpus callosum
4. 外侧裂 lateral fissure
5. 颞叶 temporal lobe
6. 脑桥 pons
7. 颈髓 cervical spinal cord
8. 颈内静脉 internal jugular vein
9. 延髓 medulla oblongata
10. 中脑导水管 mesencephalic aqueduct
11. 松果体 pineal body
12. 透明隔 septum pellucidum
13. 顶叶 parietal lobe

颈静脉孔颅外区神经的应用解剖学要点

颈静脉孔位于颞骨茎突的内侧偏前方,孔的前部为颞骨的岩部,后部为枕骨。颈静脉区除为颈内静脉的起端外,还与Ⅸ～Ⅻ对脑神经及颈段交感干解剖关系密切。

1. 舌咽神经　在颈静脉孔内位于迷走神经的前外侧,穿孔时形成两个神经节,上节位于孔内,下节位于孔外。

2. 迷走神经　与副神经包于同一鞘内,行于舌咽神经的内侧。

3. 副神经　副神经颅部离开延髓后向外行,至颈静脉孔处,加入经枕骨大孔上行的脊髓部,两者合股后穿颈静脉孔,然后又分开,颅部加入迷走神经,脊髓部在颈部下行。

4. 舌下神经　自舌下神经管出颅后,降于迷走神经、副神经的后内侧,颈内动、静脉之间,然后向外,越过颈内动脉之前进入颈部(图 2-173 ～ 图 2-179)。

应用解剖要点:

颈静脉孔位于茎突的前内侧,距茎突根部约 3.0mm。茎突位于颞骨鼓部的后下方。茎突为许多肌和韧带的起点,邻近有 4 对脑神经等重要结构。茎突根部与乳突尖相距约 18mm;与外耳门下缘中点相距约 9.0mm;与关节结节外缘相距约 30mm。颈动脉管外口在颈静脉孔之前,两孔中心点相距约 10mm。下颌神经于颈静脉孔之前走出卵圆孔,两孔中心点相距约 20mm。头颈部外科医生熟知颈静脉孔区周围解剖结构的形态、位置及排列关系,将会对颅底区、特别是颈静脉孔区疾病的诊断和手术治疗有很大的帮助。

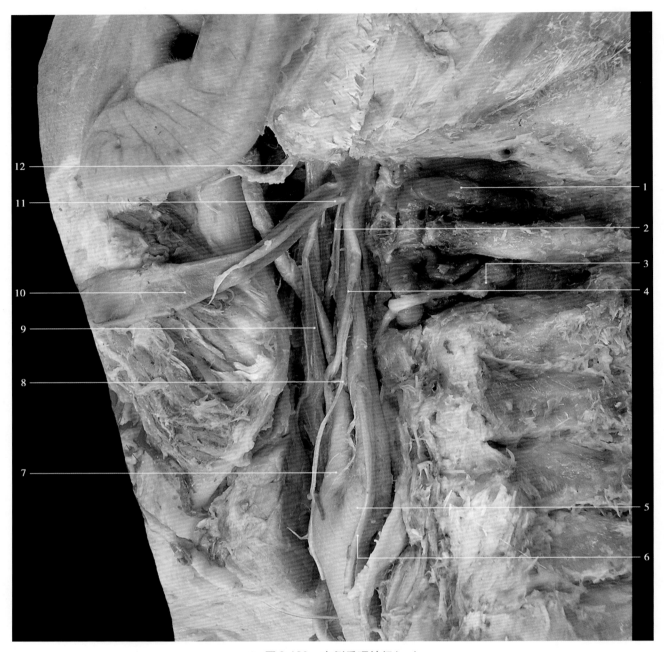

▲ 图 2-180 左侧舌咽神经（一）
Fig. 2-180 Left glossopharyngeal nerve（1）

1. 椎动脉寰椎部 atlantic part of vertebral artery
2. 舌咽神经 glossopharyngeal nerve
3. 第 2 脊神经节 the 2nd spinal ganglion
4. 舌下神经 hypoglossal nerve
5. 颈动脉窦 carotid sinus
6. 迷走神经 vagus nerve
7. 颈外动脉 external carotid artery
8. 舌下神经降支 descending branch of hypoglossal nerve
9. 茎突咽肌 stylopharyngeus
10. 颈内静脉 internal jugular vein
11. 副神经 accessory nerve
12. 面神经 facial nerve

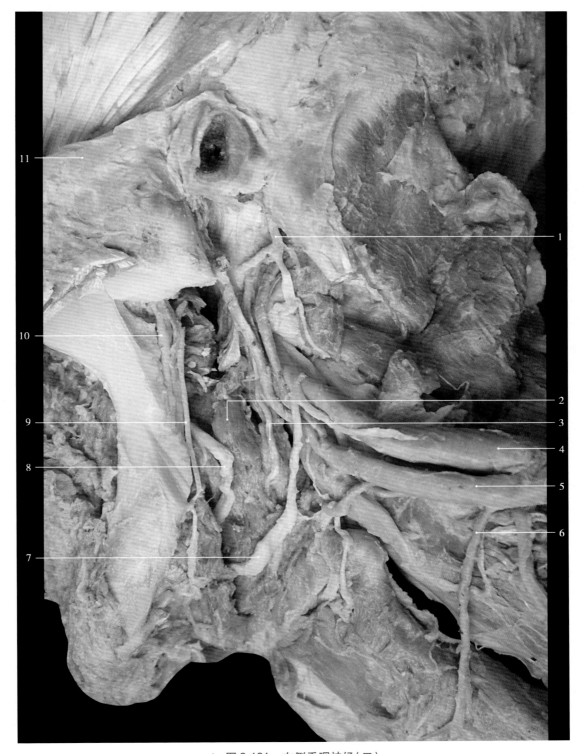

▲ 图 2-181　左侧舌咽神经（二）

Fig. 2-181　Left glossopharyngeal nerve（2）

1. 面神经 facial nerve
2. 茎突舌肌 styloglossus
3. 舌咽神经 glossopharyngeal nerve
4. 颈动脉窦 carotid sinus
5. 颈外动脉 external carotid artery
6. 甲状腺上动脉 superior thyroid artery
7. 舌下神经 hypoglossal nerve
8. 舌神经 lingual nerve
9. 下颌舌骨肌支 mylohyoid branch
10. 下牙槽神经 inferior alveolar nerve
11. 颧弓 zygomatic arch

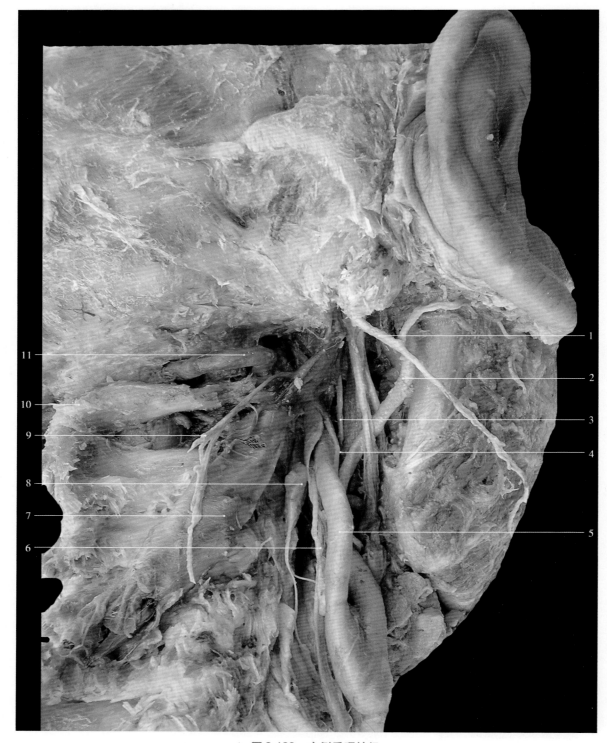

▲ 图 2-182　右侧舌咽神经

Fig. 2-182　Right glossopharyngeal nerve

1. 面神经 facial nerve
2. 颈外动脉 external carotid artery
3. 右侧舌咽神经 right glossopharyngeal nerve
4. 舌下神经 hypoglossal nerve
5. 颈内动脉 internal carotid artery
6. 迷走神经 vagus nerve
7. 颈内静脉 internal jugular vein
8. 颈上神经节 superior cervical ganglion
9. 副神经 accessory nerve
10. 寰椎后结节 posterior tubercle of atlas
11. 椎动脉寰椎部 atlantic part of vertebral artery

舌咽神经阻滞术的应用解剖学要点

舌咽神经属于混合性脑神经,含有特殊内脏传入、一般内脏传入、一般躯体传入、特殊内脏传出和一般内脏传出 5 种纤维。其中,特殊内脏传出纤维起自疑核上部,分布于咽部的横纹肌(茎突咽肌);一般内脏传出纤维起自延髓的下泌涎核,节前纤维至耳神经节交换神经元,节后纤维分布于腮腺。

舌咽神经以 3 ~ 4 条根丝走出橄榄后沟上部向外侧集中,至小脑绒球腹侧合成一干,穿颈静脉孔前部出颅,在孔内舌咽神经位于迷走神经的外侧,出颈静脉孔后,下降于颈内动脉、颈内静脉之间,内侧有迷走神经,继而向前内侧弯曲,经茎突及茎突咽肌的内侧,于舌骨舌肌内侧,向前上方横越咽中缩肌及茎突舌骨韧带达舌根:

1. 咽支(3 ~ 4 支)分布于咽黏膜(图 2-180 ~ 图 2-182)。

2. 颈动脉窦支　为颈动脉小球和颈动脉窦的传入神经,分布于颈动脉小球(化学感受器)和颈动脉窦(压力感受器)。

3. 茎突咽肌支　除了分布于茎突咽肌,此分支还接受来自面神经的交通支。

4. 扁桃体支　有数小支,在舌咽神经通过舌骨舌肌的深面时发出,主要分布于扁桃体。

5. 舌支　分布于舌后 1/3 的舌黏膜及其味蕾,司一般感觉和味觉。

应用解剖要点:

舌咽神经自颈静脉孔出颅后,在颈段主要行于茎突和茎突咽肌前内侧,呈弓形弯向前至舌(图 2-113、图 2-115 ~ 图 2-117)。

舌咽神经阻滞术的进针点常选在:乳突尖与下颌角之间连线的中点。

穿刺层次为:皮肤→浅筋膜→颈阔肌→胸锁乳突肌→茎突→舌咽神经。

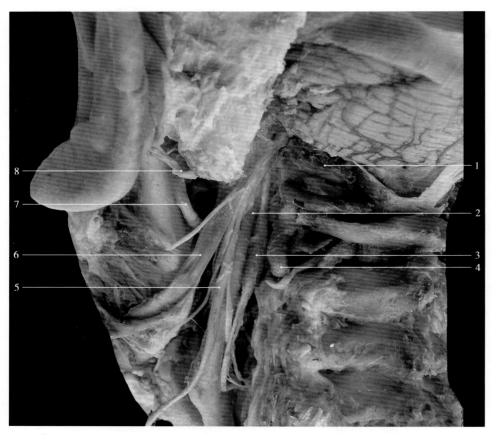

◀ 图2-183　左侧颈上神经节

Fig. 2-183　Left superior cervical ganglion

1. 枕骨髁 occipital condyle
2. 颈内动脉 internal carotid artery
3. 颈上神经节 superior cervical ganglion
4. 椎动脉 vertebral artery
5. 迷走神经 vagus nerve
6. 颈内静脉 internal jugular vein
7. 颈外动脉 external carotid artery
8. 面神经 facial nerve

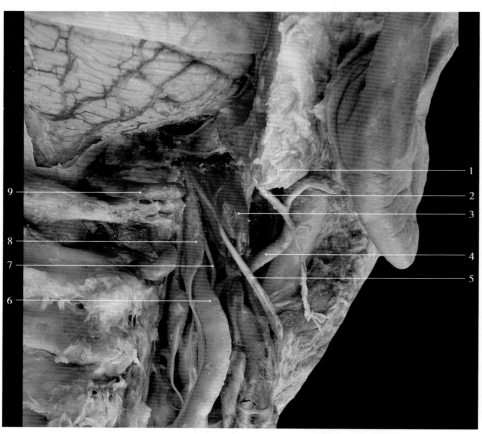

◀ 图2-184　右侧颈上神经节

Fig. 2-184　Right superior cervical ganglion

1. 乳突 mastoid process of temporal bone
2. 面神经 facial nerve
3. 颈内静脉 internal jugular vein
4. 颈外动脉 external carotid artery
5. 副神经 accessory nerve
6. 颈内动脉 internal carotid artery
7. 迷走神经 vagus nerve
8. 颈神经节 cervical ganglion
9. 椎动脉寰椎部 atlantic part of vertebral artery

颈上神经节的应用解剖学要点

颈上神经节位于第 1～3 颈椎横突的前方,节的上端有 79% 者平对第 1 颈椎横突,下端 51% 者平对第 3 颈椎横突,中国人颈上神经节的出现率为 94%,节为梭形占 88%,圆形为 10% 和肾形为 2%。节的长度为 25mm,中点处宽度为 6.7mm 和厚度为 3.2mm(图 2-183、图 2-184)。

应用解剖要点:

1. 颈上神经节阻滞术　进针点常选在枕外隆凸下方,第 2、3 颈椎棘突间隙外侧 2.5cm,乳突尖下方 1～1.5cm。

2. 进针经过层次　皮肤→浅筋膜→深筋膜→斜方肌→颈夹肌→颈半棘肌→第 2 颈椎横突→颈上神经节。

3. 穿刺注意事项　颈上神经节阻滞时有刺破椎动脉、椎静脉和将药物注入颈段蛛网膜下隙或刺伤颈段脊髓的危险。注药前一定要回抽见注射针内无回血或无回液方可缓慢推注药物。

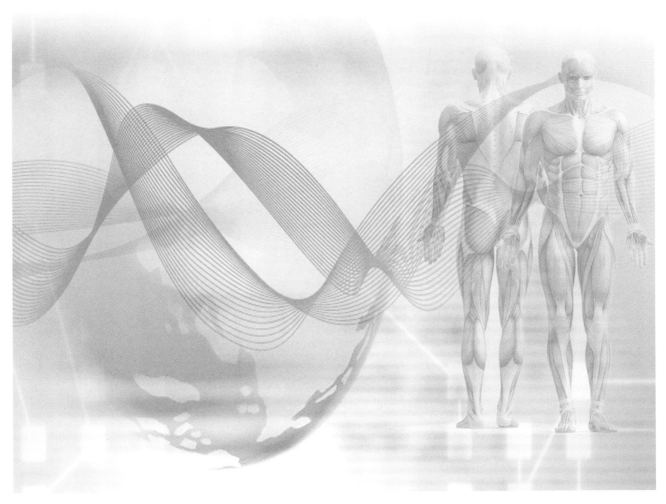

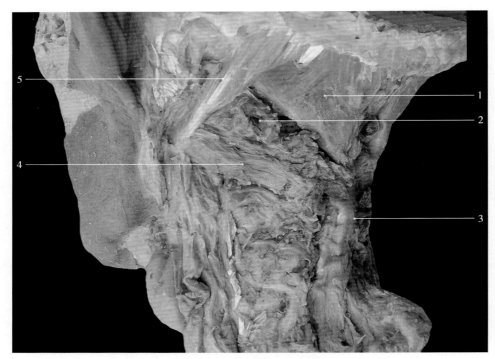

▲ 图 2-185　枕下静脉丛左侧面观
Fig. 2-185　Left aspect of the suboccipital venous plexus

1. 头后大直肌 rectus capitis posterior major
2. 枕下静脉丛 suboccipital venous plexus
3. 枢椎棘突 spinous process of axis
4. 头下斜肌 obliquus capitis inferior
5. 头上斜肌 obliquus capitis superior

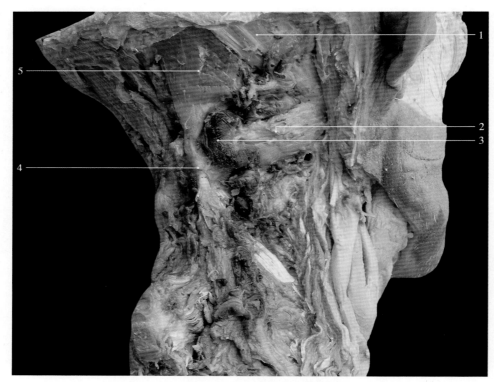

▲ 图 2-186　枕下静脉丛右侧面观
Fig. 2-186　Right aspect of the suboccipital venous plexus

1. 头上斜肌 obliquus capitis superior
2. 头下斜肌 obliquus capitis inferior
3. 枕下静脉丛 suboccipital venous plexus
4. 枢椎棘突 spinous process of axis
5. 头后大直肌 rectus capitis posterior major

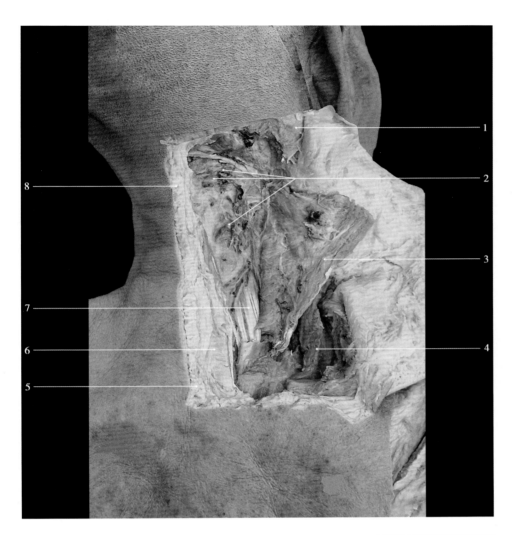

◀ 图2-187 枕下静脉丛后
面观（一）
Fig. 2-187 Posterior
aspect of the suboccipi-
tal venous plexus（1）

1. 乳突 mastoid process of
   temporal bone
2. 枕下静脉丛 suboccipi-
   tal venous plexus
3. 斜方肌 trapezius
4. 肩胛提肌 levator sca-
   pulae
5. 棘上韧带 supraspinous
   ligament
6. 深筋膜 deep fascia
7. 棘肌 spinalis
8. 项韧带 ligamentum nu-
   chae

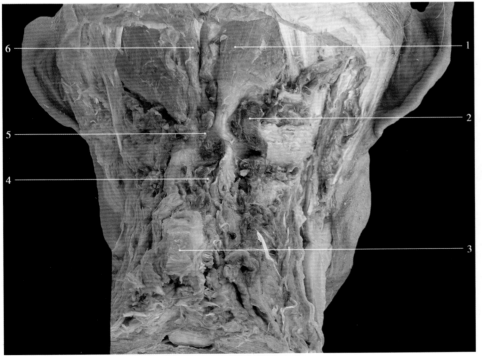

◀ 图2-188 枕下静脉丛后
面观（二）
Fig. 2-188 Posterior
aspect of the suboccipi-
tal venous plexus（2）

1. 头后大直肌 rectus ca-
   pitis posterior major
2. 枕下静脉丛 suboccipi-
   tal venous plexus
3. 第3颈椎棘突 spinous
   process of the 3rd cervical spine
4. 枕下静脉丛 suboccipi-
   tal venous plexus
5. 枢椎棘突 spinous process
   of axis
6. 头后小直肌 rectus ca-
   pitis posterior minor

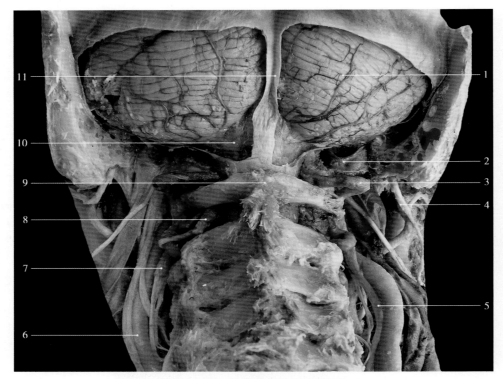

▲ 图 2-189　寰椎周围结构后面观（一）
Fig. 2-189　Posterior aspect of the structures around the atlas（1）

1. 小脑半球 cerebellar hemisphere
2. 颈内静脉 internal jugular vein
3. 椎动脉寰椎部 atlantic part of vertebral artery
4. 面神经 facial nerve
5. 迷走神经 vagus nerve
6. 颈内动脉 internal carotid artery
7. 颈上神经节 superior cervical ganglion
8. 第 2 脊神经节 the 2nd spinal ganglion
9. 寰椎后结节 posterior tubercle of atlas
10. 蛛网膜 arachnoid mater
11. 小脑镰 cerebellar falx

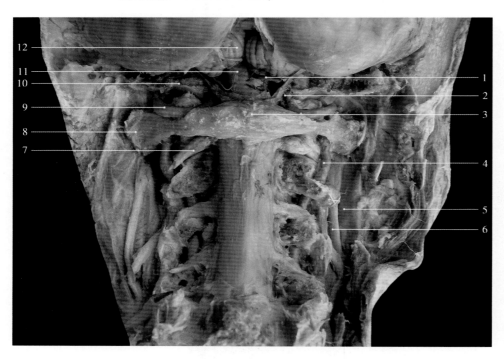

◀ 图 2-190　寰椎周围结构后面观（二）
Fig. 2-190　Posterior aspect of the structures around the atlas（2）

1. 小脑下后动脉 posterior inferior cerebellar artery
2. 枕骨大孔 foramen magnum
3. 寰椎后结节 posterior tubercle of atlas
4. 椎动脉横突部 transverse part of vertebral artery
5. 颈内静脉 internal jugular vein
6. 迷走神经 vagus nerve
7. 第 2 脊神经节 the 2nd spinal ganglion
8. 寰椎横突 transverse process of atlas
9. 椎动脉寰椎部 atlantic part of vertebral artery
10. 枕髁 occipital condyle
11. 延髓 medulla oblongata
12. 小脑扁桃体 tonsil of cerebellum

寰椎后弓、横突的应用解剖学要点

寰椎位于脊柱的最上端,与枕骨相连,寰椎整体上呈不规则的环形,无椎体、无棘突,主要由两侧的侧块及连结于侧块之间的前、后弓构成。前弓为连结两侧块前面的弓形板,前面凸隆,中央前凸的部分称前结节。后弓连结于两侧侧块的后面,较前弓长且曲度也较大,后面中部有粗糙的隆起称后结节,实为棘突的遗迹,有项韧带及头后小直肌附着。后弓下面有一浅切迹,与枢椎椎弓根上缘的浅沟相合形成椎间孔,有第2颈神经通过。后弓与侧块连结处的上面,有一深弓,称椎动脉沟,有椎动脉的寰椎部和枕下神经通过,此沟有时被一弓形的薄骨板所覆盖,此时椎动脉的寰椎部就无后凸的弓形,后弓的上缘为寰椎后膜所覆盖。

寰椎的横突上、下扁平,较粗大,末端肥厚而粗糙,为肌及韧带的附着部,横突孔也较大。

应用解剖要点:

寰椎横突距后结节右侧为47.0mm,左侧为48.3mm;后结节距后弓上面椎动脉右侧为23.7mm,左侧为21.0mm。寰椎横突孔中点距横突末端右侧为10.8mm,左侧为12.4mm。横突末端的外上方4.5mm处有面神经出茎乳孔后自内上方沿颈内静脉后壁斜向外下方,寰椎横突的前外方自外向内有颈内静脉、迷走神经、舌咽神经、副神经、舌下神经和颈内动脉经过(图2-189、图2-190)。

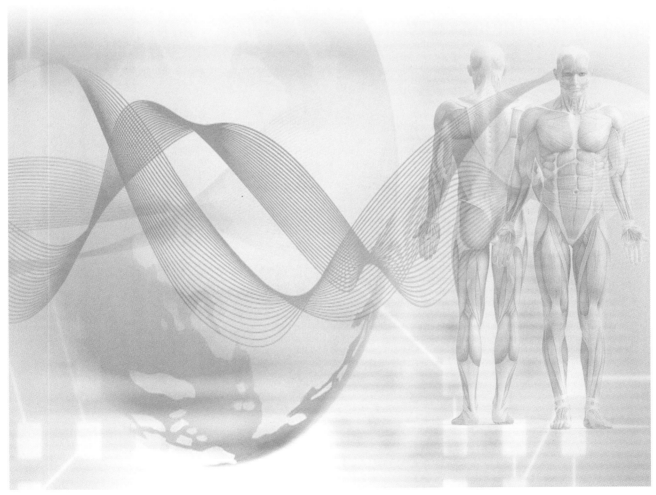

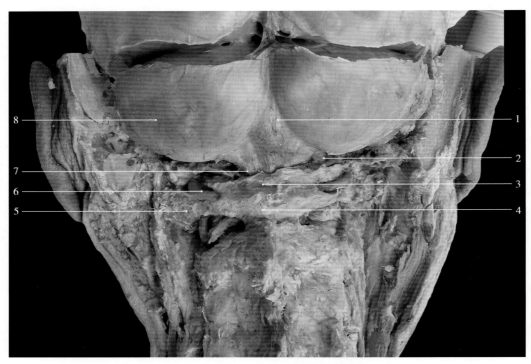

▲ 图 2-191　枕骨大孔周围结构后面观
Fig. 2-191　Posterior aspect of the structures around the foramen magnum

1. 小脑延髓池表面硬膜 dura over cerebellomedullary cistern
2. 枕髁 occipital condyle
3. 寰枕后膜 posterior altantooccipital membrane
4. 寰椎后结节 posterior tubercle of atlas
5. 寰椎横突 transverse process of atlas
6. 椎动脉寰椎部 atlantic part of vertebral artery
7. 枕骨大孔 foramen magnum
8. 硬脑膜 cerebral dura mater

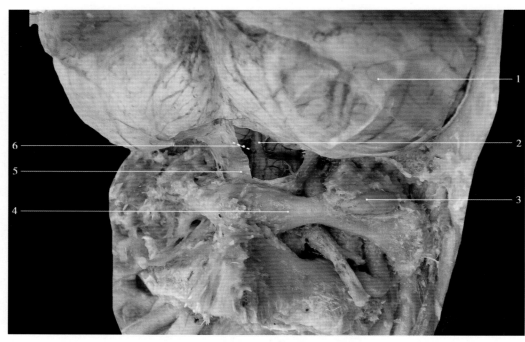

▲ 图 2-192　小脑延髓池
Fig. 2-192　Cerebellomedullary cistern

1. 硬脑膜 cerebral dura mater
2. 小脑下后动脉 posterior inferior cerebellar artery
3. 椎动脉寰椎部 atlantic part of vertebral artery
4. 寰椎后弓 posterior arch of atlas
5. 蛛网膜 arachnoid mater
6. 小脑延髓池 cerebellomedullary cistern

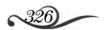

中文索引

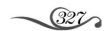

英文索引

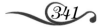

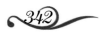

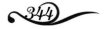

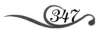

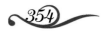

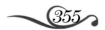